Community Prevention
Trials for Alcohol Problems

Community Prevention Trials for Alcohol Problems

Methodological Issues _____

Edited by **Harold D. Holder**
and **Jan M. Howard**

Foreword by Enoch Gordis

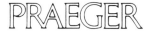

Westport, Connecticut
London

RC
564.73
.C 66
1992

Library of Congress Cataloging-in-Publication Data

Community prevention trials for alcohol problems : methodological
  issues / edited by Harold D. Holder and Jan M. Howard ; foreword by
  Enoch Gordis.
    p.   cm.
    Includes bibliographical references and index.
    ISBN 0-275-94196-5 (alk. paper)
    1. Alcoholism—United States—Prevention—Research—Methodology.
    2. Community health services—United States—Research—Methodology.
    3. Preventive health services—United States—Research—Methodology.
    I. Holder, Harold D.   II. Howard, Jan M. (Jan McDonald)
    RC564.73.C66   1992
    362.29'27—dc20   92-9804

British Library Cataloguing in Publication Data is available.

Library of Congress Catalog Card Number: 92-9804
ISBN: 0-275-94196-5

First published in 1992

Praeger Publishers, 88 Post Road West, Westport, CT 06881
An imprint of Greenwood Publishing Group, Inc.

Printed in the United States of America

The paper used in this book complies with the
Permanent Paper Standard issued by the National
Information Standards Organization (Z39.48-1984).

10 9 8 7 6 5 4 3 2 1

This book is dedicated to the pioneers in community prevention trials for heart disease, cancer, alcohol abuse, and other drug problems. They had the foresight and courage to move beyond the clinic to the community at large. Community prevention research in its earliest stages was an uncertain business that required (and still requires) the creative thinking of experienced scientists willing to take calculated risks.

The chapters and ideas in this book reflect the value of vigorous, constructive dialogue and debate among highly committed prevention researchers from a wide range of health disciplines. We are indebted to the many distinguished scientists who made this book possible.

IN MEMORIAM

David P. Byar, M.D., who died August 8, 1991, is internationally known and respected for his creative contributions to the methodology of clinical trials. His primary focus of interest was cancer research, but his influence on the design and conduct of clinical trials reaches far beyond the cancer area.

His early work in treatment research for prostate cancer established the importance of treatment covariate interactions. His later pioneering work in cancer prevention research helped lay the scientific foundation for rigorous but imaginative intervention studies in which communities are the critical units of analysis. He was the key architect of COMMIT, the community intervention trial to reduce cigarette smoking, and contributed to innovative designs for dietary intervention and cancer screening studies.

Toward the end of his life, Dr. Byar turned his attention to the knotty methodological issues in community prevention trials for AIDS. He was instrumental in negotiating collective thinking among internationally renowned statisticians which resulted in a seminal collaborative paper on AIDS clinical trials.

In the fall of 1989, Dr. Byar accepted our invitation to help brainstorm challenging methodological issues in community prevention trials for alcohol problems. His short commentary included in this volume discusses some of his initial thoughts on this subject.

Contents

Illustrations

FIGURES

TABLES

Foreword

Public concern for the large impact of alcohol abuse and alcoholism on the health, social, and economic vitality of our society has led to educational and community-based strategies, workplace programs, media-oriented efforts, server intervention programs, legal sanctions, and a variety of other programs designed to prevent these problems and their consequences. Despite growing public support for alcohol-related prevention activities, our knowledge of what actually works and for whom is still limited, a situation that must be addressed if current and future alcohol prevention activities are to have a significant impact.

While the need for alcohol prevention research is clear, it is one of the most challenging types of research to undertake. For one reason, studying real-life situations outside of the laboratory results in numerous variables beyond the researcher's control but which, nonetheless, must be considered in analyzing and interpreting findings. Also, because each individual in our society is involved in a network of relations with individuals, groups, and the larger social system, it is difficult to define activities that prevent specific alcohol-related consequences.

Community Prevention Trials for Alcohol Problems: Methodological Issues is the result of efforts by the National Institute on Alcohol Abuse and Alcoholism (NIAAA) to stimulate the development of alcohol prevention research and to help alcohol researchers understand the complexities involved in designing scientifically sound community-based studies. It examines what we know about alcohol prevention research as well as what we need to know. It also presents issues and ideas based on the experience of other health fields, such as cancer and heart disease, that have developed sound methodologies for prevention research that can be useful in alcohol studies.

Although alcohol prevention research is challenging, it is doable, as is demonstrated in this volume. Those who are considering undertaking such research should find the text a valuable source of information on community-based prevention research problems and solutions. Dr. Harold Holder and Dr. Jan Howard deserve our thanks for their efforts in bringing this volume to fruition.

Enoch Gordis

Part I

Introduction

1

Emergent Agendas for Alcohol Prevention Research

Jan M. Howard

Prevention research in the health arena has similar objectives regardless of the disease or condition targeted for intervention. The task is at least three fold: to test strategies with potential for reducing morbidity, mortality, and human suffering; to determine whether each strategy is effective; and to explain why the intervention did or did not succeed in achieving desired outcomes.

Ultimately, the goal of prevention research is to test interventions in complex, representative real-world environments. But such efforts must first be preceded by studies that answer more basic questions. Thus, in heart disease and cancer prevention research, stages or phases of research have been promulgated that provide investigators with models of logical research progression, from bench or controlled laboratory studies to the "messier" milieus of dynamic real-world communities (Greenwald, Cullen, and McKenna, 1987; Greenwald and Cullen, 1985; National Heart, Lung, and Blood Institute, 1987; Flay, 1986).

In the early phases of the research sequence, investigators may synthesize available information to develop hypotheses. They may also conduct pilot tests to determine the validity of data collection instruments, possible side effects or deleterious consequences of the intervention, and mechanisms for ensuring its adoption by critical persons in the implementation process, including so-called "gatekeepers." Investigators may consider basic components of behavioral change from perspectives such as expectancy and social learning theory, theories of social change and organizational dynamics, and economic theories relevant to consumer demand and decision-making behaviors.

In the middle range of the research phases, more elaborate controlled studies may be undertaken to test the efficacy or effectiveness of the intervention among larger samples of persons who are not necessarily representative of the target group as a whole. Eventually, the research focuses on defined population units (frequently geographically demarcated communities) that permit investigators to generalize their findings beyond the limitations of the specific study.

After an intervention proves to be effective among the defined target population, the final research phase (or phases) falls within the province of technology-transfer studies—assessing whether strategies that have proven effective in one situation have the same or similar outcomes in other contexts. These studies are frequently called demonstration projects, where "demonstration" connotes some degree of uncertainty as to outcome—particularly from a public-health perspective. There is always more that can be learned about the acceptance of an intervention, modes of delivery, benefits and costs, and effects on subgroups of the defined population. Moreover, unanticipated consequences of the intervention (both positive and negative) may not be appreciated until the number or variety of people exposed to it expands dramatically. And certain designs may permit synergistic (interactive) as well as additive effects of multiple interventions to be recognized (National Institute on Alcohol Abuse and Alcoholism & Office for Substance Abuse Prevention, 1990).

Of course, the quest for knowledge feeds on itself and challenges arbitrary boundaries—for example, time limits set by funding agencies. At some point, however, it becomes reasonable to conclude that further studies would have such diminished returns that they cannot be justified. At that point, research in any formal sense stops, and *service*-oriented demonstrations begin, assuming that the intervention deserves to be disseminated.

CONCEPTUALIZING COMMUNITY-BASED ALCOHOL RESEARCH

The phase sequence described above has not been systematically applied to alcohol prevention research. However, the National Institute on Alcohol Abuse and Alcoholism (NIAAA) is currently funding an in-depth exploration of this topic. There is every reason to believe from preliminary discussions that the phase models developed by the National Heart, Lung, and Blood Institute and the National Cancer Institute are in fact applicable to alcohol prevention research but that amendments, additions, and even exclusions will be necessary. There are also good reasons to believe that *community-based* alcohol prevention research will eventually emerge as a fertile realm of inquiry, but this expectation is still to be realized.

By the spring of 1989, when this book was first conceived, several community-oriented alcohol studies were already underway (University of California, San Diego Extension, 1990; Pentz et al., 1989); and proposals for others had been submitted to NIAAA. Concurrently, the Office for Substance

Abuse Prevention (which is responsible for funding and evaluating service demonstration projects) was actively promoting community-based "demos." Private funding bodies (such as the Kaiser Family Foundation and the Robert Wood Johnson Foundation) were similarly involved in promoting and evaluating community-based programs to reduce substance abuse. The line between program evaluation and genuine research was becoming blurred, and it was not entirely clear that the building blocks for community-based research in alcohol prevention were sufficiently in place to justify a major commitment of resources for community studies.

It seemed timely, therefore, for NIAAA to bring together several groups of scientists: those who had accumulated first-hand knowledge of community-based prevention research in a variety of health arenas including alcohol; alcohol prevention researchers who had not yet conducted community studies; and experts in research methodology. This attempt at cross-fertilization took place in Berkeley, California on December 4 and 5, 1989. Initial drafts of many of the chapters included in this volume served as points of departure for in-depth discussions of the issues.

The central task for the Berkeley meeting was to determine whether and how *community-based* research to prevent alcohol-related problems should be conducted, in light of the experiences of investigators in other health fields. Specific questions addressed by participants concerned whether available methodological tools and designs were applicable to the alcohol field; whether sufficient preliminary studies had been completed; whether appropriate outcome data could be collected; whether natural ongoing events and exogenous prevention activities would nullify scientific validity; whether case-control studies could serve as efficient alternatives to prospective intervention research; whether quasi-experimental designs could serve as legitimate substitutes for large-scale randomized controlled trials; whether interventions should focus on health problems in general or alcohol abuse in particular; and whether target groups should be determined by risk status.

It also seemed necessary to define the concept of community for the purposes of alcohol research and to review the meaning of the concept as it has been applied in health and social-science literature. Finally, it was deemed important to consider political realities since alcohol prevention programs and research are frequently defined as socio-political phenomena that reflect and threaten vested interests.

POSSIBLE INTERVENTION STRATEGIES

Over the course of history, a wide range of prevention strategies have been used in attempts to reduce alcohol-related problems. Various conceptual schemes have been advanced to classify these interventions so as to distinguish the more environmentally-oriented approaches from those that focus on individuals as individuals (Moskowitz, 1989; Secretary of Health and Human Services, 1990; Institute of Medicine, 1989). Any of the strategies can theoretically be applied in community-based research, but not all of them may be appropriate in a given situation. For example, communities may be constrained from levying excise taxes on alcohol unless they encompass whole states. However, localities may have other opportunities to affect the price of alcoholic beverages, e.g., through regulations concerning the hours and conditions of sale.

In a previous paper (Howard, Ganikos, and Taylor, 1990), the author classified alcohol prevention approaches according to a four-facet typology: selection, socialization, social control, and social support. *Selection* refers primarily to screening at the point of employment by or admission to an organization, and to certain types of drug testing. These processes constitute an emergent domain of intervention, which is eliciting debates over the right to privacy, test accuracy, and appropriate sanctions. Selection can also refer to informal group processes aimed at identifying, changing, or excluding persons who violate group norms against drinking or problem drinking. Thus, effective selection mechanisms support group homogeneity in values and behavior—in this case, support for drinking-related practices that are not deleterious.

Socialization approaches to the prevention of alcohol-related problems attempt to transfer knowledge, values, and norms from one group or person to another. If the socialization process is successful, the recipient group or individual internalizes what has been formally or informally taught and behaves accordingly, through mechanisms of self-control. Strategies described elsewhere as "measures to change *individual* behaviors" (Secretary of Health and Human Services, 1990) fall within the province of socialization. Examples of such tactics include: school-based interventions that rely on didactic instruction, training in social competency skills, and peer-group modeling; driver-education programs that rely on field experiences (such as exposure to emergency rooms); media or mass communication techniques aimed at health promotion and counter-advertising; warning labels on alcoholic beverages (which could also be considered a form of mass communication); and anticipatory-guidance by health professionals and other prestigious authorities.

Social-control strategies go beyond self-control by setting socially defined limits on human discretion. They are generally considered to be environmentally-oriented interventions that are frequently established through formal government policies. Included in this category are (a) economic disincentives to drink, to abuse alcohol, or to facilitate its abuse, such as excise taxes (whether or not the intent of the tax is prevention), liability suits against producers and servers of alcohol, and heightened insurance premiums; (b) restrictions on alcohol availability through such approaches as the legal minimum drinking age, zoning ordinances, and controlled beverage service; (c) legally established punishments and penalties for violations of laws and regulations concerning alcohol abuse; (d) enforcement of such laws and regulations; and (e) environmental safety measures to protect drinkers and other potential victims from injury (e.g., interlock devices in cars and safer highway designs).

Social support is an extension of social control, but it embodies a "helping" ideology that is in some sense amoral. Treatment strategies for alcoholism rely heavily on social support structures, exemplified by Alcoholics Anonymous and similar systems of therapy. In the primary and secondary prevention areas, a number of traditional and emergent strategies are also based on the social-support principle. These include designated driver programs that entrust the safety of drinkers and the larger society to prearranged support systems; Employee Assistance Programs that rely on social networks to identify and counsel workers with incipient alcohol problems; and peer-oriented interventions in schools that legitimize norms against drinking and support resistance behavior.

Distinctions among these four categories of interventions are sometimes blurred; and in any given situation, success may rest on the implementation of combinations of strategies that integrate two or more approaches. For example, the training of servers of alcoholic beverages (Saltz, 1989b) stresses to some extent all four types of prevention strategies: selection and exclusion of customers, socialization of servers and customers to "responsible drinking" norms, social control of abusive drinking, and social support for protective behavior (e.g., calling a taxicab for an inebriated patron).

NATURAL EXPERIMENTS

Every domain of prevention research must contend with the prospect of contamination from naturally occurring events in the community that can affect study results. These events also provide opportunities for research in the form of natural experiments. Many, if not most, of the policy-driven studies in the alcohol prevention area can be considered natural experiments because the politically-mandated intervention evolved independent of attempts to study it.

Prominent examples of these so-called experiments include retrospective and prospective evaluations of the effects of changes in the legal minimum drinking age (U.S. General Accounting Office, 1987a; O'Malley and Wagenaar, 1991); comparative studies of the impact of alcohol excise taxes (Center for Science in the Public Interest, 1990; Cook, 1981); and analyses of the effects of per se laws on drunk driving (Hingson and Howland, 1990). In a few instances, a deliberate effort has been made before the implementation of policy initiatives to collect baseline survey data.

For example, in anticipation of warning labels being required on containers of alcoholic beverages, NIAAA funded three baseline studies to assess pre-intervention knowledge, beliefs, and behavior patterns relating to risks of alcohol consumption. Follow-up studies were later conducted to measure possible post-intervention changes in these parameters. A similar approach was used to determine the potential effect of increasing alcohol excise taxes in the State of California (Gruenewald, 1990). Baseline surveys of alcohol purchase and consumption patterns and seller pricing practices were conducted before the November voter referendum on the tax issue. In this case, however, the baseline data were gathered without certainty that the intervention (increased taxes) would actually occur, because the data could be used for multiple purposes.

In natural experiments, by definition, investigators lack control over the initiation of prevention strategies, and this has important implications for the research process. It may still be possible to nest a designed experiment within the context of a natural one (e.g., randomly bringing warning labels to the attention of a community population and measuring exposure effects). But, generally speaking, natural means natural; and it may also mean that the intervention is universally applied, making it difficult or impossible for researchers to select meaningful control groups.

Even where investigators do control the experimental process, they cannot control the myriad of health-related activities that continually occur in communities and that may contaminate the study at hand. This issue is discussed in more detail later in this volume. Suffice it to say here that community-based prevention research is embedded in a dynamic environment; and in the substance abuse area, public and private funding institutions are deliberately trying to increase the amount of prevention activity. These subsidized prevention programs can become meaningful natural experiments in and of themselves, especially where geographically demarcated communities are the stipulated targets of the interventions.

SPECIAL DIMENSIONS OF AN ALCOHOL FOCUS

Although alcohol-related problems and interventions to prevent them fall within the rubric of public health, it is important to recognize certain unique aspects of alcohol. These factors can influence the direction and viability of prevention research as well as prevention programs.

First, it should be noted that alcohol is a legal drug for persons 21 years of age and over. In this respect, it differs from the majority of "other" drugs that are the concern of the National Institute on Drug Abuse. And because alcohol is a legal drug, strategies to reduce alcohol-related problems among adults must concentrate on its abuse rather than consumption per se. Among youth, the task is theoretically simpler because use is essentially tantamount to misuse.

The second distinct feature of alcohol concerns the history of its legality. Unlike the situation with tobacco products or illegal drugs, the United States once prohibited the manufacture and sale of beverage alcohol (more specifically, "intoxicating liquors" [Aaron and Musto, 1981]) and then repealed that proscription. Certain communities, including Indian reservations, still prohibit alcohol sales within their boundaries, but national prohibition is history. As a consequence, the concept of prohibition currently has invidious connotations (Aaron and Musto, 1981), and the term "neo-Prohibitionist" is frequently used to stigmatize prevention strategists. In the wake of such charges, the benefits of prohibition for the reduction of alcohol-related problems (Aaron and Musto, 1981) are sometimes forgotten, overlooked, or purposely ignored, giving the impression that strict controls on alcohol availability are not viable intervention strategies.

A number of epidemiologic studies suggest that moderate, routine use of beverage alcohol can reduce the risk of coronary heart disease (Secretary of Health and Human Services, 1990). These findings, combined with the ritualistic use of alcohol in religious services, cultural celebrations, and recreational activities, give the substance a positive image. Promotional advertising campaigns by the beverage industry reinforce that image and imprint on it symbolic suggestions of benefit, such as sexual attractiveness, peer-group camaraderie, and unbridled fun. To varying degrees, the cultural position of alcohol and the images it conveys affect the choice, acceptance, and effectiveness of prevention strategies. They may also influence the community's receptivity to some types of prevention research.

In cardiovascular and cancer research, it is assumed that the problem at hand is a disease, which gives the research face legitimacy. In the alcohol area, the situation is somewhat more complicated because the disease concept is not universally accepted. Even if alcoholism and its sequelae (such as cirrhosis and esophageal cancer) are defined as illnesses, some of the most prevalent alcohol-related problems (such as drunk driving) are frequently considered to be moral or criminal problems (Ross, 1990). These competing perspectives influence community debates about appropriate intervention strategies, particularly with respect to sanctions. They can also affect the conduct of prevention research.

Morbidity and mortality associated with heart disease and cancer are generally the result of a lengthy illness process, which often involves a prolonged "latent" or symptomless period. This is additionally true for certain consequences of alcoholism, such as cirrhosis. But it is not true for alcohol-induced trauma or mortality caused by automobile, boat, train, and plane crashes, or by homicides, suicides, and other criminal acts. These types of alcohol-related injuries and deaths occur suddenly and can have immediate, highly visible effects on communities in terms of the intensity and thrust of prevention activity and debates over prevention policy.

An overall assessment of the relative effectiveness of alcohol prevention strategies would suggest that environmental or social-control approaches have better track records than interventions that are more oriented toward individuals. The environmental emphasis might be considered somewhat unique to the alcohol area, which is laden with regulatory constraints on distribution, use, and misuse. However, environmental strategies have been gaining increasing attention in other domains of health promotion, including the heart and cancer areas. Examples are changes in the content of food products, reimbursement for screening procedures, concern over the disposition of toxic waste, and legally imposed constraints on the use of cigarettes.

Alcohol prevention advocates and researchers might wish to argue that the alcohol industry constitutes a uniquely persuasive pressure group in health policy making. However, the tobacco, dairy, and chemical industries (to name but a few) are also formidable protectors of products that can cause or exacerbate disease. Moreover, observational evidence suggests that tobacco companies (like the brewers) have established strong links to community organizations through financial support of athletic events and other activities that enhance the marketing potential of the industry (Aaron and Musto, 1981; U.S. Department of Health and Human Services, 1989; Maxwell and Jacobson, 1989).

It can *unequivocally* be argued that alcohol prevention research has a much smaller budget at its disposal than prevention research in the heart and cancer fields, where community trials are an established testing approach. Prevention *programs* in the alcohol area have attracted substantial sums of public and private monies, but prevention *research* is still in its infancy—in terms of completed studies and available financial resources. This fact has obvious implications for the design and implementation of community-based research because such studies tend to be very expensive and should be preceded by solid preliminary research.

OVERVIEW OF THE BOOK

Contributors to this book have a wealth of experience in conducting community prevention trials for heart disease and cancer or in studying the prevention of alcohol problems. Their chapters are grouped into sections with common themes.

Following this introductory chapter, the two chapters in Part II, "Definitions of Communities and Alcohol Problems," review definitions, perspectives, and issues that provide a conceptual base for the rest of the book. Also considered are the selection and measurement of alcohol problems that may be candidate outcome variables for a community intervention study.

Part III, "Lessons and Experiences from Community Trials in Other Health Fields," provides two chapters that summarize community-based approaches to such problems as heart disease, cancer, and adolescent health, because these strategies may be applicable to the prevention of alcohol problems.

The three chapters in Part IV, "Lessons from Early Community Prevention Efforts for Alcohol Abuse," discuss experiences and implications of alcohol prevention projects in Canada, Texas, and Rhode Island.

Part V, "Research Designs, Methods, and Analytic Models," contains four chapters that evaluate diverse methodologies for studying community-based alcohol interventions.

The two chapters in Part VI, "Implementing Research Designs," conclude the main body of the book by describing dynamic social and political realities that confront community prevention trials for alcohol problems and suggesting guidelines for such trials.

Part VII, "Insights, Caveats, and Alternative Research Agendas," consists of nine brief commentaries by selected experts, who elaborate on specific themes in the book.

Part II

Definitions of Communities and Alcohol Problems

2

What Is a Community and What Are Implications for Prevention Trials for Reducing Alcohol Problems?

Harold D. Holder

INTRODUCTION

The "community" can be an appropriate focus for preventing and reducting alcohol problems. At the community level, alcohol-related problems are personally experienced. There, for example, an auto fatality caused by a driver impaired by alcohol has meaning to family members and friends—the death is not just a statistic. It causes grief and anger at the unnecessary loss of life and at family disruption. Therefore, the word "community" connotes geographical and social proximity of people to each other, "localness." The cost of any single local problem resulting from alcohol misuse is not limited to the person and the event; rather, the cost includes a ripple effect of disrupted families, lost potential production and family income, and higher costs for medical care.

In early American history, drinking had a prominent role and the tavern was a center of community life. In colonial times, alcohol was often used to pay workers. The earliest temperance activities in the United States were community-based efforts to make residents and leaders aware of the threats of alcohol to home and work. The temperance movement was where a tradition of concern about the effects of alcohol abuse on the family and neighborhood was established. Drunkenness, failure to be responsible for family needs, and violence were viewed by early temperance leaders as the direct results of drinking. The temperance movement became increasingly prohibitionist in the mid- to late-1800s and culminated in American Prohibition in 1920. Even with the end of Prohibition in 1933 and return of control of alcoholic beverages to the states, most of the legislation creating state Alcoholic Beverage Control organizations carried references to the prevention of drunkenness and protection of the family in the legislative mandate (Rice, 1984).

Following the end of Prohibition, the site of the "alcohol problem" was deemed to be the individual. The idea of individual addiction to alcohol coincided with the rise of the disease concept of alcoholism. As a result, for over 40 years after repeal, the focus of prevention was on early identification of, treatment for, and public education about alcoholism. For example, when Bacon (1947) called for the mobilization of community resources to address alcoholism, his was largely a call for increased availability of treatment and social support such as Alcoholics Anonymous (AA).

In the 1970s, attention to health and social problems to which alcohol made a significant contribution (i.e., public health concerns) began to emerge, though not initially directed at communities per se (Bruun et al., 1975; Room, 1984; Holder, 1987). This shift from an alcoholism-only focus to a broader view of alcohol problems has particular import for community prevention trials.

Over the past decade, alcohol problems have increasingly become the target for prevention, which can include, but is not limited to, identification of individuals at special risk for alcohol dependency. For example, drinking while pregnant and drinking and driving are two problems involving dangerous and inappropriate use of alcohol; both are currently evoking considerable popular interest. While both could be (and have been) addressed at the national and state levels, they illustrate problems at a community level that result from drinking both by dependent persons as well as by a much larger number of nondependent drinkers.

"What is a community?" In this chapter the author considers that question and outlines how a community can become involved in a prevention trial, i.e., a well planned, well executed, and carefully evaluated program to prevent alcohol problems.

First, there is a review of definitions of community from the disciplines of sociology, political science, and social work. Such definitions provide a conceptual base for developing community prevention trials. The second part of the chapter is a discussion of two major perspectives—catchment and systems—that have been used by communities to prevent a variety of health problems. Their implication for alcohol problem prevention is explored. In the third part, case studies are highlighted. These are alcohol problem prevention projects within communities where an effort was made to evaluate the results. In the final part, the author discusses conceptual and methodological issues for community prevention trials and suggests criteria for selecting communities for alcohol problem prevention trials as well as "no-treatment" comparison communities.

HISTORICAL DEFINITIONS OF COMMUNITY

A number of definitions and characterizations of "community" have been used in the past.   Different definitions reflect discipline orientation and scholarly interests but can also reflect the use of the community as a point of reference for social, health, and economic changes. This section provides a brief overview of selected definitions that are relevant to alcohol problem prevention.

Social Science

The first use of the community as a point of reference by the behavioral sciences was motivated by scientific inquiry. While there were definitions and theories of the community in the 1800s and early 1900s, the greatest interest in theories and definitions of community appears to be from the post-World War II period up to the 1970s. Fewer scholarly books about the community were published in the 1980s, possibly reflecting a declining interest in the "community" and increased interest in urban and suburban areas. In general, the social science definitions of the community emphasize key institutions, social processes, and interaction.

One of the earliest definitions for community was derived by Tonnies in 1887 from the German word *Gemeinschaft*, which refers to the "natural will" of people to establish stable relationships with one another.   These relationships create a common bond and common expectations and destiny. A second community definition, derived from the German word *Gesellschaft*, refers to the process of rational exchanges of goods and services in which people seek those exchanges that most benefit them.   Such a "rational will" perspective does not carry with it the sentiment and attachment of the *Gemeinschaft*.   Here emphasis is on the formalizations of relationships and the development of laws, rules, and bureaucracies (Tonnies, translated 1957). Other definitions of communities were provided by Weber (translated 1964) (traditional authority vs. rational authority) and Durkheim (translated 1964) (mechanical vs. organic solidarity). Basically these historical definitions of the community were used to refer to organized collectivity for common gain within a geographical area.

Stoneall (1983) identified five discrete perspectives of the community: (a) *human ecology* using concepts of cooperation and competition; (b) *structural functionalism* characterizing the community as systems of institutions held together by shared values; (c) *conflict theory* emphasizing class struggles and the efforts of a powerful elite to control resources; (d) *social-psychological* emphasizing symbolic interaction, community symbols, attitudes, perceptions, and interaction patterns; and (e) *network-exchange* characterizing communities as the means through which goods, feelings, and social values are transmitted.

Hillery, a prolific modern day sociological theorist concerned with the community (Hillery, 1955, 1963, 1972, 1982), identified 94 definitions of community from sociological and anthropological literature and developed 16 different concepts that were most often employed within these definitions (Hillery, 1982). He observed that most definitions are in basic agreement that the community is composed of "persons in social interaction within a geographic area and having one or more additional common ties" (Hillery, 1982:15).

Poplin (1979) observes that most sociologists use the word community to refer to social and territorial organizations—where people live, earn income, raise children, and carry on most of their life activities. Freilich (1963) employs a similar definition by describing the community as "people in interaction in a geographic area."[1]

To make the concept of community useful in practice, one needs to identify the basic elements that make up a community. Rubin (1983) has defined five essential structures necessary to any community:

1. *Intermediate Size.* Structures must be small enough for people to experience them (provide a "sense of community") and large enough to provide incorporation into the larger societal structure.
2. *Presence of Significant Primary and Secondary Interaction.* Community structures must provide both a primary (directly personal) and well as a secondary (access and reference to a larger group) interaction.
3. *Key Institutional Setting.* Structures must be viewed as central and to some degree essential by the members of the community.
4. *Relative Stability.* Organizations must endure over time.
5. *Concreteness.* The organization or structure must be recognized by people as including a significant number of other people with whom they interact and identify.

Roland L. Warren (1983) defined a community as "that combination of social units and systems that perform the major social functions having locality relevance." He identified five functions that characterize these essential activities. The function of *production-distribution-consumption* concerns economics (the production and use of goods and services). The function of *socialization* involves the process through which the community or one of its organizations or institutions (such as churches and schools) transmits prevailing knowledge, social values, and desired behavior patterns to individual members. The *social control* function describes the process though which the groups influence and shape the behavior of their members to conform with group norms and values including taboos and laws as well as law enforcement. The *social participation* function is the means to provide local access to community processes and community groups and institutions. The last major function is *mutual support*, for example, caring for the ill, exchanging labor, and helping a local family in economic distress.

Community Organization and Action

Using the community as a site for social change and for mobilizing community members to make organizational and structural changes is of direct relevance to alcohol problem prevention for two reasons. First, community prevention trials focus on the entire community (or on a special subgroup). Second, the objectives of changing behavior within the population, altering community structures, and changing the environment in order to prevent or reduce targeted health problems are all consistent with the tradition of community organization.

Kramer and Specht (1983), in a brief history of community organization in the United States, conclude that, whereas the pre-20th Century charity trad- ition of volunteer organizations reflected efforts to assist individuals to adjust to existing social realities, the early 1900s settlement movement represented efforts to change society to meet individuals' needs. Examples of community members joining together for community improvement and social action include the Cincinnati Social Unit Project, a predecessor of the "war on poverty," and the "Back of the Yards" movement in Chicago, which is described by Saul Alinsky (1946). World War II stimulated the largest efforts in community organization to date when community groups organized to support the war. These early experiences and activities have established the philosophical basis for modern day community activity.[2]

Rothman and Tropman (1987) describe three approaches to community organization. The first is *locality development*, where community change is pursued though the participation of a wide spectrum of community residents in the determination of goals and subsequent action. This perspective emphasizes community initiative.

The second approach is *social planning*. The social planning approach focuses on the technical processes of problem-solving with an emphasis on rational, deliberately planned social change. The target has most often been a social problem such as delinquency, housing, or mental health. While community member participation may be significant or small, depending upon how the problem presents itself, the approach assumes the central role of experts. Experts are needed to guide large complex organizations and to provide skills and experience with the technology necessary to solve problems. Most community health-related prevention trials fit in this category.

The third approach is *social action*. This approach presupposes a disadvantaged segment of the population that needs to be organized in order to make appropriate demands for more equitable distribution of community resources. This approach may seek fundamental changes in major institutions or community practices. While the social action approach has not enjoyed much popularity in recent times, the tools and methods of the approach are considered useful by sophisticated community organizers (Rothman and Tropman, 1987).

The way a problem is characterized often establishes the operational definition of community in social action. Lauffer (1981) notes that in practice most social planners focus on problems that are inherent in consumers or community members, a service provider or network of human service providers, and/or the interrelationships between providers and consumers. If the target is consumer populations (for example, youth offenders, drug abusers, the aging) the problem is defined by such concepts as attitudes, values, and perspectives; inability of consumers to organize and effectively bring together power and influence; lack of awareness of services; or absence of necessary social and economic skills. If the target is service agencies, then the problem is defined as deficiencies in the service system including such factors as availability, accessibility, effectiveness and efficiency, and responsiveness and accountability. If the target is service/organizational networks, then the social planner is likely to define the target as uncoordinated and poorly integrated services.

Community Power Structure

One ingredient in mobilizing community members for change is concern about distribution of power. Unlike other perspectives on the community that gradually evolved over time, studies of power structure burst into the academic world (and later the popular press) in the 1950s with the publication of *Community Power Structure* by Floyd Hunter (1952) and *The Power Elite* by C. Wright Mills (1956). Both books, which described the concentration of power and control in a few (usually corporate) individuals, ran counter to the then-traditional position that power in the United States was exercised in a pluralistic fashion. Both books were criticized for drawing inferences about power arrangements from the answers of upper-middle-class professionals asked to identify the most powerful people in a city or community.[3]

More recent works by Hunter (1980) and by Domhoff (1980, 1983) have undertaken community power analyses with the primary purpose of demonstrating that there is a social upper class in the United States by virtue of its dominant role in the economy and government. See Polsby (1980) for a summary of community power perspectives.

Modern Perspectives of Mass Media and Community

Mass media and marketing are relevant to any discussion of community, alcohol use, and alcohol problems, particularly the concept of "main-streaming."[4]

"Mainstreaming" is the idea that regular exposure to television with similar if not identical programming stimulates viewers to acquire and share similar values and political perspectives. Heavy TV viewers especially are expected to share consistent values even when coming from diverse cultural, social, and economic groups (Gerbner et al., 1982, 1984). From this perspective, American society is gradually becoming homogenized or culturally leveled (Neuman, 1982).

One implication of "mainstreaming" is that a diverse society will, over time, begin to share a common set of beliefs and develop a sense of community (as shared beliefs, values, and expectations) through regular exposure to a mass medium—television. Whereas in the past community social networks were typically the means to develop shared values, in modern times not only is this function shared (if not displaced) by electronic media but the values are also more widely distributed (Webster, 1986). One could also speculate that as TV viewing increases and cultural diversity decreases, communities as organized collections of people may become more similar. Thus, mass marketing of alcoholic beverages could reinforce a popular belief that alcohol use is "mainstream" even though a sizable percentage of the population are abstainers (Wallack, 1983, 1984a). Portrayals of people drinking alcohol on prime-time television programs occur more frequently than scenes of people drinking other beverages, including water, coffee, and soft drinks (Wallack, Breed, and Cruz, 1987).

An alternate perspective on mass marketing is that, rather than behaving as a monolithic entity, American consumers actually comprise a number of overlapping market groups. This view has stimulated a variety of marketing-related applications of computer-based mapping and consumer analysis. One of these is called "geodemographics" or "geomapping," which links a population's socio-demographic characteristics to ZIP Codes. With a geodemographic data base, marketers targeting a segment of the population characterized by a particular lifestyle can prepare computer-generated maps that indicate product distribution strengths and weaknesses, desirable consumer markets, and competitive trade consumption. Such analysis is based on the premise that people with the same lifestyle and income live in the same area (Gardner, 1984; Del Priore, 1987).

A similar thrust is represented by the development of "psychographic" data bases by marketers. These data bases are derived from research on the psychological characteristics of consumers and their match with products and services. (See Riche, 1989; Rapp and Collins, 1987; Lesser and Hughes,

1986; Settle and Alreck, 1987; Townsend, 1985). The careful documentation by marketers of lifestyles and age groups suggests the importance to public health professionals of age cohorts and community stratification in any characterization of the community for prevention programming (see Osborn, 1987; Michaelson, 1988; Kinal, 1984). For alcohol problem prevention, investigators could use psychographics and demographics to understand the similarity and diversity of residents in target communities and then to customize prevention strategies for different groups. "Market segmentation" is the business term; the same approach would increase the success of a prevention trial.

WHAT ALTERNATIVE COMMUNITY DEFINITIONS OR PERSPEC-TIVES COULD BE EMPLOYED IN ALCOHOL PREVENTION?

The community, then, can be viewed both as a collection of people living in physical proximity and as a dynamic social and economic system. The community can be defined as a catchment area of people who are at risk for health problems or life difficulties involving alcohol, following the approach to community of many health problem prevention trials. The system perspective, on the other hand, describes alcohol problems as the products of the system and dynamic relationship and not the result of "high-risk" individuals only. Both the catchment area and the system perspectives deserve consideration by public health professionals designing community prevention programs.

Catchment Area

The catchment area perspective defines communities as collections of individuals who share geographical proximity and, therefore, other common-alities that make a local prevention intervention feasible and desirable. For example, if a reduction in rates of breast cancer is the prevention goal, then an increased number of breast examinations could be the goal for prevention interventions targeted at all women who live within a catchment area. Women who live within this area most likely share a number of social and economic factors and are exposed to common environmental risk factors. The incidence of the disease is not necessarily related to their social interaction.

The use of the catchment area is a cost-efficient way to define a target group that is to receive the prevention interaction—in this case, a program to encourage breast examination. This approach does not deny the contribution of the social or physical environment to the development of the disease condition. No particular changes in the social and economic structure of the community are usually proposed, other than those that make breast examination and/or mammograms available, and to change the information (awareness) level of women and, by implication, the values of women and men about the protection of women's health. Alternatively, one might target cirrhosis mortality and seek to reduce the drinking levels of heavy chronic (usually dependent) drinkers. This approach would suggest both educational strategies and various means to increase self-identification and participation in problem-drinking recovery programs. Other community members who are not directly involved with these drinkers would be unaffected. The relevance of such observations to this chapter will become clear later.

The catchment area approach is particularly useful when some of the following conditions exist:

1. The targeted condition is contained within individuals and can be treated as an individual condition or state, e.g., coronary heart disease, lung cancer, or alcoholism (defined in this chapter as a clinically diagnosable condition of chronic alcohol dependency that is life-disruptive). Even if the condition is contagious, such as AIDS or polio, it is still contained within individuals.
2. The behavior or health conditions of the individual can be identified, and preventive actions can be prescribed by health education, which, with early diagnosis, produce effective treatment or remission.
3. The condition is chronic, that is, remains with the individual over time.
4. The condition, while potentially influenced by environmental processes, appears to be largely defined within the context of the individual, his or her immediate family, and close social contacts.
5. The condition is largely disruptive of the individual's life and the immediate social network but does not usually affect directly the lives of anonymous others within the geographical boundary.

It would appear that, in most of the community health prevention trials that have occurred, one or more of these characteristics fits the target condition. While a death from lung cancer lowers overall community health, a single event does not usually directly affect the lives of many other community members.

The catchment area definition of community has a direct implication for selecting the most relevant prevention intervention. For the most part, strategies that alter individual decisions and behavior are emphasized. Education with social and physical (sometimes economic) reinforcement is the preferred strategy (for example, via messages that "everyone is doing it" or by actually paying participants). Thus, the mass media, focus groups, targeted communication, health promotion, and health awareness efforts are all excellent resources.

A System Perspective

A system perspective of prevention defines the targeted condition or event as a system product or output. The prevention target is viewed as the result of an interaction of the individual with the environment. Juvenile crime is one example of this interaction, for there is little evidence that youthful decisions about crime and the pursuit of a "youthful criminal career" are strictly individual matters. Psychological, social, cultural, economic, and physical environmental factors play a major role. To date, efforts to prevent youthful crime as a matter of individual mental health only or through law enforcement and the courts have not been very successful in reducing youth crime rates (Whitehead and Lab, 1989).

There are many public health concerns that can fit within a system perspective. Community level problems such as traffic crashes (including fatalities and injuries) as well as nontraffic death and trauma (burns, drownings, falls) have significant alcohol involvement. A major percentage of homicide victims have high blood alcohol levels. Each of these can be viewed as products of the community system. A system perspective suggests a need to combine changes in individual decisions and behavior with appropriate changes in the social, economic, and in some cases, physical environment of the community system. Holder and Blose (1983, 1987b, 1988) utilized a system perspective to develop a dynamic computer model of the community as a system of alcohol use and abuse. This model was divided into ten subsystems or sectors that emphasized the complexity and dynamics of a community. These sectors are groupings of factors and variables that research has shown to be important to understanding alcohol use and alcohol-involved problems.

The ten subsystems of the total system, as shown in Figure 2.1, can be summarized as follows:[5]

I. *Consumption*. This subsystem includes the total community population (13+ in age) represented by consumption classes and stratified by age and gender. Over time, people move from one consumption group to another in response to system changes.

IIa. *Mortality and Morbidity*. This subsystem includes the risk of illness, injury, and death related to drinking behavior, including traffic fatalities and injuries, cirrhosis mortality, etc.

IIb. *Social/Economic Consequences*. This subsystem addresses reductions in production of goods and services related to inappropriate drinking, as well as social and economic problems such as family disruption, including spouse and child abuse related to drinking.

III. *Legal Action and Drinking.* This subsystem includes crime related to or stimulated by drinking, as well as the enforcement of laws regarding public intoxication and drinking and driving.

IV. *Social and Health Services.* This subsystem includes the demand for general health care and the utilization of alcoholism treatment services.

V. *Social Control and Formal Communication.* This subsystem includes community norms as they affect drinking behavior. It also includes community pressure for increased regulation and for formal education that will affect both informal controls and individual decisions concerning drinking. Any preventive efforts to influence individual drinking behavior are a part of this subsystem.

VI. *Sales by Beverage Type.* This subsystem includes the various factors that influence the sale of alcoholic beverages and the interaction of consumption, alcohol availability, marketing and production, license outlet regulation, and price.

VII. *Production and Marketing.* This subsystem includes advertising and marketing directed at a community by producers. An effort is made to account for the effect of production and marketing at a national level that would affect a community.

VIII. *Formal Regulation And Control.* This subsystem concerns state and local government regulation of alcoholic beverages and their sale and advertising, including the minimum drinking age, hours of sale, type and density of sales outlets, etc.

IX. *Community Economic Sector.* This subsystem includes total community financial resources, including the cost of goods and services, disposable income, tax base, and tax revenue. It also includes tax dollars available for alcohol retail outlet regulation and enforcement.

PREVIOUS COMMUNITY ALCOHOL PROBLEM PREVENTION EFFORTS

Most previous community prevention efforts for alcohol problems have used either a catchment or a system perspective, as illustrated in the following case studies. However, few such efforts in the past 30 years have met even minimum conditions for scientific evaluation, i.e., can be considered a community prevention trial.

FIGURE 2.1
Model of Community Alcohol Use and Abuse

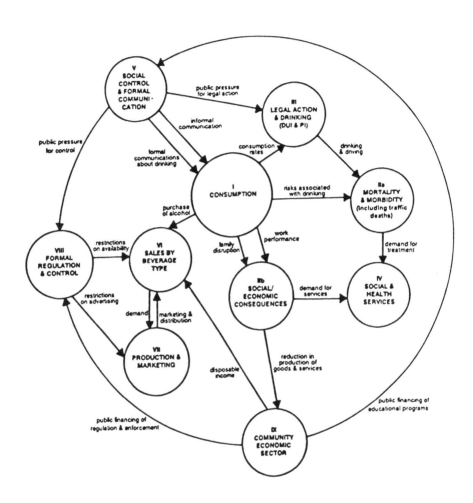

Finland

One early community experiment was undertaken in Finland between 1951 and 1953 to alter the availability of alcohol in rural areas. See Kuusi (1957) for a full discussion of the experiment and results. Since 1902 no legal sale of alcohol had taken place in rural areas in Finland; the law required that all such sales be provided by the State Alcohol Monopoly (ALKO) and then only in cities. Rural residents, for the most part, had to visit cities for their alcohol. The market towns of Ikaalinen, Nokia, and Jarvenpaa, in southwestern and central Finland, were selected as the experimental towns where a state controlled beer and wine retail bottle store would be established. Comparison towns were Ruovesi and Myllykoski.

The project evaluation found that frequency of drinking among men, but not the number of people actually drinking, increased in the test communities. The percentage of drinkers among youth and women did not increase. Both wine and beer increased in use as the beverage of choice with a corresponding reduction in spirits. Illicit alcohol use was reduced. Little change was observed in the quantities consumed per occasion and, thus, there was no reduction in frequency of drunkenness. There were declines in the number of visits to cities by residents of all experimental towns. Even with the availability of beer and wine, such beverages remained a small part of alcohol consumed leading to intoxication.

California

One of the earliest prevention efforts for community-level prevention of alcohol problems in the United States occurred in California in the mid-1970s. This program, modeled after the three-city Stanford Heart Disease Project (Farquhar et al., 1977), also called for a three-community prevention effort in which one community received community action and focus group communication/reinforcement and mass media; a second community received the mass media only; and a third control community received no special program. The budget was cut for the evaluation of this program and for political interventions, i.e., types of mass media messages that were deemed unacceptable by the State of California, which sponsored the program. The conclusions of evaluators were that there were some signs of increased awareness and knowledge about alcohol issues, that respondents in the target communities could recognize the campaign's commercials (a majority could interpret the desired preventive message), but that there was no evidence of changes in drinking behavior, particularly heavy, high-risk drinking (Wallack and Barrows, 1981, 1982-1983).

World Health Organization

Rootman and Moser (1985) and Ritson (1985) describe a World Health Organization project begun in 1977 to study ways of improving community response to alcohol problems. The project involved communities in Mexico, Zambia, and Scotland, and utilized a series of community epidemiological and social service/health agency surveys. In each study site, community organizing activities were undertaken and supported by national policy-setting activities. The local emphasis in each country differed. In the Edinburgh metropolitan area, the project contributed to the planning of an ongoing Council of Community Agencies to improve community response to alcohol problems. Some changes in service availability were documented. In a district of Mexico City, the project contributed to efforts to recruit male professionals and women's organizations to discuss alcohol problems. The efforts for males failed. The women's efforts resulted in the formation of support groups of wives of heavy drinkers. The Zambian project attempted to establish community action groups in three study communities, but these groups ceased to function when project personnel left.

San Francisco

Another American community-based prevention project was undertaken in 1983 in San Francisco, which has the third highest density of alcoholic-beverage outlets in the United States. Researchers worked with substance abuse services to convene a series of half-day community workshops attended by representatives of local agencies and interest groups including the city council, the mayor's office, the public schools, the public defender's office, alcohol and mental health treatment organizations, local newspapers, unions, the State Department of Alcoholic Beverage Control, and youth organizations. The workshops had two purposes: (1) to increase local leaders' awareness of the extent of alcohol-related problems and give them an environmental view of such problems, and (2) to develop working groups to attack specific problems with detailed action (Wallack, 1984-1985; Wittman, 1983, 1985).

As part of the campaign, the Community Substance Abuse Services compiled a *San Francisco Fact Book* detailing the history of, policies toward, and responsibilities for alcohol abuse in the city and county of San Francisco. A second product was the direct involvement of workshop participants in developing written community prevention initiatives (Wallack, 1984-1985). One working group sought to prevent a change in local ordinances that would allow the sale of alcohol to motorists stopping in gasoline stations. The work of the group stimulated members of the San Francisco Board of Supervisors to become interested in implementing a training program for bartenders and to establish server training as an essential part of the hospitality business in the city. Other task forces were created, including one to work against the sale of alcohol to minors and one to undertake a media project to disseminate prevention information. There was no evaluation of actual changes in alcohol problems associated with this community effort and, thus, such final outcomes are unknown.

Ontario

In 1981, Giesbrecht began a test of community prevention efforts to reduce high-risk drinking levels in three towns in the Province of Ontario. In the test community, the program was to reduce the drinking of the heaviest drinkers and to establish an awareness among community members of drinking levels. The results of the program, utilizing community pre- and post-project surveys and time-series analysis of alcohol sales in all three communities, showed no significant change in reported consumption among the heavy-drinking group or in community-level alcohol consumption (Giesbrecht, Holder, and Wood, 1990). See Chapter 6 in this volume for more detail.

New Zealand

A two and one-half year community prevention demonstration project was undertaken in New Zealand between October 1982 and March 1985, sponsored by the Alcoholic Liquor Advisory Council (ALAC) and the Medical Research Council of New Zealand. The program included a paid mass media campaign and use of community organizing. Four experimental communities were utilized. All four were exposed to the mass media campaign and two of the four also participated in the community organizing. Two reference communities were used as controls.

The objectives were to increase community support for relevant public health policies concerning alcohol as well as personal moderation in the use of alcohol. The program was designed to increase appropriate alcohol policies by organizations such as city councils and hospital boards. Increased voluntary use of bar-staff server training by licensed establishments and increased involvement of police in the program were undertaken. The policy areas that received the most public attention were alcohol availability and advertising. Price received less attention since it was seen as being more determined nationally. In each of the intensive intervention communities, a local person was recruited for community organizing on a full-time basis using funds from ALAC. Project evaluation, based on before and after surveys, found that public support for control policies on advertising, availability of alcohol, and prices held steady in the treatment communities but dropped in the reference communities amidst a national trend toward greater support for liberalization and reduction of government control (Casswell and Gilmore, 1989; Casswell, Ransom, and Gilmore, 1990; Wyllie, Casswell, and Stewart, 1989).

Rhode Island

Under a cooperative agreement between the Centers for Disease Control
(CDC) and the National Institute on Alcohol Abuse and Alcoholism (NIAAA),
the Rhode Island Department of Health began a five-year community
prevention trial in Rhode Island in 1984. The project had the objective of
reducing alcohol-involved trauma and violence. The treatment community was
selected randomly from three candidate Rhode Island towns. Prevention
efforts in the treatment community were targeted at retail beverage establishments, police, and the general community. (See Chapter 8 in this volume.)
The final evaluation of this program has not been published (Putnam, 1990).

Others

While not directed at the total community, a number of special
community-based prevention efforts were undertaken in the 1970s and 1980s
in the United States—for example, school-based prevention programs directed
at children from kindergarten through high school. Few have been subjected
to controlled evaluation. (See the review and assessment of school-based
programs by Moskowitz and Jones, 1988.) Positive findings in reduced levels
of self-reported initial drinking were shown in a school-based education
program in Kansas City (Pentz et al., 1989). The National Highway Traffic
Safety Administration established the Alcohol "Counter Measures" Programs
in the 1970s, which involved a number of selected cities in special Alcohol
Safety Action Programs (ASAP) to reduce community-wide drinking and
driving (Levy et al., 1978). Also, during the late 1970s the National Institute
on Alcohol Abuse and Alcoholism, through its Prevention Division, provided
funds to community-based prevention efforts to test methods, strategies, and
approaches other than treatment or rehabilitation services. One emphasis of
such projects was the college campus population. There was evidence that
these projects accomplished some of their objectives, but none was part of a
full controlled evaluation (Wittman, 1982; McCarty et al., 1983; Mills and
McCarty, 1983).

The Office of Substance Abuse was created within the Alcoholism, Drug
Abuse, and Mental Health Administration, U.S. Department of Health and
Human Services, in the late 1980s to undertake community demonstration
prevention projects to reduce substance abuse, including alcohol use, among
high risk youths. These programs, which include a number of novel
approaches, were not required to include any type of controlled outcome
evaluation (U.S. General Accounting Office, 1987b). The Office of Substance
Abuse Prevention (OSAP) has public plans to require evaluation of its newest

rounds of community prevention demonstration projects (Office of Substance Abuse Prevention, 1984).

SUMMARY AND CONCLUSIONS

A focus on the community both as a locality where people live as well as a dynamic social and economic network for exchange has a long intellectual history in the behavioral sciences.   This tradition emphasizes both the community as a relevant point to intervene in social problems and the "systemness" of the community.

Prior efforts to prevent alcohol problems in the community have either been unevaluated or, if evaluated, have shown little or mixed success. None of the previous alcohol community prevention projects can be characterized by all five of the following criteria: (1) the development of a careful baseline planning and pre-intervention period; (2) well-defined community-level alcohol-involved problems as targets; (3) a long-term implementation and monitoring period; (4) a follow-up or final scientific evaluation of changes in target problems; and (5) an empirically documented *successful result* in the target that can be attributed to the intervention.

One could conclude that there has been no community prevention project to date that has produced long-term reductions in community-level alcohol problems (see review by Moskowitz, 1989).   Some programs with target groups such as school children, alcohol beverage services, or convicted driving under the influence offenders have demonstrated changes in personal values and attitudes and specific behaviors such as initiation of adolescent drinking (Pentz et al., 1989), reductions in estimated blood alcohol concentration levels for patrons of licensed alcohol establishments (Saltz, 1989a), or re-arrest rates (McCarty and Argeriou, 1988). However, even under the best conditions, the *efficacy* of prevention trials to achieve a reduction in targeted community-level alcohol problems is yet to be demonstrated (see discussion of project phases by Flay, 1986).

In the final analysis, the community definition and perspective employed in a community prevention trial for alcohol problems is a function of the target/objectives of the prevention effort. For alcohol problems or conditions that can be easily assigned to individual residents of a community, a *catchment* area approach would be useful. In this way, at-risk individuals can be defined and prevention strategies developed accordingly.   If the targeted alcohol problem is the cumulative result of events that have time-dependent stochastic properties, such as traffic crashes or burns, then a *system* perspective that addresses individual/environmental interactions would be more appropriate. In practice, a system perspective may include the use of strategies targeted at a group of individuals with higher risk of incurring the problem event, e.g., males between 16 and 25 who have a substantially above-average risk of alcohol-involved traffic crashes. Either of these perspectives may well dictate differing forms of prevention interventions and, thus, require different research designs, measurement, and statistical analyses. Therefore, selecting the perspective for a community prevention trial to reduce specific alcohol problems should be a matter of careful planning with an understanding of the implications involved in the idea of "community."

NOTES

The author recognizes the special assistance of Kim Bloomfield in developing references on community definitions and alcohol prevention case studies for this chapter.

1. Others who have provided additional definition and background to the concept of community include Gusfield (1975) and Warren and Lyon (1983). Anthropological scholars employ similar perspectives even though the traditional study of villages and cultures provides definitions based on participant observation. See, for example, Arensberg and Kimball (1965) and Redfield (1955).

2. For other summaries of the history and process of community organization, see Blakely (1979), Grosser (1973), and Lauffer (1981).

3. A major critic of the conclusions of both books was Dahl, who analyzed decisions on specific issues to identify which persons were the most influential and what were their socioeconomic characteristics. He employed the method in a study of New Haven, Connecticut, and decided that pluralism was indeed the best description of power arrangements (Dahl, 1961). Two of Dahl's former research assistants also published books that formed a trilogy on the theoretical, methodological, and empirical bases for a conclusion that there is no special ruling class in New Haven (Polsby, 1963; Wolfinger, 1974). A later 20-year study of New Haven was a re-examination of original Dahl research materials by Domhoff (1978), who directly challenged the results of Dahl and his associates with a conclusion that those who benefit the most from specific issues (for example, urban renewal) were in formal positions of governmental power when such decisions were made, thus supporting the earlier work of Hunter and Mills.

4. The concept arose out of the "Cultural Indicators" study at the Annenberg School of Communications, University of Pennsylvania. The study monitored violence on TV in the late 1960s and early 1970s and moved on to other issues, including political orientations, sex-role stereotyping, perceptions of the elderly, and health belief and practices (Signorielli, 1986; Bryant and Zillman, 1986).

5. The subsystems are natural groupings of community factors and variables. The elements are of various levels of abstraction and aggregation but have been developed as heuristic means to organize our thinking about the community.

3

Candidate Alcohol Problems and Implications for Measurement: General Alcohol Problems, Outcome Measures, Instrumentation, and Surrogates

Robert F. Saltz, Paul J. Gruenewald, and Michael Hennessy

INTRODUCTION

The success of a community trial evaluation depends on the quality of the measures used to perform the evaluation. In this chapter we review alcohol problems that may be considered candidate outcome variables for a community intervention study.

In considering the variety of potential alcohol problem outcomes, we have identified five primary criteria for selecting of the "best" candidates:

1. Community values—does the community see a given problem as deriving from alcohol consumption? Is the candidate problem perceived as a problem by others? Is the problem seen to be "solvable"?
2. Is the candidate problem truly related to alcohol consumption?
3. Are the measures or indicators of the problem reliable?
4. Can the problem outcome be practically measured?
5. Is there a potential for amelioration of the problem through purposeful intervention?

Criterion 1, by including "community values," we are acknowledging that, in practice, the choice of candidate alcohol problems is limited by the attitudes and beliefs of key people and the general public who will be affected by the intervention (Olsen et al., 1985). There are inevitable differences in the priority one problem will be given relative to another, and some problems may not be seen as alcohol-related at all (Reinarman, 1988).

Criterion 2, the causal relationship between alcohol consumption and a problematic outcome: Obviously, it is not sufficient to observe that some percentage of those involved in, say, traffic crashes have been drinking, and then assume that alcohol was causally related to the outcome. Hingson and Howland (1987) describe four basic types of studies for demonstrating the link between alcohol consumption and a given outcome.

Type I studies are descriptive, providing the frequency of exposure to alcohol among those involved in the negative outcome (e.g., falls, drownings, motor vehicle crashes). These studies do not benefit from a comparison group that would allow calculation of the relative risk of alcohol consumption for the particular consequence of concern, and thus it is difficult to determine the causal relationship of alcohol to the problem.

Type II studies compare the frequency of involvement in an outcome for those undergoing treatment for alcohol problems with the frequency of involvement of the general population. Unfortunately, any observed elevated risk for the treated population may be spurious if some other factor correlated with being in treatment (e.g., socioeconomic status) is more directly related to the problem outcome.

Type III studies attempt to improve on the Type II design by comparing alcohol exposure of those involved in a problematic event (e.g., crash) with those who are being treated for illness or have died of natural causes (to control for biases related to medical treatment). To the degree that the comparison group's alcohol consumption is less than the general population's, the relative risk of drinking will be inflated.

Type IV studies are case-control designs (broadly defined). Here, frequency of exposure to alcohol among outcome cases is compared to frequency of exposure to alcohol among matched controls (where the match is made on both individual and circumstantial variables). Naturally, these studies are the most difficult and costly to conduct and so are rarely reported. One can see that it is often difficult to determine the actual contribution that alcohol consumption may make to a given outcome. The problem is compounded when alcohol's role is indirect or interactive.

Criterion 3, adequate reliability of the measures: Low reliability makes it difficult to detect changes in outcome relative to "noise," and serious problems with reliability would likely render the measure completely invalid.

Criterion 4, the practicality of measurement: We may well find exemplary studies that demonstrate the theoretical value of a particular outcome measure; yet we may still be unable to exploit its value in a community trial. The usual obstacles to optimum measurement are cost in personnel, inaccessibility of data collection sites, or lack of cooperation from other individuals at the specific site.

Criterion 5, potential for amelioration: Even where alcohol's causal relationship to a given problem can be demonstrated, there may be no means available either to reduce alcohol exposure or to intervene so as to "unlink" consumption and the undesired consequence.

In our review of specific problem outcomes below, we will address the suitability of each for a community trial with reference to the five criteria. Given the state of the literature on these issues, we will emphasize Criteria 2 and 3 because much less has been studied or reported with respect to the other criteria.

PARAMETERS OF INTERVENTIONS

Before turning to the specific outcomes, however, we feel it is important to clarify why we chose to emphasize selected alcohol-related <u>problems</u> rather than target groups of people or methods of intervention. Past attempts at community interventions for various problems have targeted various at-risk populations (adolescents or those with "high risk" indicators of blood pressure, alcohol consumption, or cholesterol). There are a number of tested approaches to "community intervention" in the health promotion field, and the approaches typically vary along the following dimensions: the specificity of the target group, the mechanism of the intervention, and the institutional setting through which the intervention is implemented.

For example, drug and alcohol programs often target adolescents and deliver the intervention via training as part of classroom education (Pentz et al., 1989). Interventions aimed at medical outcomes often target those in "high risk" groups, intervene through clinical screenings and medical counseling, and use community health or social service resources for intervention delivery (Benfari, 1981).

Focusing on a particular target group tends to identify only those individuals with the particular "debilitating" or "risk enhancing" characteristic as the locus of the problem. This approach systematically ignores other individuals who may also be exposed to the factors encouraging alcohol use. In addition, specifying a target group of people implicitly denotes an individually based theory of the etiology of the problem, an approach that is difficult to justify given the social factors that motivate and encourage alcohol consumption (Wallack, 1984b).

We also do not believe that any typology of prevention programs based solely on the mode of delivery is useful. Many varied program components could be used to reduce alcohol-related problems, even interventions not directly related to alcohol but rather to some other risk factor. For example, curfew programs that restrict teenage driving hours may reduce alcohol-related crashes even though the curfew policy is not explicitly designed to do so.

Finally, although school-based smoking, alcohol, and drug-use prevention programs are popular, we see no *a priori* reason that educational institutions are more appropriate for intervention delivery than are other alternatives.[1]

ALCOHOL CONSUMPTION

Alcohol use is the central focus of a number of preventive interventions. Studies of the effects of interventions on alcohol problems implicitly or explicitly address the mediating effects of alcohol use. Increases in the minimum drinking age are presumed to alter consumption patterns among youth and lead to reductions in fatal accidents involving motor vehicles (Saffer and Grossman, 1987b; Wagenaar, 1986). Increases in alcoholic beverage prices have been shown to reduce aggregate consumption (Levy and Sheflin, 1985; Selvanathan, 1988) and decrease cirrhosis mortality rates (Cook and Tauchen, 1982). Because of its association with fatal outcomes such as these, alcohol use has come to be viewed as a problem in itself, particularly among groups of heavy users.

The focus on heavy alcohol users and those characterized as "alcohol dependent" or "alcoholics" is longstanding. As the timeworn argument goes, since heavy consumers of alcoholic beverages are responsible for a substantial number of alcohol problems, these consumers should be the target of preventive interventions (Bruun et al., 1975). Concerns about heavy use and dependence have oriented the field toward establishing estimators of "alcoholism," "alcohol dependence," and "heavy" alcohol use from aggregate (Jellinek, 1959; Ledermann, 1964) and self-report (Skinner and Allen, 1982; Knupfer, 1966) data. More recently such concerns have led researchers to focus on heavy alcohol use among young people (Grossman et al., 1987) and on further definition of the heavy alcohol user (Knupfer, 1987).

These research programs have been successful in encouraging the exploration of the relationships between alcohol consumption patterns and the appearance of alcohol problems. They have not, however, clarified the primary assumption on which they were based. Other than in simple correlative ways, the specific relationships of heavy consumption to specific alcohol problems remain unknown. The vague nosological distinctions made in uses of this term, originally viewed as something of an analytic advantage (Knupfer, 1966), have become a source of confusion (Mendelson, 1987; Knupfer, 1987), obscuring the data relevant to elucidation of the relationships between consumption patterns and problems (Mäkelä, 1978; Gruenewald et al., 1990). A complete specification of the parametric relationships between any alcohol-related problem and comprehensive measures of consumption patterns has not appeared. Thus, the number of alcohol-related problems caused by heavy alcohol consumption is unknown.

It is more than obvious that alcohol use can be a problem when it interferes with the social, psychological, or physical functioning of individuals (Edwards, 1986). As Mäkelä (1978) has pointed out, the difficulty is in defining, for any given alcohol-related problem, the pattern of consumption that leads to its appearance. Mäkelä (1978) suggests that this descriptive task can best be met through the construction of parametric models of alcohol consumption that predict probabilities of problem occurrence. Although this research program has not been comprehensively pursued for any given alcohol problem, appropriate parametric models of consumption are appearing in the literature (Gruenewald et al., 1990; Gruenewald, 1989).

An example of the way such a model can improve our understanding of alcohol's role in problem behaviors is provided in recent research into consumption patterns of first offender drunk drivers (Gruenewald et al., 1990; Stewart et al., 1987). In these studies it is shown that although first offender drunk drivers consume more alcohol than the general population, the majority of first offenders are not heavy drinkers (defined by the criterion given by the National Institute on Alcohol Abuse and Alcoholism as one ounce of pure ethanol per day). The problem behavior of drinking and driving, then, is not simply related to increased consumption. While heavy alcohol consumers may be more likely to drink and drive more often than consumers who use alcohol less often, the majority of offenders look very much like the general population in their consumption patterns. Thus, preventive interventions targeted only at heavy alcohol users will miss the mark in reducing the majority of incidents of drinking and driving.

Appropriateness for Community-Level Interventions

As argued here, alcohol use is only a problem insofar as its relationships to the sequelae of its consumption have been demonstrated and are well defined. For purposes of preventive interventions, the measurement of alcohol use in a community represents a crucial mediating variable. Interventions directed at changing consumption itself, such as increasing alcohol prices, or reducing physical availability, can be expected to affect both aggregate (Levy and Sheflin, 1985) and survey measures (Grossman et al., 1987). On the basis of current data, interventions such as these can be expected to have effects on other socially significant outcomes such as motor vehicle crashes (Saffer and Grossman, 1987a) and cirrhosis mortality rates (Cook and Tauchen, 1982). Naturally occurring variations in alcohol consumption rates can be expected to confound estimates of the effects of interventions (such as roadside checkpoints) on a number of outcome measures (such as motor vehicle crashes, highway fatalities, and so on).

The validity of aggregate measures of alcohol consumption has been empirically explored and widely discussed in the literature. Aggregate measures are based on alcohol sales reported for the purposes of taxation and are subject to underreporting for tax avoidance (Cook, 1981). Reported sales may also reflect considerable variation owing to seasonal stocking. And reported sales do not include illegal sales (Smith, 1976). On the other hand, they are inflated by tourism (Nelson, 1988) and by purchases by individuals from border communities (Grossman, 1988). Despite these drawbacks, state and national studies have shown reported sales to be sensitive to changes in prices, incomes, drinking ages, spirits availability, and a number of other state level changes in access to alcohol (Secretary of Health and Human Services, 1987). Research using these data, of course, must be sensitive to these various sources of bias (Grossman, 1988).

Comprehensive investigations of the reliability and validity of survey measures of alcohol consumption in the general population have not been reported in the research literature. Arguments about the validity of self-report judgments have repeatedly appeared but have remained unresolved by empirical investigation. As Midanik (1982) has pointed out, although studies of the internal validity of a number of self-report consumption measures indicate a reasonable level of reliability in individuals' responses, these measures underestimate total alcohol consumption. Assuming alcohol sales data to be a reasonably accurate index of alcohol use, total consumption estimated in this way is some two to four times the amount estimated from self-report surveys (Manning et al., 1989). This underestimation may be due to the reluctance of individuals to report their alcohol consumption truthfully, or to a misspecification of the underlying model of alcohol use, or both.[2]

Self-reports of alcohol use patterns have nevertheless been perceived as a valuable tool for revealing differences in use between demographic groups (for example, Cahalan et al., 1969). They have been shown to be useful instruments for exploring usage patterns within subgroups of the population (Grube and Morgan, 1986), estimating the effects of interventions upon usage patterns (Stewart et al., 1987), and evaluating the relationships of use to a variety of problem outcomes (Dyer et al., 1980).

Ideally, to test the impact of an intervention upon alcohol consumption, or simply to track alcohol consumption as an intervening or confounding variable in measuring alcohol problems, both sources of data would be desirable. Community-wide surveys of alcohol consumption would provide baseline data that could be compared with self-reported rates at follow-up points in time. Aggregate sales data could be used to corroborate the self-report data and, if available over sufficient periods of time, test short- and long-term impacts of interventions upon sales.

Alcoholism and Alcohol Dependence

As in the case of heavy alcohol consumption, various definitions of alcoholism and alcohol dependence have been presented in the literature, each of which has been widely debated (Knupfer, 1987; Glaser et al., 1987; Edwards, 1986; Babor et al., 1986). Because of the ambiguities in the terms alcoholism and alcohol dependence, epidemiological approaches to these problems have generally examined the consequences of these conditions rather than the conditions themselves. Incidents of alcoholism are often taken to be reflected in the primary physiological consequence of this disease state, liver cirrhosis (Lelbach, 1974). Similarly, alcohol dependence has been dealt with in terms of deaths due to acute intoxication and other outcomes exclusive of cirrhosis (Ravenholt, 1984). Unfortunately, alcoholism and alcohol dependence are not independent conditions and liver cirrhosis does not necessarily require alcohol involvement (Crow and Greenway, 1989).

Alcoholism does appear as a unique diagnostic category in contemporary American Psychological Association diagnostic manuals (DSM-III), and reports of admissions for alcoholism can be found in the literature. Malin et al. (1982) report that 423,910 hospital discharges (or 197 per 100,000 individuals) in 1975 were attributed to admissions for alcoholism. Thus, however this term is defined clinically, the incidence of this condition can be measured using hospital discharge surveys. The reliability of this measure, however, is unknown, and the feasibility of preventive interventions acting to reduce alcoholism can only be indirectly inferred from more common studies of cirrhosis mortality rates (Watts and Rabow, 1983; Cook and Tauchen, 1982). Variations in application of the term alcoholic render use of this diagnostic category as a prevention outcome measure problematic.

As noted above, the term alcohol dependence also suffers from a number of definitional problems. Although some consensus on this term has been claimed (Skinner, 1981), measurement of a discrete state of alcohol dependence has eluded researchers. Reliable measurement of dependence has been achieved using self-report instruments (Skinner and Allen, 1982). These measurements discriminate among various clinical populations (Skinner and Horn, 1984) and have been related to alcohol use in first-offender drunk drivers (Gruenewald et al., 1990). Data on the degree of alcohol dependence among the general population is unavailable. However, if data from first-offender drunk drivers is any indicator of the general population, it is obvious that floor effects will occur in the measurement of dependence in any general survey sampling scheme. On the 48-point Alcohol Dependence Syndrome scale, the majority of first driving under the influence offenders scored four points or less (Stewart et al., 1987).

Appropriateness for Community-Level Interventions

Alcoholism

It is feasible within any community of reasonable size to track numbers of individuals treated for alcoholism on the basis of discharge surveys. Reports of admissions for alcoholism could be subject to a number of biases including the selection of this category for purposes that lie outside considerations of diagnostic accuracy (e.g., to maintain insurance copayments) or failure to use this diagnostic category in order to protect favored individuals from the socially undesirable label of alcoholic, and so on. So little is known about the validity and reliability of this diagnostic category in medical records that implementation of the measure as a prevention problem outcome would require concurrent reliability and validity studies.

Alcohol Dependence

The measurement of alcohol dependence would require the use of survey instruments appropriate to the general community. Thus, Skinner and Horn (1984) note that the Alcohol Dependence Syndrome scale was developed for and tested with populations of previously defined alcoholics. The feasibility of applying one such instrument to a very broad population of first-offender drunk drivers has been demonstrated by Stewart et al. (1987). Given the relatively high internal consistency of this scale in both clinical and first-offender samples, degrees of alcohol dependence could, in principle, be measured in the general population of any community. It remains, of course, problematic as to either what is meant by alcohol dependence or how it is related to other problem behavior measures. Although it now seems clear that one aspect of this syndrome, "loss of control" drinking defined in terms of drinking patterns, is clearly related to alcohol dependence (Gruenewald, 1989), the syndrome is also claimed to be represented by other clinically defined symptoms (Edwards, 1986). Given the current uncertain state of the notion of alcohol dependence, its ambiguous relationship to the equally vaguely defined notion of alcoholism, and its uncertain relationship to other alcohol-related problems, use of this measure as an outcome in a community prevention intervention is problematic.

SPECIFIC PROBLEM OUTCOMES

We will now review some of the other major problem outcomes that might be considered for outcome measures in a community trial. While alcohol use may be hypothesized to contribute to a wide variety of problems (e.g., interpersonal arguments), our interest here lies with those for which alcohol use is more proximal to the negative consequence and for which there exists research to support the association.

Highway Crashes

In this section we discuss general studies of prevalence, special subgroup analysis, and some research on the analysis of the covariation of accident rates with other manipulable variables that could be altered through policy changes.

Prevalence Studies

By far the most numerous attempts to quantify the involvement of alcohol in traffic crashes, injuries, and fatalities is done through the Fatal Accident Reporting System (FARS) of the National Highway Traffic Safety Administration. FARS takes the total number of crashes reported and allocates them to those in which alcohol is involved and those in which alcohol is not involved. For example, Fell and Nash (1989) report that of the total crash fatalities in 1987 (46,386) slightly over half involved alcohol; in addition to the fatalities, alcohol-involved crashes resulted in about half a million injuries. This estimate of "about half" of fatal accidents appears to be the conventional wisdom (Ravenholt, 1984) and is commonly cited in passing by investigators highlighting the drinking and driving problem (e.g., Wagenaar, 1983; Saffer and Grossman, 1987a). It is likely that the rate decreased during the 1980s; more recent estimates suggest a 40% rate of alcohol involvement (Department of Transportation, 1989).

Subgroup Analysis

Prevalence studies often discuss the different rates of "alcohol involved" crashes among subpopulations of interest, usually defined by the age and sex of the drivers, particularly younger drivers and males because these groups are overrepresented in crashes of all types (Council on Scientific Affairs, 1983; Hingson et al., 1988; Karpf and Williams, 1983; Evans, 1987). Time of day (day and night) and type of crash (single vehicle versus multiple vehicle) are other categories. Younger drivers have high rates of alcohol-related crash involvement, even though they tend to drive fewer miles annually and are typically less impaired than older drivers (Department of Transportation, 1989:Table 25; Williams and Karpf, 1984; Pelz and Schuman, 1971; Williams, 1985; Mayhew et al., 1986). In relation to time of day and type of crash, alcohol involvement appears to be higher on weekend nights, when most teenage driving takes place (Williams, 1985) and for single-vehicle crashes. These findings have obvious implications for the design of prevention programs (Council on Scientific Affairs, 1983).

A smaller number of subgroup studies estimate the rates of alcohol involvement in crashes not through the use of official statistics (which have associated measurement problems) but through the use of general population surveys eliciting self-reports of drinking and driving behavior (which have a different set of measurement problems). These studies concentrate on teenagers (e.g., Pelz and Schuman, 1971) and show rates of teenage drinking and driving that are quite variable across studies. Teenage drivers have generally lower rates than do respondents in the early twenties (see Wagenaar, 1983; Mayhew et al., 1986; Elliot, 1987) but higher risk of crash involvement (of any type) even after controlling for miles driven (Cameron, 1982; Hingson et al., 1982; Williams, Lund, and Preusser, 1986) and BAC level (Mayhew et al., 1986).

Policy Studies

At the most general level, these studies look at the covariation between crash rates (sometimes alcohol-involved crashes in particular) and other variables, some of which could be used to reflect actual or potential policy changes. For example, Colon and Cutter (1983) relate 1976 state data on fatal accidents and fatalities (not necessarily alcohol related) to a set of independent variables reflecting state driving policies, alcohol regulation, alcohol consumption measures, and driver characteristics. They suggest that limiting outlets may increase drinking and driving while reducing liver cirrhosis rates. Using a similar approach, Rush, Gliksman, and Brook (1986) found a positive association between retail availability of alcohol, alcohol consumption, and alcohol-related morbidity and mortality and concluded that government policies that restrict the availability of alcohol will reduce per capita consumption and, indirectly, lower alcohol-related damage. Mann and Anglin (1988) also found a positive relationship between per capita consumption and the number of alcohol-related crashes and single-vehicle and nighttime fatalities.

Looking at different regulation and control policies, Preusser et al. (1984) examined the effects of curfew laws restricting teenage driving and found them generally effective in reducing teenage crashes. Robertson (1980) compared crash rates of 16- and 17-year-olds in towns that had eliminated driver education and found lower crash rates due to the effect of reducing the pool of young, inexperienced drivers. Saffer and Grossman (1987a) compared the expected effects on teenage crash mortality of changes in driving age versus increases in excises taxes on beer. They concluded that tax policy has the potential for greater influence on fatal crashes of teenage drivers than do minimum age laws. Finally, a review of many studies evaluating the effects of changes in minimum drinking age can be found in Wagenaar (1983).

Thus all these studies, while varying dramatically in choice of policy instrument to control alcohol-related crashes and fatalities, examined the aggregate relationship among different policy instruments in affecting alcohol-related crashes and/or fatalities. Many of them highlight the potential of policy changes to affect such outcomes.

Measurement Problems in Alcohol-Related Crash Literature

The measurement problems relating to alcohol-related fatalities and crashes include the reliable measurement of Blood Alcohol Concentration (BAC), the accuracy of the established community reporting system for fatalities and accidents, and the use of the appropriate proxy measure for estimating the effects of policy changes specifically designed to reduce drinking and driving. Each of these issues is discussed below.

Measuring BAC

This problem has two separate components. First, there is a bias using the FARS data because selective testing for BAC inflates the estimate of alcohol involved crashes and their victims (Zylman, 1974; Noordzij, 1983; Public Health Service, 1983; Heeren et al., 1985). For example, Williams et al. (1988) report a BAC testing rate of over 70% of deceased drivers in 1986 but a test rate of only 23% for surviving drivers. In addition, other more local crash handling procedures (e.g., autopsy policies of county coroners) may also tend to inflate the apparent rate of alcohol involvement (Mason and McBay, 1984). Precisely because of the problem of incomplete BAC reporting, the FARS reporting system attempts to estimate statistically the BAC levels of drivers using data on driver, crash, and vehicle characteristics (Klein, 1986). We know of no validation studies of this *post hoc* approach.

The second problem with BAC lies with its measurement at the individual level. Standard formulas for estimating BAC are based on average or composite estimates that may not apply to specific individuals and may mask the variance inherent in the test itself (O'Neill et al., 1983; Hume and Fitzgerald, 1985). Moreover, specific methods of test administration and subject response (such as breathing patterns) can produce erroneous results (Jones, 1982).

Assessing the Accuracy of Archival Records

Since most published research uses only a single source of data, the quality of archival information on crashes and the characteristics of victims appears to be unknown. The few existing studies provide examples of approaches to data validity but tend to focus on events that are specifically noncrash related (Agran and Dunkle, 1985), are performed in an organizational environment dissimilar to that found in the United States (Maas and Harris, 1984), or do not focus on alcohol-related issues (Bull and Roberts, 1973).

Proxy Measures for Drinking and Driving

Because of the problems with BAC testing, there has been a search for archival data that could be used as a proxy to estimate the effects of policies designed to reduce drinking and driving. Using two states with relatively complete FARS BAC testing,[3] Heeren et al. (1985) suggest the use of total nighttime fatalities (out of five alternatives) as the best proxy measure in the absence of complete BAC testing.

Appropriateness for Community-Level Interventions

Alcohol-related highway crashes probably do have potential as outcome measures for community interventions because they can be affected at the community level by various regulatory and enforcement interventions. Furthermore, such crashes represent a well documented domain of alcohol research with both basic and applied components of many interventions already tested.

However, some preliminary work would be necessary in a particular community before complete confidence would be warranted in the validity of the outcomes measured. Comparisons of police and hospital recording systems would be mandatory to assess the accuracy and crash coverage percentages of normal community level crash data collection. This assessment should also include a review of the BAC testing procedures in the community, which may in turn require BAC testing of all crash participants to rule out systematic selection effects present in past studies.[4] Such on-site coding has been done in great detail for motorcycle crashes, for example, and could be done for all vehicular crashes if the community crash catchment area is small.

Falls, Drownings, and Burns

Falls, drownings, and burns are the second, third, and fourth leading causes of accidental death in the United States. With an aggregate rate of 11 deaths per 100,000 annually, these causes of death trail behind the leading cause of accidental death, traffic-related fatalities (18.2 per 100,000, Aitken and Zobeck, 1985). As with traffic-related accidents, a major research concern has been to determine alcohol involvement in these three causes of death and injury. In contrast to studies of traffic-related accidents, however, evidence regarding alcohol involvement is scarce.

Deaths and Injuries Due to Falls

Deaths due to falls occur at an annual rate of 5.5 per 100,000 individuals. Injuries are estimated to occur at the much higher rate of 6,700 per 100,000 (Howland and Hingson, 1987). Of the three sources of accidental injury and death discussed in this section, alcohol involvement in the case of falls is best documented.

Three basic types of studies have been used to ascertain the involvement of alcohol in deaths and injuries due to falls: (1) coroner studies of deceased individuals (Haberman and Baden, 1978; Waller, 1972); (2) emergency room studies of people hurt in falls (Stephens, 1987; Cherpitel, 1988); and (3) studies comparing rates of death and injuries due to falls between the general population and samples of treated alcoholics (Thorarisson, 1979).

Each of these three types of studies presents unique methodological problems that render their estimates of alcohol involvement somewhat suspect (Howland and Hingson, 1987). In the case of coroner studies, the use of autopsies to ascertain BACs of some but not all deaths, the confounding of estimated BACs with time since death, and the absence of a control group with which to compare alcohol involvement in these deaths, makes estimates from these studies biased and difficult to use. Emergency room studies have attempted to establish an adequate comparison group by relating rates of alcohol involvement among emergency room entries for injuries due to falls to the alcohol involvement in other illnesses at entry. Unfortunately, since individuals entering emergency rooms do not constitute a representative sample of the general population and alcohol use may interact with other reasons for emergency room admission, population-based estimates of alcohol involvement from these studies are also biased.

Because of the methodological limitations of these studies, Hingson and Howland (1987), in their review of the literature, estimated alcohol involvement in fatal falls to range from 21 to 77%. Similarly, their estimate of alcohol involvement in nonfatal falls ranged from 17 to 53%. Thus, depending on one's reading of the literature, alcohol involvement in deaths and injuries due to falls may be low or high.

Some of the problems confronted in obtaining an accurate estimate of alcohol involvement in fatal and nonfatal falls were resolved in a Finnish study. Honkanen et al. (1983) established an estimate of alcohol involvement in injuries due to falls using a case-control study. Adults seeking emergency care for falls were compared to similar adults selected from the sites at which the original falls took place.[5] Thus, the comparison group was composed of selected individuals who did not fall at the accident sites. The authors found that alcohol was involved in 60% of the fall cases they examined. They were also able to establish the relative risks of alcohol exposure for falls at various BACs. They found that at BACs of 50 mg/dl, the relative risk of falls was not elevated. However, the relative risk of falls climbed dramatically at higher BACs. At 50-100 mg/dl the relative risk was 3, at 100-150 mg/dl the risk rose to 10, and at BACs of 160 mg/dl and higher the risk rose to 60.

On the basis of this study it appears that increasing levels of alcohol use are related to increasing relative risks of injury due to falls. However, on the basis of studies conducted in the United States, the incidence of alcohol involvement in injuries and deaths due to falls in this country remains unclear.

Deaths Due to Drownings

Deaths due to drownings occur at an annual rate of 3 per 100,000 (Howland and Hingson, 1988). Studies of this cause of death have focused upon four water sport activities: swimming/surfing (Cairns et al., 1984; National Transportation Safety Board [NTSB], 1985), boating (Mogford, 1983; NTSB, 1985), fishing (Cairns et al., 1984; Press et al., 1968) and scuba/skin diving (Pleuckhahn, 1982).

Coroner studies have been exclusively used to establish the level of alcohol involvement in drownings. In addition to the previously mentioned problems in regard to these types of studies, Howland and Hingson (1988) point out that the degree of ascertainment of cases in studies of drowning varies widely, aggravating selection bias. The studies also vary substantially in reports of submergence (a confounder in estimating BACs at injury), methods for determining alcohol exposure, and reports of the sociodemographic characteristics of the subjects observed. Thus, comparability among studies is at a minimum.

Based on their summary of the literature, Howland and Hingson (1988) hazard a guess that some 25 to 50% of all drownings may involve alcohol. However, they note that "without data on the frequency of alcohol consumption among nonvictims engaged in aquatic activities, the causal role of alcohol in drowning is uncertain." The absence of any case-control studies renders any causal attribution regarding the role of alcohol difficult.

Deaths and Injuries Due to Burns

Deaths due to burns occur at an annual rate of 2.5 per 100,000. Injuries are estimated to occur at the rate of 423 per 100,000 (Howland and Hingson, 1987). Coroner studies (Mierley and Baker, 1983; Trier, 1983), emergency room studies (Stephens, 1985), and comparisons of deaths and injuries due to burns between alcoholic subjects and the general population (Combs-Orme et al., 1983) have been used to ascertain alcohol involvement in these accidents. The same criticisms of these studies apply here as with falls and drownings. Coroner studies indicate an involvement of alcohol in from 37 to 64% of deaths due to burns. Emergency room studies suggest that alcohol involvement in burn injuries can be found in about 18% of cases. Comparisons of the relative risks of death due to burns between alcoholics and members of the general population suggest odd ratios ranging from 9 to 98 (Howland and Hingson, 1987). No case-control studies are available with which to determine alcohol's causal involvement in death and injuries due to burns.

Appropriateness for Community-Level Interventions

The rates of fatalities due to falls, drownings and burns, regardless of alcohol involvement, eliminate these measures as candidate outcomes for any community level intervention. While interventions may affect the incidence of these fatal accidents, the base rates for these events are too low to use them as evaluative criteria. The high rate of reported injuries for falls and burns (7,123 per 100,000), on the other hand, suggests that these outcomes may be profitably measured at the community level. Unfortunately, as noted above, our knowledge of alcohol's role in these accidents is sketchy.

Investigations of the role of alcohol in nonfatal falls and burns is currently at a somewhat primitive stage. For example, while it is feasible to track emergency room admissions for nonfatal falls and burns, the determination of alcohol's causal involvement in these cases is difficult. Current procedures seem to be accompanied by too many flaws to be relied upon without ancillary studies of alcohol's causal role in these accidents.

Medical Outcomes

First, we will discuss the general literature on morbidity and mortality that looks at the negative consequences of long-term alcohol use and is usually based on samples of alcoholics or participants in clinical intervention and/or health promotion programs. Then we focus specifically on four specific medical outcomes: liver disease, blood pressure, types of cancers, and heart disease.

"Heavy" Alcohol Consumption and Mortality or Health Problems

Most of these studies are derived from clinical reports from special populations or from cohort data collected during general health-promotion programs (e.g., Poikolainen, 1983; Petersson et al., 1984). Virtually all reports show heightened relative risk of mortality or years of potential life lost (YPLL) (Public Health Service, 1985) from many sources including accidents, suicide, traffic crashes, burns, and health problems, given membership in the heavy drinking group, which is variably defined (Schmidt, 1980).

Liver Diseases

Liver cirrhosis is the ninth leading cause of death in the United States with an estimated alcohol-related age-adjusted prevalence of 4.4 cases per 100,000 in 1985 (Williams et al., 1988) and an overall rate (that is, not necessarily alcohol-related) of about twice this number (Grant et al., 1986; Williams et al., 1988). Although this case is one where the "etiological importance of long-term heavy alcohol use . . . has been established beyond doubt," (Schmidt, 1980; see also Hasin et al., 1990; Popham et al., 1984), there has been little advance in the medical treatment of fully developed liver cirrhosis during the last two decades (Saunders et al., 1981; Schenker, 1984).

High Blood Pressure

As in the case of cirrhosis, the relationship between alcohol and high blood pressure has been consistently established and appears to be causal, since it responds positively to experimental dosages of ethanol and is highest in heavy drinkers compared with moderate and light drinkers (Livingston, 1985; Gleiberman and Harburg, 1986). Note, however, that blood pressure in clinical alcoholics does not seem especially elevated (Gleiberman and Harburg, 1986).

Cancers

Alcohol's role in cancer appears to be relatively limited to specific cancers of the respiratory and upper digestive tracts, with considerable physiological and social confounding because of the positive relationship between individuals who both drink and smoke (Popham et al., 1984; Schmidt, 1980). Indeed, the combination of these two risk factors may interact to produce greater combined risk than would be expected given the effects of each activity alone (Ravenholt, 1984). Other types of cancers are not conclusively implicated with alcohol use (Olsen et al., 1989; Lowenfels and Zevola, 1989).

Heart Disease

There appears to be evidence for a "protective effect" against heart disease of moderate alcohol consumption (Moore and Pearson, 1986). Even more surprising, many studies conclude that the risk function is U or J shaped, with abstainers and heavy drinkers experiencing higher probabilities of heart disease than those who consume at moderate levels (Marmot, 1984). To many public health professionals this is not unequivocal.[6] As a result, the published research is more comprehensive (as well as less neutral in tone, see Goplen,

1982) than in other health areas. There appears to be basic agreement on only two points.

First, many reports suggest that there is a plausible physiological basis for the "protective hypothesis" due to ethanol's effects on high density lipoproteins, which have been extensively studied in clinical and quasi-experimental research (Fraser et al., 1983; Thornton et al., 1983; Gruchow et al., 1982; Ferrence et al., 1986; Marmot, 1984; Barboriak et al., 1983). Second, because the results are so unexpected, researchers are invariably careful to control for numerous other confounding risk factors. Almost uniformly, however, the negative relationship between moderate consumption and heart disease remains unaffected by these controls (Kaufman et al., 1985; Ferrence et al., 1986; Marmot, 1984; Stampfer et al., 1985; Colditz et al., 1985; Gruchow et al., 1982; Siscovick et al., 1986; Moore and Pearson, 1986).

Schmidt and Popham (1981) suggest diet and Kaufman et al. (1985) suggest "Type A" behavior as alternative explanations.[7] One result that would conclusively show that the observed negative correlation between moderate alcohol consumption and heart disease was spurious: differential heart disease rates between consumers of different types of alcoholic drinks.[8] Unfortunately, most studies do not address this issue and the few studies that do so find inconsistent results (Marmot, 1984; Popham et al, 1984; Stampfer et al., 1985).

Measurement Problems with Health Outcomes and Alcohol Literature

In their medical context, there are few apparent measurement problems. Most studies use fatalities as the outcome (verified through medical exams and/or the collection of death records). Others performed on living subjects use already developed medical measurements (i.e., "occlusion scores"). The studies that utilize individual respondents (as opposed to archival data) are typically very comprehensive in collecting data that can be used as mediating or control variables (such as diet, self-reports or spousal reports of alcohol consumption, and extensive medical measurements).

Appropriateness for Community-Level Interventions

While there is an impressive number of health outcome and alcohol studies performed on a wide variety of populations, it appears that two factors could prevent them from being particularly appropriate for community-level interventions: (1) prevalence rates are low for any medical outcome, even those unambiguously linked to alcohol consumption such as cirrhosis and (2) the length of time necessary to test a significant effect may exceed available resources for evaluation.

CRIME AND ALCOHOL

Of all the candidate outcomes for a community trial study, the link between alcohol consumption and crime is probably the least well-developed, though not through lack of interest in the topic. There exist several excellent overviews of research in the area (Pernanen, 1976, 1981; Roizen and Schneberk, 1977; Roizen, 1982). Our purpose here is not to update those reviews but rather to consider the possibility of targeting alcohol-related criminal acts (or some subset of them) through a directed intervention and the adequacy of measures that might be used to evaluate that effort.

Several working models address the alcohol and crime relationship. Early explanations postulated that consumption of alcoholic beverages could be a sufficient cause of violent and criminal behavior. Drinking was also seen as an activity to bolster one's courage before committing an illegal act. Later, alcohol was postulated to "disinhibit" antisocial behavior through its effects on the "higher" mental processes. These explanations are now out of favor (Pernanen, 1976; Room and Collins, 1983). Current theories are more apt to include social and cultural factors (MacAndrew and Edgerton, 1969), as well as individual attitudes and expectancies regarding alcohol and violence (Lang et al., 1975). Researchers are also more likely to see alcohol consumption as a mediating or interactive variable in settings likely to give rise to violence. There are also a handful of studies that examine the role of alcohol in one's likelihood of becoming a victim (e.g., by being an easy target when intoxicated), or that see alcohol consumption as a likely outgrowth of criminal lifestyles (e.g., having periods of inactivity, having large sums of cash, being unmarried) (see Cordelia, 1985).

Most of the empirical research done in this area is of Type I (Hingson and Howland, 1987) in that it concentrates on the prevalence of drinking in association with various criminal acts. One finds, for instance, that either the offender or the victim or both were drinking in 36 to 70% of homicides, 37 to 48% of assaults, 31 to 50% of sex offenses, and 12 to 64% of robberies (interquartile ranges given in Roizen, 1982). These studies typically provide no comparison groups from which to calculate "expected values" (Pernanen, 1981) for these proportions.

In addition, the research is handicapped by the various definitions used for alcohol involvement and crime. With the exception of homicides, for which the victim is available for blood alcohol testing, alcohol involvement derives from either a police officer's judgment or the offender's self-report.

There is, as well, a disproportionate emphasis on crimes against a person as opposed to property crimes.

Numerous potential sources of bias and unreliability exist in these data sources (Greenberg, 1981). In the case of police reports, there are seldom standards for defining alcohol involvement. It sometimes includes evidence of any drinking, excessive drinking, or someone's being under the influence. Sometimes the setting alone (e.g., a bar) may be used to establish alcohol involvement. Another problem with police reports lies in the relatively low priority police officers have for establishing the role of alcohol in the crime. This would be especially true in cases where some time has elapsed between the event and locating the alleged offender. Finally, what evidence there is seems to suggest a lack of agreement between police officers and participants regarding drunkenness (Bard and Zacker, 1974).

Self-reported drinking by offenders during the crime may be biased in several ways. The offender may believe that his or her drinking excuses the act. The investigating police officer may be more or less likely to arrest someone in a personal assault if either or both parties have been drinking. Drinking offenders may, through either acute or chronic impairment, be more likely to be caught, and those with a history of alcohol problems may be sent to residential treatment centers in lieu of prison, where offender surveys are typically conducted.

These biases are further compounded by police practices for investigating a crime. Police officers will most often attempt a reconciliation rather than invoke official action (Gove et al., 1985) for non-serious personal crimes (e.g., not involving injury or threat to life or the use of a weapon), especially when the alleged offender and the victim are known to one another. Since most personal crimes involve family members, friends, or acquaintances, this means that many of these incidents will be negotiated without an arrest. These settings are precisely those most likely involving alcohol (Welte and Abel, 1989).

A real possibility exists that the relationship of alcohol consumption to crime is spurious. On a gross level, both activities are predominantly engaged in by young males and both may derive from features of the male role in a given culture (Zucker, 1968; McCord and McCord, 1962). The association could derive from the fact that alcohol is available and consumed in many of the social settings for personal crimes without its being causally related.

There are, nevertheless, two particularly intriguing studies conducted by Lenke (1975) in Sweden and Takala (1973) in Finland, in which rates of violent crime dropped during reductions in the availability of alcohol. A 1972 strike in the Finnish alcohol monopoly stores, for example, reduced consumption by an estimated 30%, "cases of assault and battery were reduced by some 20 to 25 percent," and there were reductions in other crimes as well (Mäkelä, 1980, quoted in Room, 1983).

These last examples suggest that interventions relevant to the availability of alcohol could be efficacious in reducing violent crime. The results are only suggestive, however, given that a community intervention is not likely to involve such severe changes in alcohol availability. Furthermore, generalizing from other cultures to the United States is risky. And, as others have pointed out, the drop in alcohol supply may have affected crime by reducing social interaction that would normally have occurred in drinking places or in other informal settings.

Appropriateness for Community-Level Interventions

The empirical evidence suggests that there is an alcohol/crime association and that the relationship is most likely in violent crime against the person (homicide, aggravated assault). Further research is needed to raise confidence that the apparent association is not spurious.

It is difficult to conceive of a community-level intervention directed at violent or criminal behavior. The most likely approach would be server intervention to reduce the incidence of intoxication, which would presumably lower interpersonal conflict among those drinking in licensed establishments. We might then expect the incidence of bar fights in particular to decline, although bar fights are probably not prevalent in the community as a whole and probably occur at bars and restaurants that would be least likely to participate in a server intervention program.

The other likely avenue of prevention would be much less direct; it would be the possible change in community norms concerning intoxication per se. If a community intervention program emphasized the varied risks of intoxication and altered the public's reaction to drunkenness, there might very well be some intervening to reduce intoxication (in ways other than server intervention) or to take action with someone who is intoxicated.

The measurement of alcohol-related crime is difficult at best. One would likely limit measurement to serious cases of aggravated assault and homicide (the two are usually different only in the circumstances of the weapon used or the availability of medical treatment) so as to limit the reporting bias of both citizens and police officers. But even here one would probably have to rely on the officer's report of alcohol involvement. These data could be improved through the routine use of passive breath testing devices in the field, but the use of such devices would be problematic because of questionable legality and the previously mentioned lack of interest among police in establishing alcohol involvement. The success of measurement, then, becomes dependent on the particular community's willingness to cooperate and the resources they are willing to commit.

CONCLUDING REMARKS

Several alcohol-involved problems can be considered candidates for community-level intervention. Our choice of candidates and criteria for evaluating them obviously reflect our perspective on alcohol problems generally.

We have deemphasized alcoholics or problem drinkers in our discussions, not only because of the vagueness these labels carry but also because a large proportion of alcohol-related problems derive from episodes of acute impairment, and that impairment is distributed across the drinking population. While some drinkers (including alcoholics and problem drinkers) are no doubt at higher risk themselves for problems, at the community level, many more problems involve those whose drinking is quite infrequent and often light or moderate. We would nevertheless expect that interventions targeted at the community level would affect the drinking of chronic and heavy drinkers in addition to all others.

Our emphasis on drinking *events* leads us to look at outcomes related to particular occasions of alcohol consumption. Thus, we have focused more on trauma, for instance, than on long-term financial difficulties related to heavy alcohol consumption or dependency. Specific outcomes such as trauma lend themselves to more reliable measurement, despite the difficulties previously cited.

Finally, the quality of any measure seems strongly related to the seriousness of the outcome. A death through traumatic injury or homicide, for instance, is much more likely to be categorized as alcohol-related or not than is a slight injury. On the other hand, because the most serious outcomes are the least prevalent, investigators have to weigh the inherent quality of measurement against the prevalence of the phenomenon it measures. Furthermore, investigators should select the test community in conjunction with the targeted outcome to optimize the tradeoff between the quality of measurement and its power (related to prevalence) in a given setting.

The review of candidate outcomes provided here serves as a reminder that a successful community trial research project represents an artful blend of research design, scientific rigor, informed judgment, fertile ground, and blind luck. Our hope is to minimize dependence on the last of these.

NOTES

1. We would emphatically disagree that " . . . prevention is essentially an educational process." (Pentz et al., 1986:390).

2. Gruenewald (1989) suggests that the mathematical model used to calculate total consumption estimates from self-report data (e.g.,

quantity-frequency judgments) is misspecified; it will always underestimate total alcohol use, even when confronted with perfectly accurate data.

3. It is no coincidence that the two states selected were Delaware and Vermont.

4. At the very least, detailed crash data would need to be collected to model the selection process of those participants tested and not tested.

5. The availability of government funded medical services at emergency rooms in Finland substantially alleviates biases in sample representativeness among fall victims. Few accident victims seek private care. To test for sample bias, two sets of comparison subjects were selected to match characteristics of the accident group. Estimates of relative risk using the two comparison groups were found to be quite stable.

6. It should be pointed out that all researchers who find evidence for the "protective hypothesis" emphasize that alcohol consumption leads to other, negative, consequences (e.g. Colditz, et al., 1985:889; Stampfer et al., 1985:272; Criqui, 1990:856).

7. It is also suggested that this result is an artifact of inappropriately classifying ex-heavy drinkers as abstainers in certain samples (Fraser et al., 1983:321-322; Popham et al., 1984:156, Shaper, 1990); but Marmot (1984) finds little evidence for this explanation, and when Stampfer et al. (1985:268-269) reanalyzed their data to adjust for this, they found no difference.

8. This finding would not, of course, identify the important confounding variable; it would simply demonstrate that the observed negative relationship was invalid.

Part III

Lessons and Experiences from Community Trials in Other Health Fields

4

Phases for Developing Community Trials: Lessons for Control of Alcohol Problems from Research in Cardiovascular Disease, Cancer, and Adolescent Health

John W. Farquhar and Stephen P. Fortmann

INTRODUCTION

In this chapter we examine experiences in comprehensive community-based approaches to solving health problems in cardiovascular disease (CVD), cancer, and adolescent health in order to derive lessons applicable to the prevention of alcohol-related problems. The theory, design, implementation, and evaluation of the growing number of large community projects are described. Special attention is paid to the stages of research that preceded their field application in these projects to examine whether community studies are now appropriate in the alcohol field.

RATIONALE FOR COMMUNITY-BASED STUDIES

The goal of public health is to control disease and injury in entire populations through comprehensive treatment, effective prevention, or a combination of the two. Such an ideal health policy can be seen as the end result of a logical sequence of research proceeding from basic science through clinical investigation and field research to implementation. Community studies come near the end of such a sequence, testing the generalizability and effectiveness of treatments introduced on a scale that could lend to comprehensive control. As such, community studies carry a number of advantages that will be outlined

Research and preparation for this chapter was supported in part by Grant 5R01 HL21906 13, National Heart, Lung, and Blood Institute, United States Department of Health and Human Services.

below. First, however, we will elaborate on this idealized sequence as a context for understanding both the community studies described in this chapter and the implications for controlling alcohol-related problems.

Both the National Heart, Lung, and Blood Institute (NHLBI) and the National Cancer Institute (NCI) have developed definitions of the various stages in an idealized sequence of research (Tables 4.1 and 4.2). For both, community studies are shown as the final phases for testing the applicability of interventions (including prevention) developed in the early stages. Flay (1986) describes a more elaborate model with eight phases. He denotes studies in Phases II and III of both the NHLBI and NCI models as efficacy trials, which determine if a treatment works under optimum conditions (when a treatment is *delivered* to all individuals and is *accepted* by them). Effectiveness trials, in contrast, test interventions in more realistic settings that accept greater variability in both delivery and acceptance. Flay describes three levels of effectiveness trials, ending with demonstration studies in whole systems, such as cities, states, and nations.

TABLE 4.1
The National Heart, Lung And Blood Institute Research Spectrum

Phase	Description
I.	**Basic research.** Research seeking new knowledge about normal and abnormal functions of the heart, lungs, and blood and the etiology and pathogenesis of their diseases.
II.	**Applied research and development.** Research seeking to develop new ways of using basic research results to achieve specific practical goals.
III.	**Clinical trials.** Trials to determine the efficacy and safety of clinical interventions in samples of patients drawn from larger population groups.
IV.	**Prototype studies.** Small-scale tests of refined programs using component suggested by Phase II research to be efficacious (and further development of methods for future research).
V.	**Demonstration and education research.** Tests of the effectiveness of interventions designed to promote health or prevent disease in defined populations. The interventions selected for such testing should be those that have already been found to be efficacious in other studies and include, but are not limited to, education strategies and modifications in health care and health-related practices.

Source: National Heart, Lung and Blood Institute, 1983. "Guidelines for Demonstration and Education Research Grants." National Heart, Lung and Blood Institute, Washington, DC.

TABLE 4.2
The National Cancer Institute Cancer Control Research Phases

Phase	Description
I.	**Hypothesis development.** Identifies and synthesizes available scientific evidence about a specific cancer. A testable hypothesis is then formulated about the effectiveness of applying an intervention.
II.	**Methods development.** Characterizes the variables that must be controlled or monitored in subsequent intervention studies, and ensures that accurate and valid procedures are available before the actual study is begun.
III.	**Controlled intervention trials.** Test hypothesis developed in Phase I, using methodology validated in Phase II. Phase III studies test the efficacy of an intervention. Case-control methodology is generally used.
IV.	**Defined population studies.** Quantitatively measure the impact of an intervention in a sizable, distinct, and well-characterized population.
V.	**Demonstration and implementation.** Application of the intervention in a community at large to measure the public health impact.

Source: Greenwald, P. and Cullen, J. W., 1984. "The Scientific Approach to Cancer Control," *CA: Cancer Journal for Clinicians*, *34*, 328-332.

While useful, these idealized linear models have limitations. At times, public policy moves more rapidly than research, and some phases are often skipped. For example, the National High Blood Pressure Education Program was implemented before large-scale community studies confirmed the generalizability of clinical trials of antihypertensive treatment. Also, trials of single components of what will become a comprehensive community effort may not indicate the true potential of each component because together the components may perform differently. Finally, there are components of community intervention that cannot be modeled in more limited studies that seek organizational, environmental, and political changes.

The principal rationale for conducting community studies is that they are necessary to validate interventions suggested by earlier stages of the research process. Community studies have other rationales, particularly in the context of behavior-related health problems such as heart disease, cancer, and alcohol use. Community interventions are able to affect individuals directly through education and indirectly through social and environmental changes, leading to the potential for synergistic interactions among components of the intervention. For example, both an education program and a new law might increase seat belt use in separate ("efficacy") studies. Together, however, they might achieve more change than expected from summing their separate effects.

Community studies allow the use of multiple channels for communicating with individuals, such as the mass media, health professionals, schools, and worksites. Some such channels, particularly the mass media, are inherently cost-effective.

In summary, the rationale for community trials is that they provide for the development and evaluation of health interventions of appropriate scope for implementation as public health policy. These trials provide for the testing of programs among diverse populations, and they also develop methods, such as those useful in community organization, that can only be developed in the entire community. Examples of community organizing tasks include: forming health promotion coalitions (overcoming territoriality), training community groups in health promotion methods (technical training), and facilitating passage of legislation favorable to health promotion (political action). These community trials frequently represent a *nonlinear* progression from earlier basic research. They are usually *adaptive*, as the quality of interventions improve during the trial, and they represent an *interactive* model because of synergism among intervention components.

STUDIES IN CARDIOVASCULAR DISEASE

We report on two CVD prevention programs in California to describe lessons learned from almost 20 years of community studies designed to achieve measurable risk reduction for CVD in total populations. Next, selected examples from other primary prevention efforts in cardiovascular disease, cancer, and adolescent health are reviewed, both to report on successes and to identify principles for possible application to alcohol abuse prevention. The placement of these studies within the spectrum of research phases of Tables 4.1 and 4.2 are also described.

The Stanford Three Community Study and Five City Project

The Stanford Three Community Study (TCS) began in 1971 and showed that community-wide health education involving mass media and supplemental face-to-face instruction was very effective in changing knowledge, attitudes, and behavior, thus reducing CVD risk factors (Farquhar et al., 1977). Education in the TCS was carried out in one town through mass media (including electronic media, newspaper, and printed self-help booklets), and in another town through mass media supplemented by a ten-lesson face-to-face program of intensive instruction for high-risk individuals. A third town served as a comparison community.

A significant reduction was achieved in a composite risk score for CVD as a result of significant declines in smoking, blood pressure, and cholesterol levels. This score decreased about 22% for the media-only community and almost 30% in the community in which media were supplemented by face-to-face instruction (Farquhar et al., 1977). We concluded that considerable success was achieved when mass media programs were supplemented with intensive instruction, but exposure to mass media alone was also quite success-ful (Maccoby et al., 1977). The results strongly suggested that health status at the community level can be improved significantly through a low-cost but well-designed educational program carried out over two years using both media and interpersonal channels.

The Stanford Five City Project (FCP) is an outgrowth of testing the TCS model in larger communities over a longer time. Beginning in 1978 and continuing until 1993, it involves 350,000 people and employs multiple methods of education and community organization. During the first five of six years of intervention, about 26 hours of multi-channel education and skills training in nutrition, exercise, and smoking was provided involving schools, worksites, hospitals, voluntary health agencies, the health department, and the media.

Results of the FCP showed that the risk-factor reduction achieved was nearly comparable to those of the TCS. For example, the proportion of smokers in a cohort sample of the two treatment communities declined 15% more than in two control cities. Significant net decreases in blood cholesterol and blood pressure also occurred. Estimates derived from risk factor changes of future disease events for total mortality and for coronary heart disease were reduced significantly in treatment communities by about 15% during four time periods from two to five years after education began (Farquhar et al., 1990).

Environmental and regulatory changes have been incorporated in restaurants, schools, and worksites. In studies on smoking cessation it was shown that low-cost self-help booklets for smoking cessation are more cost-effective than either classes or contests (Altman et al., 1987). In Flay's terminology (1986), studies of different components of a broad campaign are examples of tests of *efficacy* done within the community trial, which itself is a Phase V demonstration trial testing *effectiveness*.

Lessons from the Stanford Community Studies

Successful reduction of risk factors for CVD suggest that it is possible to change the health habits of entire communities and to mobilize existing community resources to achieve those changes. While better methods of community health education are still needed, particularly for minority and poorly educated groups, it is also appropriate to learn how to replicate these results in other fields (Farquhar, Fortmann et al., 1985; Farquhar et al., 1977; Farquhar, 1978; Farquhar et al., 1990). Based on our experience in the Stanford studies, several keys to success are described below. These can insure that programs are well planned, implemented, and evaluated.

Theory Should be Used as a Basis for Program Planning, Implementation, and Evaluation

Theory-based planning is essential for interpreting the results of evaluations and hypothesis testing. Without a theory or a model for change, outcome evaluation results are difficult to explain.

Theories and models used in community CVD prevention include the communication-behavior change model, the social marketing framework, and the community organization model (Farquhar et al., 1991). The communication-behavior change model draws on Bandura's social learning theory, McGuire's communication-persuasion model, and Rogers' diffusion theory (Farquhar, Maccoby, and Solomon, 1984) to identify a series of steps for behavior change:

    a. Creating awareness of the need for behavior change
    b. Producing a change in attitude toward the behavior
    c. Increasing motivation to change
    d. Learning skills for change
    e. Learning maintenance and relapse prevention skills.

A Comprehensive, Integrated Program is Needed

Primary prevention approaches used in effective programs have sought to address the entire population, rather than just high-risk individuals. Because complex health problems involve individual and institutional behavior, social norms, and family modeling influences, a comprehensive integrated program is required for program success. The "comprehensive" feature embraces the notion of Holder and Wallack's system, which they have advocated for prevention of alcohol-related problems (Holder and Wallack, 1986). The integrated feature implies that components of the system, inadequate when initiated singly, are more effective when they are integrated and when they are delivered in the right sequence (Farquhar, Flora et al., 1985; Green and McAlister, 1984). Comprehensive health promotion programs are those that actively involve all of the following:

    a. Multiple channels of influence and communication, such as media
        and face-to-face contacts. Regulatory change and environmental
        change are additional "channels" of influence.

    b. Multiple target audiences, such as minorities, youths, families, health professionals, institutions, and adults. For example, high—risk individuals or families, "hard-to-reach" individuals, highly-motivated "early adopters," and less knowledgeable adults are common subgroups. Also, groups or organizations such as schools or worksites may be targeted.

    c. Multiple outcome objectives, such as knowledge gain; changes in behavior, policy, and physical environment; and media promotion. These different objectives reflect the use of different interventions, for example, using advocacy activities to change organizational or community policy.

    d. Multiple levels of evaluation, including formative, process, and summative evaluation, applied to individuals, groups, organizations, and communities.

An integrated program is one that insures that each program component reinforces and strengthens other components. For example, a smoking cessation program may rely primarily on self-help booklets and classes but also reinforces its message through a campaign at local worksites, publicity in the local media, and collaboration with other local agencies or events, such as a quit-smoking contest or legislation to restrict smoking in public areas.

Formative Evaluation and Process Evaluation are Needed for Success

Three general categories of formative evaluation were employed in the Stanford programs: needs analysis, pretesting of education programs, and analysis following the introduction of education programs into the field. These three categories of formative research are based on the elements of social marketing and are analogous to methods used in product marketing (Kotler and Zaltman, 1971). In the California programs, a needs analysis discovered the interests, educational needs, media use, and other characteristics of different community subpopulations. This formative research helped determine the proper name, location, and time for educational activities and the cost and acceptance of any educational material developed. Prototypes of educational programs were tested to determine the appropriate content and method of delivery of the message. The pretest data were used to revise the message or program prior to use so as to insure effectiveness.

Process evaluations, or analysis of education programs following their introduction into the community, also were employed to revise programs and examine content issues. Process evaluation identified event or program attendance, learning, and behavior change in various community groups. These data were also used to revise programs, at least in the earlier intervention years. From this example it is clear that the definition of the type of evaluation (i.e., process or formative) depends on the objective of the experimenter.

Extensive Outcome Evaluation is Essential

Cardiovascular disease prevention programs in the United States and other countries have invested considerable resources in evaluating outcomes. For example, the FCP involved two intervention and three control communities. Periodic cross-sectional and cohort household surveys were conducted in these communities. Epidemiologic data on CVD morbidity and mortality were also collected.

In addition, the efficacy of specific risk-reduction strategies, such as smoking cessation and dietary counseling, was evaluated to determine their effects on individual knowledge, attitudes, and behavior. For example, outcomes of one "quit smoking" contest with 500 participants were evaluated based on several outcome measures: a mail survey of contest finishers, a telephone survey of selected nonrespondents, expired-air carbon monoxide assessment of contestants who quit, and a one-year follow-up (King et al., 1987). Such data revealed both successes and shortcomings. The quit rate for contestants was twice as high as the general adult population in the control communities, and the cost of the program was lower than that of traditional classes. Program planners concluded that the contest could be strengthened by preventing relapse through extending the program's length and by use of incentives to maintain abstinence. The contest was repeated the next year and again evaluated. These iterations of formative studies provided tests of efficacy within the context of an effectiveness trial of multiple components.

The TCS and FCP attempted to change both individual and organizational behavior. Individual change was most studied in these two projects and had the strongest basis in theory. Limiting analysis to the individual, however, makes artificial distinctions between the individual and his or her environment. Therefore, changes in organizations, including social service agencies, restaurants, grocery stores, hospitals, and worksites were examined in a second level of intervention analysis. Community change—for example, changes in law, regulations, taxation, and environments—was considered in a third analytical tier. Each change level required somewhat different evaluation strategies.

Research Phase Sequence of the Stanford Studies

As demonstration projects involving the total populations of entire communities, the Three Community Study and Five City Project are properly considered Phase V studies (Tables 4.1 and 4.2). In Flay's more elaborate scheme of eight research phases, the TCS would fit Phase VII (an implementation effectiveness trial) and the FCP would be Phase VIII (a demonstration study).

In practical terms the TCS also functioned as a pilot study and, therefore, an efficacy trial precursor for the FCP. Alternatively, to the extent that goals, methods, and outcome measures overlapped, the FCP was a replication of the TCS (although the FCP communities were larger and more complex and the methods used were more advanced).

If the TCS, which was carried out between 1972 and 1975, is properly identified as a Phase V demonstration project, did it have an adequate background of efficacy trials preceding it? For one component—the intensive instruction provided in group settings—a satisfactory efficacy trial in a worksite near Stanford was completed in 1971 and the methods were applied subsequently in the community using a local church as the education site (Meyer and Henderson, 1974). However, the mass media component had not had a prior efficacy trial, and the prevailing opinion among communication researchers was that mass media campaigns generally *failed* to accomplish any goals other than minor shifts in knowledge and attitudes (Hyman and Sheatsley, 1947). The TCS did apply prior research in mediated learning to prove how television, radio, and print mass media could succeed in training in particular behavior change skills rather than being channels for exhortation alone. As an example, participatory learning was achieved in an hour-long television program that asked viewers to score their own cardiovascular risks in the context of providing specific instructions on how to lower those risks (Farquhar, Maccoby, and Solomon, 1984). The TCP showed a surprisingly large effect for the media-only condition as compared to the control condition, an effort only slightly increased by addition of the intensive face-to-face instruction (Farquhar et al., 1977).

The FCP was then able to adopt these mass media methods and to refine them by adding elements in keeping with new findings on human learning. For example, the more recent emphasis placed by Bandura on the role of self-efficacy as a determinant of behavior change (Bandura, 1986) led to a set of media-based programs to instruct ex-smokers in skills of relapse prevention.

An important feature of the FCP is that ongoing formative research allowed adoption of better methods for achieving risk factor change, as mentioned previously for the FCP quit-smoking contest (King et al., 1987). Therefore, not only are *interactive* models appropriate (interactions among components may increase the effects of each) but *adaptive* models are also advisable. The history of the TCS and the FCP provide evidence that incomplete prior efficacy testing can be coupled successfully with an adaptive process of improving the quality of the intervention during the course of the health promotion trial.

The Finnish North Karelia Project

A growing movement to create comprehensive studies in CVD prevention is clearly underway, and ten such projects that began between 1972 and 1982 were recently reviewed (Farquhar et al., 1991). The Finnish North Karelia Project, which began in 1972 (Puska et al., 1981), is the best known of such projects outside of the United States. Risk-factor changes in the North Karelia Project were comparable to those of the Stanford TCS. The Finnish Study continued for ten years, allowing its impact on cardiovascular disease morbidity and mortality to be studied. Decreases in these outcomes were found in comparison not only to the adjoining county but also in comparison to the trends in the remaining part of Finland (Tuomilehto et al., 1986).

The North Karelia Project, clearly Phase V, began with the advantage of strong local support generated by the results of a large epidemiologic study. The Seven Country Coronary Disease Study targeted the province of North Karelia as having the highest heart disease death rate in the world (Keys, 1980). Accordingly, Finnish national health service personnel became an integral part of the Project. Much of the program's success, however, stemmed from diligent formative research, which provided efficacy tests of components over the course of the project.

Other Cardiovascular Disease Prevention Projects

Three other community-based studies using analogous methods to the TCS and the North Karelia Project have published their results. One study, which took place in three small rural South African towns, reported significant changes in cholesterol levels and blood pressure control as well as in smoking cessation (Rossouw et al., 1981). Two others, in four towns in Switzerland (Gutzwiller et al., 1985) and a three-town study in Australia (Egger et al., 1983), reported a 6% and a 9% drop in smoking rate, respectively, but no other risk factor changes. These three projects were patterned after the Stanford TCS, and brief technical assistance was provided to them by our group.

Two additional studies comparable to the Stanford FCP are nearing completion in the United States: the Pawtucket Heart Health Program in Rhode Island involving two cities with a total population of 173,000 (Lasater et al., 1984) and the Minnesota Heart Health Program involving six communities with a total population of 356,000 (Blackburn et al., 1984). Results from these two studies provide more data on the feasibility of such studies and on methods of community recruiting, as well as on education methods. For example, the Minnesota study reported that food labeling, nutrition education, and environmental change at "point of purchase" in grocery stores and restaurants have been shown to be effective (Mullis et al., 1987; Mullis and Pirie, 1988; Glanz and Mullis, 1988). The three studies (Stanford FCP, Pawtucket, and Minnesota) now all use "point of purchase" components in their overall program. As another example, the Pawtucket Program has reported considerable success in mobilizing volunteers and in use of local churches (Lasater et al., 1984).

One large study, the German Cardiovascular Prevention Study (GCP) began its planning in 1982 under a bilateral scientific agreement between the U.S. and the Federal Republic of Germany; considerable amounts of technical assistance were provided by Stanford and Pawtucket investigators (GCP Study Group, 1988). Intervention began in 1984 and major federal funding was extended through 1991. Five regions are involved with a total population of 1,230,000. Test sites will be compared to the balance of what has heretofore been "West Germany." A study of comparable design, the New York Healthy Heart Program, began in 1987 with eight intervention communities to be compared to the rest of the state. This project is funded by the State Health Department and is designed as an initial phase of a statewide program (Shea, 1992).

Given the proliferation of CVD projects, one may rightly ask why the alcohol field has relatively so little in the Phase V research stage. The scientific consensus that CVD risk factors are causal for CVD has been reasonably high since the early 1960s, although a greater case for cholesterol has emerged recently. In contrast to the alcohol field, a reasonably strong consensus emerged in CVD as to the feasibility of intervening on the major risk factors through educational means. By many measures, however, this type of consensus is now stronger in the alcohol field (Institute of Medicine, 1989), so the time for community alcohol interventions may have arrived.

RESULTS FROM PRIMARY PREVENTION STUDIES IN CANCER

The CVD prevention studies just described are relevant to cancer prevention through their cigarette smoking and nutrition change elements, and success stories from some other health fields also provide evidence of lifestyles change. Unfortunately, there are as yet no completed examples of comprehensive community-wide programs in fields other than cardiovascular disease. However, there is one national mass media program and two promising comprehensive programs in cancer prevention underway. These programs are described below.

The Cancer Prevention Awareness Program of the National Cancer Institute (NCI), now in its fifth year, is a nationwide program that seeks to change the American people's knowledge, attitudes, and behavior to prevent cancer. NCI's plans include launching a mass media campaign on cancer prevention, producing and distributing print materials for the general public, and educating health professionals about cancer prevention. A part of the campaign is intended especially for black Americans because of the relatively high incidence of cancer in the black population (National Cancer Institute, 1986).

One component of the NCI program reported at least short-term changes in dietary behavior. This resulted from a collaboration with Kellogg's cereal company to publicize a low-fat, high-fiber message in the national media, and to promote Kellogg's new bran cereal. The two-year cereal advertising campaign included NCI's diet message and telephone number in television ads and on the back of cereal boxes. It produced more than 20,000 telephone and 30,000 written inquiries to NCI, and sales of all high-fiber cereals increased in the Washington, D.C. area (Freimuth et al., 1988).

The study found that consumers were able to generalize the health message resulting in the purchase of all types of high-fiber cereal. In response to campaigns to encourage substitution of nonalcoholic beverages, this could mean that promotion of one particular nonalcoholic beverage could increase consumption of *many* types of these beverages. Further research on consumer behavior is necessary before firm conclusions can be drawn.

The NCI/Kellogg campaign is difficult to place in the hierarchy of the five research phases. Most appropriately, it as an efficacy trial of a mass media component. Its success, though assessed in a manner to test only a short-term effect, may well be attributable in part to a considerable pre-existing heightened awareness of the American people to a "fiber is good for you" message.

The influential role that private industry can play in health promotion was demonstrated by this campaign. NCI reached an audience of millions through the cooperation and financial backing of Kellogg's cereal company. This observation could be relevant to the alcohol-problem field, because the food and nonalcoholic-beverage industry could promote their products as healthful alternatives to alcoholic beverages. However, cooperation between health promotion agencies and the private sector may not be readily achieved. The alcohol industry is not likely to assist in any attempt to *reduce* sales, although a move to lowered-alcohol-content products could have greater appeal. Furthermore, some large companies have integrated production, distribution, and sales of food, nonalcoholic beverages, and alcoholic beverages, respectively. These integrated companies could have greater resistance to campaigns on alcohol use than would companies that do not market alcoholic beverages.

Programma a Su Salud

A second program designed to prevent cancer entitled "Programma a Su Salud" (Program for Your Health), began in 1985 in a low-income Mexican-American border community in Texas (Ramirez and McAlister, 1988; Amezcua et al., 1989). See Chapter 7 in this book.

This unique Phase V project addresses many health topics (cardiovascular disease risk, alcohol use, cancer, and injury prevention) and various social needs (unemployment and social service counseling) (Amezcua et al., 1989).

Programma a Su Salud was begun in a county on the border with Mexico with the highest unemployment rate in the nation, a county whose residents were over 93% Mexican-American and whose alcohol use and nutrition patterns conferred very high risk (Amezcua et al., 1989). The creation of culturally specific educational materials was achieved during the early phases by Spanish-speaking scientists (Ramirez and McAlister, 1988), another example of formative research carried out during the course of a Phase V trial. Therefore, some of the components had prior efficacy testing, but considerable unexplored territory was present here as well as in the previous CVD phase V trials.

The COMMIT Trial

A third project begun with NCI funding involves 22 matched pairs of cities randomized to compare comprehensive intervention on smoking with a control condition (Pechacek, 1987). This ambitious Phase V trial involves more communities than any of the previously described Phase V CVD trials. It relies on evidence from efficacy trials of various components, such as classes and mediated or self-help programs for adult smokers, and it is carried out by many investigators, including the Phase V CVD community trials. Intervention began in 1988 and will continue through early 1993.

STUDIES IN ADOLESCENT HEALTH

The Midwestern Prevention Project (MPP), also referred to as Project STAR, is an example of a study having broad goals to decrease substance abuse among adolescents. It is an ongoing demonstration project that involves various cities in Kansas, Missouri, and Indiana. The project staff developed a school-based curriculum and supplements classroom instruction with media messages, vendor education, police patrols, and alternative activities. This project has reported significant use reductions in three drugs (tobacco, marijuana, and alcohol) in a two-year follow-up of 15 communities near

Kansas City, Missouri (Pentz et al., 1989). MPP is probably the most ambitious and comprehensive program to date that includes an alcohol-use prevention component. Although it is restricted to adolescents, many insights relevant to comprehensive community-based prevention of alcohol problems will result.

The MPP is a comprehensive Phase V study in young adolescents carried out by a team experienced in prior smoking prevention research in adolescents (Flay, 1985; Hansen et al., 1988). Other groups have also been successful in delaying the onset of smoking among early teens, increasing confidence in the generalizability of what Killen (1985) has called the "social pressure resistance training approach" (McAlister, Perry, and Maccoby, 1979; Telch et al., 1982; Botvin, 1982; Best et al., 1988; Hansen et al., 1988). The resistance training approach alerts young people to the various pressures that may encourage smoking and teaches specific skills for use in resisting these pressures.

SUMMARY OF LESSONS LEARNED FROM COMPREHENSIVE PREVENTION TRIALS IN CVD, CANCER, AND ADOLESCENT HEALTH

Important lessons from community-based programs noted above are summarized as follows:

1. Although efficacy testing preceded some of the comprehensive projects reviewed here, they all relied on adapting program elements to needs and opportunities discovered during field operations. This lesson suggests that an adaptive model is preferred to one that attempts to have all elements of the intervention defined in advance.
2. All large-scale comprehensive Phase V trials have been quasi-experimental in design, conducted by single research groups on a reasonably limited number of communities. Phase V alcohol studies may need to avoid complex multi-site trials until one or more demonstration studies patterned after the CVD model have been carried out. Researchers would thus fulfill Flay's (1986) recommendation that success be demonstrated both for the delivery and for adherence to an intervention.
3. Theories of change are an important part of all successful interventions. Theory should guide the development of both the intervention and the evaluation, as well as the interpretation of effects.
4. Extensive formative, process, and outcome evaluations are needed for the development of the program, monitoring of the implementation process, and determination of effects over time.

5. Needs assessment and audience segmentation are essential ingredients of formative evaluations. Much of the content of the intervention flows from this information.
6. There is a potential beneficial synergistic effect of combining approaches across different levels of intervention.
7. It is important to establish multiple outcome objectives and to match outcome objectives to the level of intervention in order to increase our understanding of change. For example, few school, worksite, or community programs measure organizational change along with individual change.
8. Because primary prevention strategies are particularly important for adolescents, attention to high-risk subsets of adolescents is important. Strategies that include delay of onset of a particular behavior, minimizing use of harmful substances, or preventing entirely initiation of a behavior are important components to any population-wide strategy for prevention in adolescents.
9. Extension of these principles to the alcohol field should be a carefully planned endeavor involving scientific consensus formation, definition of hypotheses, efficacy trials, careful assessment of scientific resources available, and a critical review of past research.

Table 4.3 presents a matrix display of studies (cited by author and year) done in various health fields covering such aspects as worksites, schools, regulatory change, and comprehensive community studies. Efficacy trials are presented in the two columns on the left and effectiveness trials in the three columns on the right. Table 4.3 is presented only as an example of how a matrix can display the types of research that have been done. In designing comprehensive programs for prevention of alcohol problems, the special roles of taxation, law enforcement and other regulatory changes, and server-intervention studies, as well as the role of mass media in altering attitudes to prevailing social norms regarding alcohol, are examples of components for which efficacy trials might be done.

Implications for Prevention of Alcohol Problems

Significant implications for preventing alcohol problems can be derived from the studies described above. The first, and perhaps most important, is that community-level prevention is possible. Beyond that, applying each lesson to preventing alcohol problems raises challenging questions, such as:

TABLE 4.3
Matrix of Successful Primary Prevention Interventions in Three Health Areas

Research Phase

Efficacy Trials <------ | -------------------- > Effectiveness Trials

Focus of Intervention

Health Problem	School-based Education	Worksite Education	County or State Regulatory Change	Comprehensive Community Studies for Subgroups	Comprehensive Community Studies, Total Populations
Cardio-vascular Disease Risk	Killen, '88	Brownell, '84 Felix, '85 Sallis, '86 (a review) Kornitzer, '85			Farquhar, '77, '90 Puska, '81 Rossouw, '81 Egger, '83 Gutzwiller, '85 GCP Study, '88**
Cancer Risk			(Pechacek, '87)	(Smokers) COMMIT Trial**	McAlister, '90* (includes CVD risk)
Adolescent Health (Smoking)	McAlister, '79 Botvin, '82 Luepker, '83 Flay, '85 Best, '88 Killen, '88 Hansen, '88		Flay, '87 Altman, '89		King, '87
Adolescent Health (Alcohol and Drug Use)	McAlister, '79 Telch, '82 Hansen, '88 Telch, '90			(Adolescents) Pentz, '89 (includes smoking and drug abuse)**	

* McAlister, A., personal communication. This ongoing study is relevant to both cardiovascular disease and cancer risk.
** These studies are incomplete, Pentz et al. have reported interim results, 1989.

1. Is there a sufficient scientific consensus to support comprehensive projects that focus on changing entire populations, not just high-risk groups, toward a markedly changed social norm of both decreased general alcohol use and increased abstinence?

2. Should comprehensive integrated trials for prevention of alcohol problems be carried out, or should policies toward alcohol be derived entirely from replication of efficacy trials of various components of education or regulation that may play a role in a national program?

3. What theories have been used in alcohol-problems prevention planning, and how thoroughly have they been tested?
4. What is the extent of research experience in efficacy trials needed for components of multicomponent demonstration trials before such trials should be attempted in the alcohol field?
5. Is it possible to integrate various seemingly unrelated prevention strategies into one multicomponent prevention program?

The techniques from one prevention program will never fit exactly the needs and goals of another program. However, it would be imprudent to disregard the years of experience in comprehensive CVD prevention and the lessons learned from the failures and successes in other smaller pilot studies in primary prevention of other health problems.

5

Designs Employed in Community Heart Disease and Cancer Prevention Projects

Thomas M. Lasater

INTRODUCTION

This chapter reviews the key designs of major heart disease and cancer prevention projects. In order to be reviewed here, a project had to be:

1. Targeting a highly prevalent health disorder
2. Considering multiple risk factors
3. Including community involvement in program design and delivery
4. Targeting all persons in a defined geographical area as opposed to a high-risk only approach
5. Having a research or evaluation design with at least one reference area to control for secular trends.

The definition of community as a defined geographical area is primarily for evaluation purposes because it allows unambiguous designation of "eligible" or "ineligible" for all potential respondents. Many people around the borders of the target areas are attracted to the programming and are not excluded for two basic reasons—they are part of the social environment of the target communities and it would be impractical to systematically identify and refuse them services.

The largest number of projects that are comprehensive enough to fit this definition of community interventions are concerned with the primary

Research and preparation for this chapter were partially supported by Grant HL23629 (Pawtucket Heart Health Program) from the National Heart, Lung, and Blood Institute, United States Department of Health and Human Services.

prevention of cardiovascular disease (CVD). CVD has the advantage of clearly established risk factors (e.g., high blood pressure, smoking, high blood cholesterol) that are both strongly influenced by behavior and measurable in accurate and precise ways. Moreover, CVD is a highly prevalent disease with large numbers of both morbid and mortal events occurring in virtually all communities. In cancer prevention, the most comprehensive and largest community approach targets smoking, a major risk factor.

As a prelude to considering designs for community interventions in the primary prevention of CVD and cancer, very brief overviews of some of the larger studies that meet the definition for community interventions will be discussed. These will be followed by descriptions of several design issues common to all those studies.

There are a number of intervention (or educational) elements that all of the studies have in common.

1. All studies utilize the concept of reciprocal influence; that is, the individual is viewed as able to influence as well as be influenced.
2. All include both individual and systems approaches. They target individuals, organizations, the community at large, and the social and physical environments within which individuals and organizations exist.
3. The studies take a population-based approach to prevention, the high-risk approach being subsumed under a general strategy.
4. The studies include a health professional (including physicians) education.
5. And they use existing community resources, including volunteers.

While all of the programs are funded by government agencies for three to six years of active intervention, they share the major aim of achieving permanent change in the social structure so that at least some types of primary prevention efforts remain after outside funding for the specific study has ceased. None perceive themselves or the behavior change process as being short-term. Finally, all of the interventions are dynamic. They are expected to evolve by discarding specific programs and approaches that do not work and piloting, refining, and adopting those that do.

SUMMARY OF STUDIES

Following is a brief overview of community heart disease or cancer prevention projects that meet the five criteria above. More detail on each program can be obtained from the references cited.

North Karelia Study

The first two of the true community CVD primary prevention studies began at roughly the same time in the early 1970s—the North Karelia Project (NK) and the Stanford Three Community Study (TCS). The most active phase of the North Karelia project was conducted between 1972 and 1977 (Puska et al., 1983). The program was described in this volume in the previous chapter by Farquhar and Fortmann. A baseline cross-sectional risk-factor survey of North Karelia's 180,000 inhabitants and a matched reference area (a neighboring county with 250,000 residents) was conducted with a total random sample size of approximately 11,000 individuals between the ages of 25 and 59. A second random sample survey of approximately the same size was conducted again in 1977. Some aspects of the program have continued, and long-term evaluation results based on CVD morbidity and mortality are released at regular intervals (Puska et al., 1985). The five-year follow-up survey was on the same "birth cohort," which was then ages 30 to 64 but was a cross-sectional random sample of all those eligible. Because of the large samples drawn, a number of the post-program survey respondents ($N=700$) had also been selected and measured for the baseline survey. Thus cohort analyses were possible on this smaller group.

Stanford Three Community Study and Stanford Five City Project

The Three Community Study (Farquhar et al., 1977) began with a random-sample risk-factor survey ($N=2,151$) of residents ages 35 to 59. The TCS was described in the previous chapter by Farquhar and Fortmann. The three cities had a total of approximately 42,000 residents. The original baseline sample was retested twice at yearly intervals. There was also a small cross-sectional survey of participants not in the initial baseline survey of approximately 100 per town; they were selected and tested in 1975. As well as being a pilot test of the feasibility of a community approach, the research design also included different interventions between the two education communities.

Based upon the encouraging results of TCS, the Stanford Five City Project (FCP) began in 1978 with the initial risk-factor surveys in four communities with a total population size of approximately 350,000 (Farquhar et al., 1990). Farquhar and Fortmann describe the FCP in more detail in the previous chapter in this volume.

The outcome evaluation included both cross-sectional ($N=650$) and cohort population-based risk-factor surveys. Measurements were at approximately two-year intervals and were based on those 12 to 74 years of age. These surveys were carried out in the two education communities and in two of the comparison communities. The third comparison community received only epidemiologic surveillance for CVD morbidity and mortality to control for the possibility of the risk-factor surveys themselves affecting the risk factors and, thus, morbidity and mortality. Morbid and mortal events in all five cities were ascertained from death records, reabstracting of medical records, and key informant interviews for out-of-hospital deaths. All hospital records were reabstracted using a common protocol developed in both the Minnesota and Pawtucket programs (e.g., McKinlay et al., 1989).

Minnesota Heart Health Program

The next U.S. study to be funded in early 1980 by the National Heart, Lung, and Blood Institute of the National Institutes of Health (NIH-NHLBI) was the Minnesota Heart Health Program (MINN) based at the University of Minnesota (Blackburn et al., 1984). It included three intervention and three comparison communities with a combined population of approximately 400,000. The intervention used all available channels (e.g., mass media, face-to-face interactions, worksites, religious organizations, schools, libraries, health-related agencies, health-care professionals, point of purchase) with a heavy emphasis on community organization and on screening at least 60% of the adult population at the beginning of the intervention in each of the cities. CVD morbidity and mortality surveillance began in 1980 with reabstraction of hospital medical records of all potential cases and with informant interviews for out-of-hospital deaths. Risk-factor surveillance was carried out through annual population-based samples of 500 adults aged 24 to 74 in each of the three education and three comparison communities. Periodic cohort surveys were also conducted in all communities. All types of process evaluation plus extensive formative research were an integral part of the project. One important evaluation technique was the random digit dial telephone interview.

Pawtucket Heart Health Program

In July 1980, the Pawtucket Heart Health Program (PAWT) began with NIH-NHLBI funding (Carleton et al., 1987). The first baseline risk-factor survey was completed in March 1982, and the early intervention efforts began. A grassroots community activation approach was taken, and all sectors of the community have been actively involved, with the planned exception of electronic media. A major emphasis of PAWT has been to involve volunteers in all aspects of the intervention. In addition, the community hospital of the intervention city received the grant, became the base from which all activities have been carried out, and thus has been identified by the public as the organization most associated with the program. Social marketing techniques (Lefebvre and Flora, 1988) and extensive utilization of mobile screening, counseling, and referral activities have also characterized the intervention.

The combined population of the two communities is approximately 180,000. Risk-factor measurement is conducted on a sample of adults aged 18 to 65, of whom 1,200 to 1,400 are randomly selected from each of the two communities. These surveys are conducted biennially with all measurement taking place in the homes of the respondents. The baseline survey, completed in March 1982, has been converted into a cohort with the first remeasurement being completed in 1987 and the third measurement beginning in March 1990. Process and formative evaluation are assisted greatly by a tracking system that allows every person who participates in an active program to be followed by telephone interviews throughout the entire study period and to be linked with the risk-factor surveys and the morbidity and mortality surveillance (McGraw et al., 1989).

New York State Department of Health

The New York Healthy Heart Program (NY) began in the state of New York in 1987 and involves eight intervention communities with the balance of the state acting as the reference area. The major emphasis is on community organization and use of volunteers and other endogenous resources to augment the intervention budgets provided by the state. The most distal outcome measurement will be restricted to publicly available mortality data. Risk-factor status is assessed through random sample telephone surveys similar to the Centers for Disease Control-sponsored Behavioral Risk Factor Surveillance System. The baseline survey was conducted in 1989 with a target of approximately 3,500 respondents. Intervention activities began simultaneous with the baseline survey. Process measurement will rely heavily on the PAWT tracking system.

The German Cardiovascular Prevention Study

The largest of the CVD studies is being conducted in Germany (GCP Study Group, 1988). Intervention began in 1984 immediately after a baseline population based risk-factor survey. The survey was repeated (separate random sample) again in 1988 and in 1991. Respondents include 25- to 59-year-old resident German citizens. The initial survey yielded approximately 11,594 completed surveys in the study regions and 4,836 in the reference sample. The second and third cross-sectional surveys completed in 1988 and 1991 were somewhat smaller. The German Cardiovascular Prevention Study

(GCP) also uses a process tracking system developed cooperatively by the FCP, MINN, and PAWT staff. Mortality surveillance utilizing existing records is also underway.

In addition to its size, the GCP is distinctive for its testing of two different approaches. One resembles the U.S. studies in that it involves all organizations, aggressive programming, mass media, and volunteers. The second approach is restricted to working through the physician community by eliciting physician volunteers. The volunteer physicians then help establish lay leadership committees that help all those in their particular subregion reduce their risk factors using any techniques they believe will be effective.

South Carolina Cardiovascular Disease Prevention Project

The South Carolina Project (FSC) was funded by the Centers for Disease Control in 1987 (Wheeler et al., 1991). It builds on the earlier studies to test the feasibility of a community approach in a public health setting rather than a research setting. A small staff introduced a community organizing approach relying almost exclusively on existing community resources for program delivery. Existing programs and materials were emphasized, rather than the development of new ones.

The evaluation design includes one intervention and one comparison community of approximately 60,000 population each. Process measurement includes recording of the number of participants in each event and maintaining records by name of all participants in screening events; extensive files are kept on each organization worked with, and detailed staff activity logs are kept.

The major outcome measurement relies upon a random digit dial telephone survey of those 18 and older plus an invitation for face-to-face physiological measurement of risk factors. Remeasurement of these 5,491 respondents is planned for 1991-92.

COMMIT

The cancer project, COMMIT (COM) (Pechacek, 1987) was initiated in 1986 through funding by the National Cancer Institute of the National Institutes of Health. The original target group was heavy smokers which has since been modified to include all tobacco smokers. The total population of the 22 communities is well over 1,500,000. This study is also unique in that the intervention and comparison cities were determined by random assignment: one of a matched pair of cities to intervention and the other to comparison for each of the 11 pairs. The interventions use comparable protocols, but each site is free to pursue opportunities as they arise. Volunteers and organizations are being recruited from all sectors of the communities, and all forms of media are being utilized. Basic outcome measurements depend both upon baseline and post-trial cross-sectional population sample surveys and upon a remeasurement of a designated cohort. Intervention began in October 1988 and is scheduled to continue through February 1993. The entire baseline survey was completed in May of 1988 and will be repeated again in 1993.

DESIGN FEATURES

All of the community studies developed or adopted a model (either explicitly or implicitly) of the causal chain of factors that results in the problem (e.g., CVD). The sets of assumptions contained in such a model determine both the specific interventions and the most appropriate evaluation techniques. The assumed causal links for CVD are fairly universal and are illustrated by the Pawtucket Heart Health Program's experimental model as presented in Figure 5.1. This explicitly places variables in an assumed causal chain from independent through intervening and impact variables to motivated activity, which in turn is assumed to influence physiological risk factors and finally morbid and mortal events. Along the base are illustrated the domains of variables covered by the basic types of process and formative and outcome evaluation.

Once the model is adopted, a number of design decisions arise. The balance of this chapter will concentrate on some of these issues and the ways they have been resolved by the studies described earlier. Table 5.1 summarizes many of those major decisions.

Intervention and Comparison Areas

In all the studies the reference areas used to control for secular trends are comparison rather than control populations, as it is not possible to prevent some level of activities similar to the intervention from being delivered in these reference areas. For example, the National High Blood Pressure Education Program and the National Cholesterol Education Programs were not only being received by all the CVD reference communities, but the National Heart, Lung, and Blood Institute was also immediately disseminating knowledge being gained from the studies through these national programs.

A related question is selection of intervention and reference areas. Only one of the studies (COM) has randomly assigned communities to reference or intervention, in matched pairs.

FIGURE 5.1
Pawtucket Heart Health Program Research Model

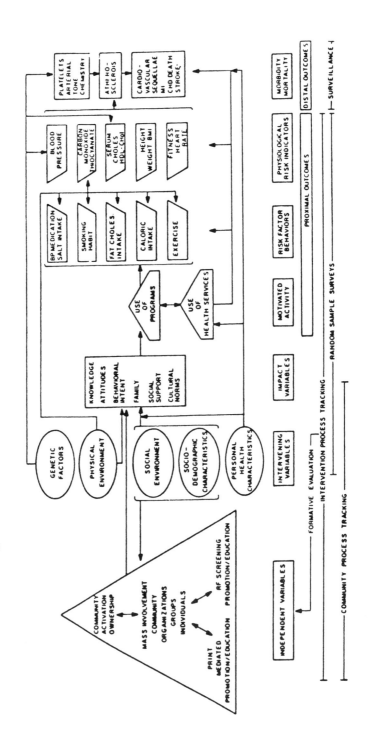

Reprinted from: Carleton, R.A., Lasater, T.M., Assaf, A., Lefebvre, R.C., and McKinlay, S.M. (1987). The Pawtucket Hearth Health Program: I. An experiment in population-based disease prevention. *Rhode Island Medical Journal, 70,* 533-538. Reprinted with permission.

TABLE 5.1
Studies by Design Features

DESIGN FEATURE	TCS	FCP	NK	MINN	PAWT	GCP	NY	FSC	COM
Mortality		X	X	X	X	X	X		
SURVEILLANCE									
Morbidity		X	X	X	X	X			
Year Began	1972	1978	1972	1980	1980	1982	1987	1987	1986
Cross-Sectional		X	X	X	X	X	X	X	X
RISK FACTOR SURVEYS									
Longitudinal	X	X	X	X	X	?			X
Number of Education Sites	2	2	1	3	1	5	8	1	11
Area(s)	X	X	X	X	X	X		X	X
COMPARISON									
Rest of Country (State)	X	X	X	X	X	?			X

Distal Outcome Measurement

Another early decision for each study was the selection of outcome measure(s). To a large degree this choice has been based on available resources as well as scientific grounds. While CVD morbidity and/or mortality are obvious choices, there are problems when only mortality is considered. The existence of death certificate data of moderately high accuracy in the United States makes this a feasible measure of effectiveness (National Heart, Lung, and Blood Institute, 1984), albeit at a rather gross level. For studies tracking moderate size populations, the number of mortal events in a particular category is quite small, which greatly reduces statistical power. In order to increase statistical power and at the same time take advantage of all manifested CVD (i.e., myocardial infarctions and strokes sufficiently severe to result in hospitalization or death), morbidity must be added to mortality. Morbidity, because it has major negative effects apart from mortality, is also included as an important outcome in its own right. In addition to death certificates, hospital records must also be reviewed.

Hospital and death records are often inaccurate and even potentially influenceable by the intervention itself. For example, a major emphasis on

CVD could lead members of the medical community to look for and record signs of the disease. Also, potential bias can come from differences in hospital requirements and even differences among physicians. Hospital records become more useful the larger the number of individuals under surveillance. Larger numbers of physicians and hospitals help reduce bias of individual physicians and hospitals and are more likely to reduce artificial differences between populations under study. Conversely, the smaller the populations and the fewer events that occur in any unit of time, the more the need to increase the accuracy and precision of this outcome measure. However, such increases are expensive to achieve.

At the same time resources are being expended to increase accuracy and precision, it is also important to do everything possible to maximize cross-study comparisons. Limited numbers of community studies are likely to be funded because of their expense. Also, the knowledge base is most likely to be advanced when multiple investigators study a common problem in ways that allow maximum comparability across studies. One important way to do this is to measure common variables in the same way.

The studies described in this chapter have achieved comparability in three important ways. First, investigators designing a new study considered existing studies in all of these projects. For example, investigators made numerous site visits and employed experienced staff from early studies to design the evaluation of the new studies. This was particularly the case for the GCP and NY studies. Second, whenever possible, investigators adopted existing measures rather than "reinventing the wheel." The willingness of all the CVD studies to share their survey instruments has helped others, particularly MINN, PAWT, GCP, NY, and FSC. Finally, there has been extensive cooperation among investigators in ongoing studies to develop new measures that can be used across studies. An example is the cooperative development by the NHLBI studies (FCP, MINN, PAWT) of a common procedure for abstracting hospital records and the algorithm with which those data are converted by computers into one of three designations—"definite," "probable" or "non" CVD event. Thus distal outcomes can be compared with confidence across these studies.

One difficulty, even with accurate CVD morbidity and mortality surveillance, is that the time between behavior changes and expected changes in morbid or mortal events is usually longer than the traditional research-granting agency is willing to fund. This problem leads to a greater reliance on measuring the risk factors themselves or, even earlier in the assumed causal chain, measuring behavior assumed to affect the risk factor values. The anticipated changes in CVD are then computed using one of a number of predictor equations developed on other populations for which risk-factor measurement and later morbid and mortal event information are both available (e.g., Truett, Cornfield, and Kannel, 1967). The logical difficulties include the necessity of assuming that the intervention and comparison populations are similar in all important (but sometimes unspecified) ways to the populations upon which the predictors were based and that the relationships observed over a previous period of 10 to 20 years will be the same for the next 10 to 20 years.

Risk-Factor Measurement

One way to minimize error in predicting the correct amount of effect on morbid and mortal events is to measure variables in the causal chain as close to the CVD event as possible. For virtually all of the studies except NY this has meant physiological assessment of the key risk factors. These measurement procedures are neither free from error nor automatically comparable across studies. For example, the measurement of blood cholesterol has been known to vary widely across methods and across laboratories (U.S. Department of Health and Human Services/NCEP, 1988). This has made it difficult in the past to combine cholesterol data across studies. Potential measurement differences are more important in making absolute value comparisons than in comparing relative change across projects. For example, a systematic error of plus 5 mg/dl in the PAWT laboratory and a minus 5 mg/dl in the MINN laboratory would mean that all absolute value comparisons would indicate that PAWT respondents are 10 mg/dl higher than they actually are in comparison to MINN respondents. On the other hand, if both achieve a 10 mg/dl drop in their intervention versus their comparison communities, the change values would be the same regardless of the laboratories. Any systematic error is algebraically cancelled in the computation of change scores.

Even with comparisons of changes over time, there is the important problem of differential laboratory drifts that could make even change scores difficult to rely upon. Fortunately, there is a way to estimate and correct for both systematic error and laboratory drift: that is to use an outside and stable referent. For cholesterol the referent has become the Centers for Disease Control standardization program. They send out samples with known (by CDC) values to all participating laboratories. The resulting analyses in each laboratory provide a good estimate of any systematic error present in that laboratory. These samples are furnished every four months.

While it is still possible to make gross comparisons of cholesterol values and changes between projects without a common and stable referent, the loss of precision and the inability to combine data greatly reduce the progress in understanding that multiple studies should bring to any field. This flaw is easily avoided by planning, when a stable referent exists.

In other types of measurements such as blood pressure, the problem is even more complex, as a number of measuring "instruments" are involved. Again, the objective is to reduce the difficulty of cross-project comparisons through a commitment to producing maximally comparable data on the part of all those involved in community studies.

Risk-Factor Surveys

All of the studies attempt to measure periodically the risk-factor status of both intervention and reference populations. Along with physiological assessment of risk factors, risk-factor surveys also include self-reports by respondents concerning all of the variables in Figure 5.1 from intervening variables through recall of personal morbid events. Risk-factor reporting is another important area to target for maximum cross-study comparability. Comparing even such sociodemographic variables as income, marital status, and education can be a problem unless a thorough knowledge of measurement in other studies is a part of the planning process for new studies. Psychosocial variables (e.g., personality, stress, social support) are even harder to measure and compare.

Another important set of decisions has to do with whom to measure and when. None of the projects has the resources to include every eligible person in its risk-factor surveys. For this reason, subsamples are selected and measured to estimate population values. Thus, two important concerns have had to be addressed—sampling and whether or not to include longitudinal (cohort) remeasurements.

With respect to sampling, the necessary size is usually specified by degree of hypothesized change, power considerations, and fiscal constraints. However, another issue is the sampling unit. For example, should all members from a sampled residence be encouraged to participate in the survey measurement (TCS, FCP) or should only one household member be selected for measurement (all others)? Any sampling approach raises important statistical issues that are beyond the scope of this chapter. An additional source of variation among studies is the lists from which respondents are selected. These range from telephone numbers selected at random (NY) to lists of all residents of a community (GCP). The most common starting points are addresses provided by city directories or area sampling from maps or census blocks.

The second question is whether to select a separate random sample of the population for each survey (cross-sectional) or to remeasure some or all of the same respondents over time (cohort). When resources permit (FCP, MINN, PAWT, COM) both types of design options are selected, as they have very different advantages and disadvantages. There are two advantages of using a cross-sectional design. First, the samples remain representative of the community over time even if the composition of the community changes.

Second, the possible effect that the measurement process itself may have on subsequent behavior (reactivity) is avoided.

Measurement reactivity is particularly important because there is an ethical requirement to notify respondents if they are found to have one or more elevated risk factors. Unfortunately, from a research perspective, this source of measurement reactivity cannot be considered controlled for by simply warning all respondents of the intervention and comparison areas in the same manner. The treatment community has more opportunities for change through its social and physical environments. Measurement reactivity is more likely to lead to program participation by survey respondents in that community than by either nonsurvey respondents in the intervention community or survey respondents in the comparison community.

A disadvantage of the cross-sectional approach is the difficulty of adjusting for differences in baseline values among communities if these are found. At least the longitudinal design allows each subject to act as his/her own control and does not have potential differential sampling problems at time one and again at time two to deal with. The cross-sectional design also includes new immigrants in the community who have not been fully exposed to the treatment. Also the use of between-subject rather than within-subject error terms in statistical analyses of changes over time requires a larger sample size to achieve the same statistical power as a cohort. There is another disadvantage faced by the longer studies, such as PAWT, which sample for cross-sectional surveys without replacement (eliminating as ineligible anyone previously surveyed): that is the potential for survey saturation as more and more households are "used up."

Cohort designs do allow for more precise statistical adjustments for baseline differences. They also allow the exploration of potential predictors of change and other interactions between baseline characteristics and follow-up values as the use of the same respondents allows the linking of time one measurements to later values. Finally, cohort designs have a higher statistical power for a given sample size. On the other hand, the cohort design is subject to major loss of respondents through migration and death. Loss increases directly with the length of the study. The passage of time also continues to make the cohort being followed less representative of the total population, since the loss cannot be assumed to be random. Those who die tend to be the older respondents, and those who migrate tend to be the younger. New citizens who immigrate to the area are not represented. And the cohort as a whole ages since no new respondents can be added through birth and aging.

The problem of measurement reactivity potentially increases even more the differences between the cohort and the rest of the population. The cohort that was pretested is becoming smaller with respect to the population it represents. Also, the cohort has had more time to be differentially affected because the members have been exposed longer than the average resident they represent.

Process and Formative Evaluation

Process evaluation is defined to include measurement of the application of intervention; the changes that occur in community structures over time; the types and numbers of individuals, groups, and organizations that become involved; and changes that occur all along the causal chain from independent variable application to final outcome occurrences. Formative evaluation is defined as those data collection efforts that result in changes in program elements to make them more effective. The distinction between these two types of evaluation is based on the use and the purpose of gathering the data. For example, a program might keep a very accurate record of the age and gender of all participants to measure rates of involvement (process evaluation). However, if a large percentage is found to be young females, program elements might be added to appeal to other segments of the target population (formative evaluation).

Obviously it is extremely difficult to draw sharp distinctions. For example, in the PAWT study there is very thorough tracking of all actively participating individuals. This data collection documents the "independent variable" but is also being used in a social marketing framework to refine components and to target underrepresented subgroups. A second distinction is between community process evaluation and implementation process evaluation. The term "community process evaluation" is used to describe measurement of community level variables such as organizations and their structure, function, and "behavior"; social and physical environments; laws and regulations and their enforcement; and all activities similar to the intervention program activities. The measurement of all activities (whether under study personnel control or not) throughout the community that are a direct part of the intervention is referred to as "implementation process evaluation".

Community Process Evaluation

Community process tracking occurs at some level in all of the studies, particularly health-related agencies within the community and their delivery of services over time. These are tracked at PAWT with annual interviews of the directors of all agencies within both communities that provide services related to any of the risk factors. Other key informants are also used in other studies. Part of the risk-factor surveys discussed earlier are usually dedicated to this assessment as well. For example, questions concerning CVD prevention programming conducted by organizations that the respondent belongs to, diffusion from secondary schools, degree of urging others to make risk-factor changes, employment opportunities, social networks and norms, and health care utilization data are all gathered in this way.

A major issue with community process tracking is whether or not to conduct tracking in the comparison communities as well as the intervention communities. The decision is influenced both by available resources and by hypothesized reactivity of such assessments. Some of the studies (e.g., COM, NY) have opted to assess only organizations within the intervention communities, while others (e.g., PAWT, MINN, FCP, GCP) have elected to conduct these assessments in both communities simultaneously. It could be argued that such assessments are reactive and thus become part of the intervention. However, failure to gather comparison data makes tenuous the attribution of observed changes to the intervention rather than to secular trends.

Another common tracking procedure is newspaper content analysis for any risk-factor-related articles including such topics as cigarette advertisements, legislative initiatives, and major events such as a mayor or other leading citizens suffering a heart attack or stroke. Perhaps the most ambitious of all these community process tracking efforts has been attempted by the GCP, with many sociocultural dimensions being included. Because of the relative lack of knowledge concerning the impact of community process variables on the major outcome variables, compared with individual variables like program participation, the community processes to be tracked are less consistent across studies and are often quite vague in their conceptualization and measurement.

Implementation Process Evaluation

Implementation process measurement is related to another important design decision: the degree to which the intervention will be allowed to change over the course of the study. Unlike a clinical trial for a new drug, where the exact composition of the substance to be ingested is known and stays exactly the same from the first day through the last, chronic disease prevention designs include evolution as experience and data accumulate throughout the active intervention phase. This change is not restricted to the intervention; there are usually important measurement developments occurring as well. For example, the development of the portable desktop analyzer for the measurement of cholesterol allowed both rapid feedback for intervention utilization and greatly increased the ability of process and formative evaluation components to gather actual blood cholesterol measurements on large numbers of participants. The fact that all of the studies selected the changing option increases the importance of implementation process evaluation.

Secondly, community approaches are complex and often influenced by unanticipated barriers and opportunities, e.g., the decision of a major worksite to start participation, changes in laws, interest of the mass media, and labor strikes. The more thorough the documentation of the actual activities that together make up the "intervention," the greater the opportunity to understand more about the links between specific types of activities and outcome changes. In a single study this is very tentative, but as data accumulate across studies more and more confidence accrues to these types of analyses. To further cross-study analyses, the three NIH-NHLBI studies in the United States (FCP, MINN, PAWT) have adopted a more general implementation process measurement procedure that, while not as comprehensive and extensive as the individual studies tracking systems, greatly facilitates generalizations. The system is also being actively considered for all the study regions of the GCP, and the extensive tracking system of PAWT has been adopted by NY, allowing later adoption of the NIH-NHLBI system.

Virtually all of the studies have procedures for documenting the community organizing efforts and results and the organizational changes that occur in the community. These data are usually collected through file review and staff diaries.

Without comprehensive process measurement it is difficult to make cost-effectiveness statements. These data, important for policy makers who consider wide-scale replications of successful models, are being increasingly incorporated into the studies as investigators become more confident that the knowledge base is sufficient to support wide-scale replications. At present the most extensive efforts seem to be in the COM and PAWT studies, but FCP and MINN are also conducting these types of analyses.

Formative Evaluation

Most community projects have been designed to test hypotheses and to generate new hypotheses. In all the projects reviewed here, a small number of hypotheses have been stated in general terms for the intervention (e.g., volunteers can be effective change agents), but very specific criteria have been stated for hypothesized changes in the more distal outcome variables (e.g., the mean cholesterol level can be lowered by 6 mg/dl; morbidity and mortality can be reduced by 15%). At the same time each project is generating (and often testing) a large number of more specific hypotheses (e.g., contests are an effective method of enlisting large numbers in the change process; immediate feedback of cholesterol results facilitates change). These ideas are often testable in a shorter time-frame than are the overall hypotheses, which rely on outcome assessment pre- and post-trial. These types of studies tend to concentrate on testing hypotheses concerning the links between variables illustrated in

Figure 5.1 and the effect upon a variable closer to distal outcomes (i.e., formative research). Thus any individual study uses formative research to take advantages of the cost savings of conducting multiple studies in the same setting; enjoys the access already established for the overall effort; and can utilize the overall data concerning the community and its subpopulations to plan, implement, and interpret the results of each specific formative study. Such research has resulted in increased knowledge about such things as how to work more effectively with various groups (e.g., the prevention of smoking among school children, as represented by the work in MINN; the utilization of volunteers at PAWT; and communication through electronic mass media at FCP). The studies described in this chapter have resulted in hundreds of articles in scientific journals based on this type of formative research.

SUMMARY

A number of major community interventions have been conducted in the primary prevention of CVD and cancer since the early 1970s. These have been large, extensive, expensive, and productive. While the specific approaches have varied, the efforts have benefited from a great deal of communication and cooperation among studies. The emphasis has been on having a well-defined design with a wide variety of evaluation techniques and on assuring as much comparability across studies as possible. This allows valuable cross-study comparisons that potentially advance the field more than simply a sum across each study.

Part IV

Lessons from Early
Community Prevention Efforts
for Alcohol Abuse

6

Focusing on the Drinking Environment or the High-Risk Drinker in Prevention Projects: Limitations and Opportunities
Norman Giesbrecht and Ann Pederson

INTRODUCTION

In this chapter we explore the relative merits of community-based prevention efforts directed at either the general population in the drinking environment or at high-risk, heavy drinkers. While there is evidence to suggest that the most effective mechanisms to reduce alcohol problems may be those directed at the general population, limits on the legal and regulatory powers of communities constrain their ability to act at this level. Furthermore, because higher levels of government resist implementing population-level approaches, it is important to determine effective and feasible strategies within community jurisdictions. To illustrate the challenge of conducting demonstration projects that attempt different levels of preventive action, we briefly describe a community-based prevention project conducted in southern Ontario in the mid-1980s. We hope that this discussion encourages other investigators to adopt innovative approaches to preventing alcohol-related problems.

THE PREVENTION PARADOX

In comparing the relative merits of two basic prevention strategies to curtail cardiovascular disease—a "high-risk" versus "mass" approach—Geoffrey Rose (1981, 1985) describes a prevention paradox that may apply to current deliberations on preventing alcohol-related problems:

> In the "high-risk" prevention strategy we go out and identify those at the top of the distribution and give them some preventive care—for example, control of hypertension or hyperlipidaemia. But this "high-risk" strategy, however

successful it may be for individuals, cannot influence that large proportion of
deaths occurring among the many people with slightly raised blood pressure
and a small risk . . .

We are therefore driven to consider mass approaches, of which the simplest
is the endeavour to lower the whole distribution of the risk variable by some
measure in which all participate. (Rose, 1981:1849)

Thus, "the prevention strategy that concentrates on high-risk individuals
may be appropriate for those individuals, as well as being a wise and efficient
use of limited medical resources; but its ability to reduce the burden of disease
in the whole community tends to be disappointingly small . . . ," whereas "a
measure that brings large benefits to the community offers little to each
participating individual" (Rose, 1981:1850-1851).   In other words, dealing
with the immediate, pressing problems of specific individuals through
secondary or tertiary prevention measures may have little benefit for the
overall incidence of problems; conversely, broader prevention measures, such
as public policies, may have little apparent benefit for specific individuals.
    Earlier, reflecting on public health generally and alcohol problems in
particular, McGavran had argued that real control of any public health problem
is unlikely to come through early diagnosis and treatment:

We must face the fact that the health of individuals is dependent upon the
health of communities—communities as entities, not as mere aggregates of
individuals. We must at least quit kidding ourselves in believing that early
diagnosis and treatment programs will accomplish much control. Our almost
complete absorption in the individual approach has deterred progress.
(McGavran, 1963:59)

Building on this broadening view of alcohol problems, Kreitman (1986)
and Kendell (1987) examined Rose's prevention paradox in light of both
clinical and survey data from the alcohol field.   Kendell summarizes the
findings and poses the central empirical and practical question:

We have firm evidence that reducing per capita consumption reduces a wide
range of ill effects. The crucial issue is—whose consumption ought we to be
trying to reduce?   Should we simply be trying to persuade the heaviest
drinkers to drink less, or should we try to persuade everyone to drink less
including, of course, modest drinkers like you and me? (Kendell, 1987:1282)

Both Kreitman and Kendell come to similar conclusions: individually
oriented approaches have limited general efficacy.   Specifically, both argue
that educational messages that seek to proclaim "responsible" or "safe"
drinking thresholds may have much less impact than policies or campaigns that
reduce consumption overall. They note that a minority of people are currently

drinking above the levels advised in British campaigns, and although the rate of problems per person is higher in this "at-risk" group,[1] a substantial proportion of drinkers below the so-called "safe limit" also encounter problems. Since the overall number of persons in the latter group is much larger than in the at-risk group, a dramatic lowering of the overall rate of problems is unlikely unless the behavior of the larger group of consumers is altered.

Extending Rose's analysis, Kreitman and Kendell conclude that encouraging *everyone* to drink less would have far greater impact than encouraging higher-risk drinkers to cut back on their consumption. Implicit in this discussion is the view that problems (e.g., drinking and driving, family violence) are caused by low- as well as high-risk drinkers. Both individual and mass change are difficult to achieve, however, and there is likely to be tremendous resistance to mass or population-oriented approaches that aim to reduce overall consumption rather than curb the behavior of the high-risk user. It has been demonstrated, however, that while targeted interventions may have limited impact on overall alcohol-related problems, they may be effective in reducing the consumption of high-risk users (Kreitman, 1986). And, for individual communities aiming to reduce alcohol-related problems, including crime, domestic violence, and illness, targeted approaches may be the most feasible, given both limited resources and limited regulatory powers. Kreitman and Kendell have thus raised important questions as to the appropriate focus for intervening to prevent alcohol-related problems.

LIMITATIONS OF FOCUSING ON THE HOST

The epidemiological trilogy of agent, host, and environment reminds us that there are three key dimensions in disease etiology. In the alcohol field, the agent and the environment have been used less often as pathways to prevention than has the host. The majority of efforts have tended to focus on the individual, saddling the individual drinker with responsibility for broader social changes (Mäkelä and Room, 1985). As summarized by Holder and Giesbrecht,

> [It is] curious that behavior, such as alcohol or other drug use, that is highly social, organized in groups, typically takes place in institutional contexts, and has strong cultural restraints and inducements, is usually confronted via prevention programs which focus on the individual. (Holder and Giesbrecht, 1990:8)

This individualistic perspective in part arises from Western liberal traditions that support individually oriented solutions to social problems, but it has also been encouraged by the alcoholic beverage producers (Maloy, 1984). The legacy of Prohibition, the fear of stigmatizing labels such as neo-

Prohibitionist, and the prominence of alcohol in contemporary culture together challenge prevention initiatives that focus on alcoholic beverages. Not surprisingly, environmentally oriented interventions that focus, for example, on the availability of alcohol, the number and distribution of outlet locations, the atmosphere and serving practices in drinking establishments, or mores and norms about drinking and drunkenness are perceived as serious threats to the sales of the alcoholic-beverage industry, as well as the related service industries. Concern about individual liberties has also contributed to a reluctance to implement environmental strategies.

While some have estimated that there are about 10.4 million alcoholics in the United States—about 5% of adults (Williams et al., 1987; see comment by Hilton, 1989)—this population is not necessarily the primary contributor to the frequency of a wide range of drinking-related complications (e.g., drinking and transportation events, worksite accidents, domestic problems, leisure and recreational incidents). Nonaddicted, relatively heavy consumers of alcohol, who are more numerous than dependent drinkers, appear to be involved in the lion's share of what are conventionally labelled as alcohol-related problems (see Cahalan, 1987; Room, 1977, 1980b). Individual nonaddicted heavy drinkers will, on the average, have fewer and milder drinking-related complications than alcoholics; however, because they constitute a relatively large proportion of the population, they are major contributors to the frequency of observed alcohol-related problems. It thus appears prudent to attempt to lower the consumption levels of those drinkers in order to reduce the incidence of alcohol-related problems. However, powerful vested interests (see Morgan, 1988) continue to seek to limit the definition of alcohol issues more or less exclusively to alcoholism and addiction.

Directing intervention and prevention efforts at the host presents other difficulties, including determining who specifically constitutes the target population. For many individuals, current drinking practices and related problems are neither permanent phenomena nor particularly accurate predictors of more severe problems in the future (Cahalan, 1987). For example, higher rates of trauma or certain social problems (e.g., violence, property damage) are typically associated with the teenage or early adult years but tend to decline with age and associated changes in lifestyles; risk-taking is reduced with age and responsibility increases (Cahalan and Room, 1974). Similarly, declining rates of drinking as well as spontaneous remission from alcoholism have been noted among some individuals reaching retirement age (Fillmore, 1987). Thus the nature of the high-risk population changes both temporally and cross-sectionally, and seeking to reduce the overall rate of problems through interventions that target the individual can be an elusive target.

BROADER FOCI IN PREVENTION INITIATIVES

One potential approach to prevention is to target the general population with measures directed at the culture of drinking; these include institutional arrangements for alcohol manufacturing, distribution, and consumption. International studies have documented higher rates of consumption in jurisdictions with high rates of certain alcohol-related problems (Bruun et al., 1975). This finding has been supported by investigations of changes over several decades (1950 to 1980) in seven countries (Mäkelä et al., 1981). The general levels and patterns of drinking in society are powerful but often underestimated dynamics in generating alcohol-related problems (Skog, 1985, 1989). Modifications of the environment, particularly through measures that influence pricing, have been shown not only to affect overall rates of consumption but also to reduce the number of addicted drinkers (Cook, 1987; Moskowitz, 1989). Furthermore, studies in a number of countries have noted positive correlations between availability of alcohol, rates of consumption, and drinking-related problems (Seeley, 1960; Terris, 1967; Bruun et al., 1975; Mäkelä et al., 1981; Moore and Gerstein, 1981). Increasingly, we are witnessing policy initiatives at all levels of government (see Mosher and Jernigan, 1989; Room, 1980a, 1989) based implicitly and explicitly upon a broader, environmental approach.

Another approach to alcohol problems has arisen from Ledermann's (1956, 1964) distribution-of-consumption model. The research following Ledermann's work has contributed significantly to the debate on how the drinking habits of the majority (moderate or light drinkers) have a bearing on the minority (heavy drinkers or alcoholics), and vice versa (Bruun et al., 1975; Schmidt and Popham, 1978; Parker and Harman, 1978). Ledermann observed that the distribution of alcohol consumption in general populations with widely different average consumption is approximated by a lognormal curve. This distribution implies that the relationship between moderate consumers and heavier consumers is a dynamic one, with the proportion of each being related to the other. Furthermore, the distribution curve points to a gradual transition from light to heavy consumption rather than a bimodal distribution or two independent distributions that would reflect underlying differences in the two types of drinkers.

Ledermann (1956) proposes "snowball" or "contagion" mechanisms in which an increase in the number of heavy drinkers is geometric. Others have elaborated his model more precisely. Bruun et al. (1975) suggest an interaction in which increased consumption by one heavy drinker will potentially influence a number of drinkers, in part because heavy drinkers participate in more drinking occasions than lighter drinkers and also tend to be the pace setters. Skog (1983) has developed hypotheses based on network models and the expectation of multiplying effects to elaborate on the relationships between overall rates of consumption and proportion of heavy consumers.

These lines of research suggest that the association between the drinking environment and average rates of consumption, on the one hand, and rates of heavy consumption, on the other, is more than a meaningless anomaly. One expects that a change in the general climate of drinking should have an effect upon the habits of the heavy drinker. The research thus provides a basis for unraveling the prevention paradox. Ledermann's model challenges Rose's prevention paradox by postulating that it may be possible to obtain a general population impact through a focused intervention directed at the high-risk drinker. Beauchamp's interpretation is in line with this orientation:

> The heavy user or alcoholic cannot be considered apart from the larger social environment. Even in his own immediate environment, most of the individuals the heavy consumer will encounter use substantially less alcohol than does he. The crucial issue is the structure of norms and sanctions that restrict alcohol use; a rise in consumption is to be taken as indicating a relaxation of existing norms and supporting sanctions (especially prices and control, or broad economic circumstances or cultural forces that have the same effect). (Beauchamp, 1980:111)

In our view, the Ledermann model suggests two complementary approaches to prevention. The first is to influence aggregate consumption levels and thereby, theoretically, the proportion of heavy drinkers in the population. This goal might be accomplished through regulatory measures affecting overall alcohol availability or by raising public awareness as to the relationship between the availability of alcohol and general patterns of alcohol consumption and the attendant public health risks of heavy drinking (Schmidt and Popham, 1978; Nörstrom, 1987). The second approach is altering the behavior of heavy drinkers with the expectation of reducing overall consumption—that is, subsequently moving the entire population to the lower end of the consumption curve.

There are, therefore, at least two distinct targets for prevention initiatives: drinkers in general and heavy drinkers or high-risk consumers. In considering these targets, we should remember that, for individuals, membership within either of these categories may vary throughout the lifespan. As previously noted, patterns of consumption vary with age, and thus high-risk is not a permanent characteristic for a given individual.

A TRI-COMMUNITY PREVENTION PROJECT

An example of a prevention project that employed both approaches is a community project undertaken in southern Ontario, Canada, in the 1980s. The project was specifically framed as a test of the distribution-of-consumption model articulated by Ledermann (1956, 1964) and elaborated by others (de Lint and Schmidt, 1968; Bruun et al., 1975; Schmidt and Popham, 1978; Skog, 1980). Previous research on this topic (Ledermann, 1956, 1964; de Lint and Schmidt, 1968; Bruun et al., 1975; Skog, 1980) suggested that if sufficient numbers of heavy drinkers were to reduce their consumption, there would be a decrease in the number of drinking role models and a concomitant reduction in pressures to drink heavily, which together would result in lighter drinkers subsequently modifying their consumption—a ripple effect.

The central hypothesis guiding the study was therefore that a decrease in the number of heavy drinkers would be accompanied by a comparable reduction in consumption among lighter drinkers. The goal was to reduce overall average consumption by focusing primarily upon the heavy drinker.

Study Design

A quasi-experimental design of the pretest-posttest nonequivalent comparison groups form was employed in the study. Three small, southern Ontario communities (8,000 to 12,000 inhabitants) were selected based upon similarities in patterns of alcohol sales by season, stability of rates of consumption, and existing services for heavy drinkers. One of these communities served as the intervention community, one was a pure control, and the other served as the regular control.

Aggregate trend data on alcohol sales, hospital admissions with drinking-related complications, and police charges were collected in all three communities. In addition, the study community and the control community were each surveyed before and after a multifaceted intervention was offered for 17 months in the study community (Giesbrecht, Pranovi, and Wood, 1990).

Intervention

A key component of the study was an education and counseling service for heavy drinkers. Developed from the behavioral modification literature (Sanchez-Craig, 1984; Marlatt, 1982), this service was available to both males and females. The overall goal of the counseling/educational program was to reduce the amount of drinking by the participants, thereby reducing the social and personal risks of heavy drinking. Clients were encouraged to reduce their alcohol consumption to less than 20 standard drinks[2] a week and no more than 4 per occasion, essentially changing their style of drinking (Giesbrecht and Pranovi, 1986).

The intervention also included broad educational and community development efforts aimed at increasing overall community awareness of alcohol-related problems. This aspect was thought to be particularly important for fostering a receptive climate for those people seeking to reduce their alcohol consumption, not only those involved in the counseling service but also other individuals in the community who independently wished to cut down.

Community awareness was promoted by making presentations on the prevention of alcohol problems, offering training workshops to health and social-service professionals, providing advice to the town council on local alcohol policy matters, organizing server-intervention workshops and meetings for regular and occasional servers of alcohol, and initiating union activities concerning workplace alcohol issues. In addition, project staff took part in a number of ongoing committees working on alcohol issues or broader health and social problems in the intervention community (Giesbrecht, Pranovi, and Wood, 1990).

Preliminary Findings

For the purposes of this chapter, it is important to note only the general trends found within the control and intervention communities. Both the pretest survey and alcoholic-beverage sales data indicate heavy drinking in these communities (Giesbrecht, 1987). In the intervention town, the seasonally adjusted rate of consumption was 18.02 liters of absolute alcohol per adult (aged 15 and older) in 1983, prior to the study.

The baseline survey of adult males found that alcohol use was acceptable under various circumstances within the intervention community (Community One), and many respondents also alluded to complications related to alcohol consumption. For instance, the importance of alcohol use in the social life of the intervention community is suggested by the baseline survey. One-third (34.7%) of the adult males reported consuming at least four or more standard drinks on drinking days, and 37% admitted to having been "a bit intoxicated" once a month. Almost 82% of the respondents had taken a drink in the 7 days prior to the survey, and 14% admitted to drinking more than 21 standard drinks over the last 7 days. In addition, a substantial proportion of all respondents to the pretest in Community One admitted to the following over the last 12 months (responses to "frequently," "occasionally," "seldom" options combined): driving a motor vehicle after drinking a lot of alcohol (46%); drinking in a car (35%); getting into arguments after drinking (31%); upsetting their wife or girlfriend in connection with drinking (30%).

Although relatively few heavy drinkers participated in the counseling and educational component of the intervention ($N=50$), it appears that on average there was a reduction in alcohol consumption in the course of their participation (Table 6.1). In view of the social pressures in the community to drink, many clients welcomed our efforts to increase the visibility and awareness of alcohol issues in the community through newspaper stories, media announcements, and presentations to service groups and clubs (Giesbrecht, Pranovi, and Wood, 1990).

There is evidence of slightly reduced consumption in the intervention community (One) as compared to the control community (Two) (Figures 6.1 and 6.2). In summary, the intervention was largely unsuccessful at demonstrating a reduction in aggregate alcohol consumption levels.[3] What can we learn from this study in relation to our initial question on the appropriate focus for prevention efforts: high-risk groups or the drinking environment?

TABLE 6.1

Overview of Changes in Client Consumption of Alcohol During Participation in the Alcohol Educational and Counseling Program

ESTIMATED NUMBER OF STANDARD ALCOHOLIC DRINKS PER WEEK		
WEEK BEFORE FIRST SESSION	WEEK AFTER FIRST SESSION	WEEK BEFORE LAST SESSION
Range:		
Low 0.0	0.0	0.0
High 91.0	74.0	52.0
Median 20.1	14.7	9.0
Mode 0.0	0.0	0.0
Mean 15.0	7.5	7.0

ESTIMATED PROPORTION OF PARTICIPANTS DRINKING HEAVILY PER WEEK		
WEEK BEFORE FIRST SESSION	WEEK AFTER FIRST SESSION	WEEK BEFORE LAST SESSION
More than 14 drinks (%) 54.1	43.3	21.2
More than 28 drinks (%) 27.0	17.3	4.2

NOTE: These data are based on information available from 47 of the 50 clients who participated in the program.

FIGURE 6.1
Alcohol Consumption Standard Drinks in the Past Week (Q4) at Times 1 and 2—Community One

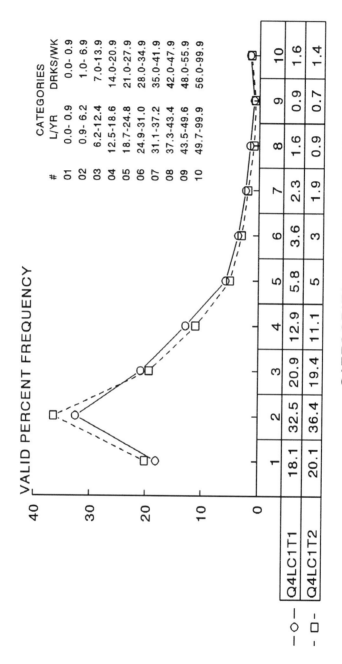

	1	2	3	4	5	6	7	8	9	10
Q4LC1T1	18.1	32.5	20.9	12.9	5.8	3.6	2.3	1.6	0.9	1.6
Q4LC1T2	20.1	36.4	19.4	11.1	5	3	1.9	0.9	0.7	1.4

CATEGORIES OF CONSUMPTION

CATEGORIES

#	L/YR	DRKS/WK
01	0.0- 0.9	0.0- 0.9
02	0.9- 6.2	1.0- 6.9
03	6.2-12.4	7.0-13.9
04	12.5-18.6	14.0-20.9
05	18.7-24.8	21.0-27.9
06	24.9-31.0	28.0-34.9
07	31.1-37.2	35.0-41.9
08	37.3-43.4	42.0-47.9
09	43.5-49.6	48.0-55.9
10	49.7-99.9	56.0-99.9

VALID PERCENT FREQUENCY

VALID CASES: C1T1 = 1346   MISSING CASES: C1T1 = 7.2%
C1T2 = 989   C1T2 = 8.6%

106

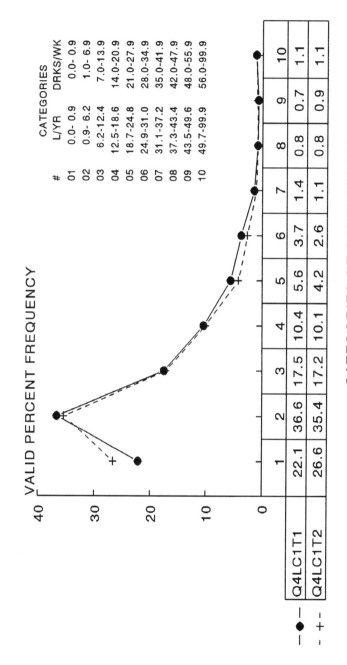

	1	2	3	4	5	6	7	8	9	10
Q4LC1T1	22.1	36.6	17.5	10.4	5.6	3.7	1.4	0.8	0.7	1.1
Q4LC1T2	26.6	35.4	17.2	10.1	4.2	2.6	1.1	0.8	0.9	1.1

CATEGORIES OF CONSUMPTION

CATEGORIES		
#	L/YR	DRKS/WK
01	0.0- 0.9	0.0- 0.9
02	0.9- 6.2	1.0- 6.9
03	6.2-12.4	7.0-13.9
04	12.5-18.6	14.0-20.9
05	18.7-24.8	21.0-27.9
06	24.9-31.0	28.0-34.9
07	31.1-37.2	35.0-41.9
08	37.3-43.4	42.0-47.9
09	43.5-49.6	48.0-55.9
10	49.7-99.9	56.0-99.9

VALID CASES: C1T1 = 1437   MISSING CASES: C1T1 = 4.9%
C1T2 = 1322   C1T2 = 6.8%

107

MULTIPLE-LEVEL PREVENTION FOCI IN COMMUNITY-BASED INTERVENTIONS

In the community study, the focus of intervention was the heavy drinker, primarily through the education and counseling service. As noted, this activity was supplemented by efforts directed at the population of the community as a whole in order to support the efforts of people attempting to reduce their drinking, whether as participants in the education/counseling service or independently. These activities diffused somewhat the focus of the project, transforming it from a fairly narrowly targeted approach to a more general one. In Rose's terminology, the project thus attempted to combine both a high-risk and a mass approach, although primary emphasis was on the former. This combined approach, however, while successful in assisting participants in the education/counseling service, was unable to demonstrate dramatic changes in indicators of aggregate consumption.

Several factors probably contributed to this inability to alter overall alcohol consumption levels. Although data such as overall alcoholic beverage sales records may provide indications of heavy drinking, a community may not perceive excessive alcohol consumption to be a problem. Furthermore, it is possible that although changes occurred among some individuals in our study, these changes may not have been enough to influence rates at the community level. Perhaps a longer intervention term would have demonstrated greater impact. Both lifestyle practices and attitudes change slowly, and the effects of interventions such as the one used here may not be readily apparent for some time.

Another contributor to the difficulty in changing the behavior of community members may have been the genesis and structure of the project itself. This project was community-based but not community-initiated, a distinction that may prove fundamentally important (see Pederson, Roxburgh, and Wood, 1990). As Room (1990:2) has suggested, local concerns may not coincide with the agenda of prevention workers or researchers:

> By and large, local communities are more concerned with the immediate consequences of drinking events than with the cumulative health or social-role toll of long-term heavy drinking . . . .
>
> Community-level actions also tend to have particular aims and forms. Taxes on alcohol are usually set at other levels, as is the general criminal code. Local governments may have some power to criminalize, and to pass local alcohol control measures, but these powers are conditional on and constrained by state, provincial or national legislation. Community-level organizing may, of course, be directed at changes at other levels; for instance, in the U.S. a local chapter of Mothers Against Drunk Driving may lobby the state legislature for a change in the drinking-driving laws.

This quotation highlights important distinctions between immediate local concerns and longer term, more broadly based agenda. As a research project initiated by the investigator, the project was less likely to have community support and commitment than one that was developed in consultation with the community and as a result of community concern.

It is possible that, given the larger social context of alcohol issues, interventions focusing on the environment or agent would be more effective in making the changes sought. Such measures are likely to involve health protection and/or regulatory strategies (Wallack and Wallerstein, 1987; Ashley and Rankin, 1988). Unfortunately, many of these measures, such as regulation of alcohol sales, lie beyond immediate community control, are too controversial to be readily undertaken by a single community, or are next to impossible to incorporate into studies (e.g., random assignment of communities to experimental conditions, such as raising the legal drinking age, is not feasible). Jurisdictional boundaries and the apparent simplicity of focusing on the host rather than on the environment or agent probably enhance a community's readiness to accept interventions directed at high-risk drinkers rather than at the community as a whole. Perhaps most significantly, targeting the high-risk drinker does not blur the line between conventional and problematic alcohol consumption patterns, and thus is not a threat to the mores or institutions linked to drinking in our cultures.

Environmental interventions are still fairly novel and run counter to postwar trends in alcohol policy, which have tended toward liberalization of availability (Bruun et al., 1975; Mäkelä et al. 1981). Experience with evaluated projects in regulating alcoholic beverages or drinking environments is not yet extensive; many programs and projects have emerged through trial and error or are derived from "natural experiments" such as reduced access to alcohol resulting from strikes or lockouts. This lack of experience with environmental approaches and their controversial nature suggest that introducing such a strategy may require extensive negotiation and promotion with community leaders.

Interim interpretation of field notes during the community study (Giesbrecht and Pranovi, 1986) concluded that community members were unsympathetic to an environmental view of alcohol problems and tended to translate references by project field staff to community-wide prevention agenda into treatment "by another name."

The multidimensional nature of the intervention, that is, the fact that it included a community awareness-raising strategy, the counseling and education service, and policy initiatives, may have contributed to people interpreting the project in terms that did not challenge in any fundamental way their current patterns of consumption. The comprehensive, integrative nature of the program and its overall aim to reduce consumption in the community was apparently not widely accepted.

In short, alcohol-related problems and preventive interventions are difficult to match.[4]   Modest, short-term, single-strategy interventions (constrained by local agenda, vested interests, and narrow perspectives) are often the main preventive action taken against long-term, deeply-rooted, and multifaceted drinking-related problems. Our community study represented an attempt to adopt a more multidimensional approach although its primary focus, derived from its theoretical basis, was on the high-risk drinker.

CHALLENGES OF COMBINING PREVENTION AND EVALUATION

There may be fundamental difficulties with fostering social change in the manner attempted in the community study. In part, these challenges reflect the traditional tension between the academy and the field: What may be valued for basic knowledge development may be less significant when viewed from a societal or community perspective. Thus, the desire to test hypotheses, while of interest to researchers, may be less important to communities that are interested in solving practical problems. Assuming that it is possible to meet both sets of priorities, we are confronted with the challenge of designing projects and trials that are effective and efficient, given scarce resources.

We need to accumulate experiences on how best to combine the multiple components that are being advocated as important to efficacious projects. Multicomponent interventions are difficult to both implement and to evaluate (Holder and Blose, 1987b), in spite of being likely to have a greater impact and being closer to how things typically happen in communities when special prevention trials are not underway. When we attempted in the tri-community project to act on several fronts simultaneously, we had to rely on our own sense of how to proceed because there was little support from the literature on how to actually put together such a multidimensional project.

Our interpretation of the community study suggests another dilemma arising from the attempt to demonstrate significant social changes with short-term, research-driven projects: Combining prevention efforts with the need for careful evaluation may constrain the possibility of having a powerful impact. Combining the two may also constrain our ability to assess that impact (Giesbrecht and Douglas, 1990). In the community project, we supported our more limited, focused intervention with community-level activities, such as policy discussions and awareness raising. Incorporating multiple foci, however, confounds interpretation of the impact of the intervention while possibly increasing its effectiveness.

Is it realistic to attempt broad approaches within demonstration-type projects? Is it possible to make the kinds of environmental manipulations desirable to attain maximum impact within the context of a research trial? If not, what are the implications for community-oriented research? Would researchers, communities, funding agencies, and politicians be willing to use projects as pilots for regional or national policy changes? Furthermore, without a realistic opportunity for extensive policy initiatives at the regional level, can we really hope to have any impact on alcohol consumption or on drinking-related problems in the community?

At the outset we posed the prevention paradox discussed by Rose, by Kendell, and by Kreitman. The paradox suggests that the choice of prevention foci is between individual actions with limited broad effectiveness or mass actions that have an aggregate impact but little direct bearing on individuals. Thus, the selection of foci for prevention projects seems to imply a choice between a narrow focus, such as high-risk drinkers or certain alcohol-related problems, or a broad prevention agenda. Ledermann's work has extended our view of possible foci for intervention in the context of alcohol-related problems. Through the interactions between the high- and low-risk consumption groups, the model implies, at least theoretically, that our choice of focus may be more flexible than the prevention paradox implies; namely, in targeting whichever group—either high-risk drinkers or the general population—the intervention may also have an impact on the other group. Our options in selecting targets may therefore be diverse, but the challenge remains to satisfactorily demonstrate the impact of prevention efforts, particularly those combining multiple interventions in action research.

NOTES

We are pleased to thank a number of people who contributed in various ways to the preparation of this chapter. Ken Allison, Mary Jane Ashley, and Roberta Ferrence drew attention to background literature. Jenet Bogles and Lucia Farinon located key articles and prepared material. Comments by Ron Douglas and Robin Room about demonstration projects had a bearing on the orientation of the chapter. Harold Holder suggested the topic and encouraged an exploration of environmental agenda. Finally, we appreciate the detailed and thought provoking comments by Harold Holder and Jan Howard on an earlier version of this chapter. The views and opinions expressed in this chapter are those of the authors and are not necessarily those of the Addiction Research Foundation nor the University of Toronto.

1. "Drinking Guidelines" referenced in Kendell's paper are: "up to 21 units a week for a man, or 14 for a woman, is a safe level of consumption, and that over 50 units a week for a man, or 35 for a woman is definitely harmful" (Kendell, 1987:1281). These are not necessarily Kendell's guidelines but are drawn from the UK College of Psychiatrists, London College of Physicians and the Health Education Council. According to our calculations, a 12 ounce bottle of beer containing 5% ethanol by volume would represent 1.37 units.

2. A "standard drink" is defined as one 12-ounce bottle of beer (5% alcohol by volume), a 5-ounce glass of table wine (12% alcohol), or a drink of spirits containing a 1 1/2-ounce shot (40% alcohol).

3. For a discussion and interpretation of the findings of the tri-community study, see Giesbrecht, Pranovi, and Wood (1990).

4. While we have alluded to some of the factors that contribute to this divergence, extensive interpretation would require an examination of cultural and political forces and is beyond the scope of this chapter (see Beauchamp, 1980; Room, 1980a; Cahalan, 1987).

7

Integrating Alcohol Abuse Prevention into Community Programs for Other Health Problems: Issues and Experiences

Alfred McAlister and Elizabeth Edmundson

INTRODUCTION

The purpose of this chapter is to discuss how theory-based and problem-specific alcohol abuse preventive interventions can be integrated within community-based public health strategies designed to address a wide range of health problems. There has been increasing concern in recent years that preventive programs may be unnecessarily fragmented when they are organized by diseases or risk factors (McAlister and Green, 1985). Large-scale, community programs differ from smaller, institutional-based programs by more than just an additive effect. Conceptually and pragmatically, community-wide programs employ a multi-faceted public health approach to health promotion and disease prevention. In community programs the mass media are used along with interpersonal and community support to facilitate diffusion of risk-reduction health behaviors to large numbers of individuals (Green and McAlister, 1984). Moreover, in a preventive health model, health is viewed as wholeness, with components (spiritual, physical, mental, etc.) in a dynamic balance (Weil, 1988). Those aspects of balance and wholeness permeate most public health programs (e.g., the messages of eating a balanced diet, exercising routinely, and drinking in moderation).

Because many chronic diseases share some basic precursors (smoking, imprudent nutrition, alcohol abuse, neglect of preventive health care), separate programs for common risk factors are not warranted. Similarly, because public education about different risk factors uses basic channels of communication (mass media, community volunteers, organizational settings such as health care institutions, work places, and schools), separate programs for each risk factor may divide efforts that might be better coordinated under a single administrative and theoretical framework. Thus, rather than competing with one another for the attention of media and community "gatekeepers," efforts to address different risk factors should be coordinated synergistically.

Alcohol abuse is a particularly interesting candidate for the "integrated" approach to prevention because its impact cuts across numerous other risk factors and disease categories. Alcohol can contribute to cardiovascular and cerebrovascular disease, cancers in several forms, and accidents—in addition to its better-publicized relationship with chronic liver disease. For example, more than 100,000 people died of alcohol-related causes in 1987— approximately 5% of the total national mortality (Massachusetts Medical Society, 1990).

Furthermore, heavy alcohol use is correlated with cigarette smoking, imprudent nutrition, failure to receive preventive care, and other forms of self-neglect. Alcohol misuse often precedes relapses in smoking cessation, weight-loss, maintenance of therapeutic regimens, as well as the maintenance of risk-reducing behavior among persons at risk of HIV infection. Alcohol abuse is related to the disintegration of families and the disruption of education and employment, factors which profoundly influence the full spectrum of health conditions and health-related cultural practices (Cahalan, 1987; Fingarette, 1988).

The mortal and economic cost of alcohol abuse is not disproportionate to that of cigarette smoking, but its impact is more immediately observable and also observable at younger ages (e.g., years of life lost from an alcohol-related motor vehicle crash). From the standpoint of a policy activist, local forces in opposition to alcohol abuse are not easily linked with those concerned with cigarette smoking, AIDS prevention/control, nutrition, etc. Citizen interest in alcohol policy is typically mobilized by those connected to its most dramatic victims (e.g., relatives of victims of drunken driving). On the other hand, one might argue that such emotional forces are less dependable than forces generated by a larger coalition of interests with a broader public health perspective.

UNIFYING THEORETICAL CONCEPTS

A notion of how to combine mass media and interpersonal communication effectively can be derived from social learning theory (Bandura, 1977, 1986). The key concepts are modeling and social reinforcement. Modeling refers to the learning that occurs when a person observes and copies the behaviors of others. Social models are those people who influence observers to changes in attitudes, beliefs, and decision making, and to acquire new patterns of behavior. Models derive their potency from attributes—in the eyes of observers—such as attractiveness, social competence, expertise, and credibility.

Peers are often the most influential models in everyday social learning. For modeling complex behaviors and skills to be learned by observers, the most salient factor in whether the skill is learned is the model's demonstration of complex sequences in a gradual, systematic manner. Modeling of difficult behavioral patterns is most effective when persons are shown coping realistically with predictable problems. Social models can powerfully influence addictive behaviors (e.g., when celebrities enter alcohol treatment).

Many policy-activists and researchers have expressed concern about the representation of alcoholic beverages in advertising and on television programs. The effect of advertising and alcohol drinking scenes on television is difficult to determine. However, several studies have demonstrated that alcohol is severely over-represented among beverages seen during television programs. The frequency with which alcohol is seen on television may contribute to an unrealistic conclusion, particularly among youth, about the frequency of drinking in the "real world" (Secretary of Health and Human Services, 1990).

Social reinforcement is best understood by considering the distinction between acquisition and performance of new behaviors learned from role models. New behaviors may be acquired from mediated communication (e.g., from television), but they will not be performed unless the environment is one in which those behaviors will be reinforced. A powerful source of reinforcement is found in interpersonal communications, particularly apparent in verbal praise from peers or other significant persons. A key psychological element in social learning theory is the development of self-efficacy expectations. If a learner does not expect to do well, performance will be delayed. Verbal information from others is a powerful source of the learner's expectations, as are the reactions of others to the learner's initial efforts. Participant learning, as in participant modeling or role playing, can be combined with social reinforcement to provide both skills training and a persuasive influence on self-perceptions and perceived norms.

An example of social reinforcement and norm-setting is server training. Although the evaluation of server-training programs is just beginning to appear in the scientific literature, such programs appear effective, particularly if they are supported by management. Trained servers may be more influential than public service announcements, because their "front line" efforts are directed at specific drinkers immediately prior to driving (Secretary of Health and Human Services, 1990).

Recognizing that alcohol use may be influenced by environmental factors such as sales hours, marketing practices, price, police action, etc., our theoretical approach also includes how social change can be accomplished through media and community programs. To stimulate social change, theory calls for expressions of interest through collective behavior (e.g., Olson, 1965). Organizing voters, consumers, workers, and other groups can change the behavior of policy-makers and, ultimately, environmental factors that influence behavior. For example, price manipulation through taxation can be stimulated by organized advocacy, as can limits on advertising or increases in resources for treatment.

There is evidence that an increase in the real price of alcoholic beverages, resulting from higher federal or state excise taxes, can decrease highway fatalities. For example, an increase of as much as $1.50 per 24-limit case of 12-ounce cans may decrease fatal traffic accidents by 27 percent among 18-21 year-old drivers and by 18 percent among 15-17 year-old drivers (U.S. Department of Health and Human Services, 1990). Furthermore, the increase in the minimum drinking age from 18 to 21 years appears to have decreased fatal traffic accidents from drunk driving, particularly among those 18-20 years old.

Administrative license-revocation programs also offer opportunities to reduce crash-related fatalities. The constraints on the effectiveness of license-revocation programs include resistance to enforcement by law officers and the unanticipated creation of delays, postponements, and avoidance of punishment in the courts. However, there is some evidence that a reduction of 10 percent in alcohol-related crash fatalities can be obtained from license-revocations (Secretary of Health and Human Services, 1990). The impacts of alternative policies need to be carefully considered from both a theoretical and practical standpoint; however, there are no theoretical barriers to combining efforts to influence alcohol policy with efforts involving tobacco, nutrition, or health services.

An approach to the integration of mass media and interpersonal communication was presented by Green and McAlister (1984). They noted several distinctions between early and late adopters of public health messages. Early adopters and innovators are usually affluent or middle class, are well-educated, and have more knowledge of and access to health care. Yet, because of their affluence, these people actually do not need many of the products and/or services they purchase for health. According to Green and McAlister, national mass media programs, without auxiliary social, governmental or clinical support, are adequate for diffusing health-related interventions and policies for early adopters.

In contrast, the majority of potential adopters of public health campaigns are less affluent and have less interest than early adopters in national health matters. The interests of the majority lie more with local media, organizations, and interpersonal dialogue. These are the people targeted by comprehensive public health programs to adopt lifestyle changes that will reduce risks of common causes of morbidity and mortality (e.g., cardiovascular risk reduction). Therefore, the influence of nationally-based mass media is limited with the majority of people. Social modeling (locally-based) and social reinforcement appear to augment mass media efforts to encourage health behavior change for late adopters.

The most frequently targeted groups for public health interventions are also the most difficult to reach. They are typically characterized by social alienation, low socio-economic status, low education levels , little or no health insurance, and in need of basic health services such as immunization and maternal and child health care. Mass media are primarily a source of entertainment for these groups. Therefore, the most successful strategies for public health interventions with them include interpersonal communication and labor-intensive community outreach (Green and McAlister, 1984).

Depending on their ideological perspective, different researchers of addiction recommend various preventive measures. A common theme presented by several prominent researchers (Cahalan, 1987; Fingarette, 1988; Peele, 1989; Weil, 1988) is that addiction is a symptom, not a cause of poor health. Rather than send an "abstinence only" message as the main preventive effort, they recommend interpersonal, community support of basic values and the acquisition of "life skills." For example, Fingarette (1988) and Peele (1989) have suggested that heavy drinking be treated in the same manner as poor dietary and exercise patterns, as an activity that is likely to cause illness. Indeed, Goodstadt has proposed the following:

> The non-use of drugs is not merely the absence of drug use, but is the choosing of an alternative set of behaviors as a source of gratification . . . . [Drug] education should also be seen as complementary to noneducational strategies, which fashion an environment that discourages undesirable drug use and promotes healthy behavior. (Goodstadt, 1989:208)

Peele (1989) has proposed the inclusion of alcohol abuse in a comprehensive risk-reduction program as part of promoting individual responsibility and respect for ourselves. He also argues that a sense of community responsibility and community efficacy enhances an individual's sense of self-efficacy, which in turn increases the abuser's ability to regulate his/her drinking behavior.

Although the special interests of activists may vary across risk factors, two common themes are their desire to *prevent* rather than to treat and their willingness to impose costs on consumers and controls on commercial enterprise. That is, they advocate reducing short-term personal gratification or corporate profit in favor of anticipated future gains in health and the equitable distribution of comfort and resources across social classes.

Social learning theory and diffusion theory can guide the design of combined mass media and interpersonal campaigns to promote behavioral change across risk factors. Role model stories should be emphasized. Mass media may effectively inform, persuade, and train their audiences, but lasting change will not be achieved without a supportive social environment, for example, via community volunteers. Research suggests that adding interpersonal support and reinforcement for behavior change through community organization can double the effects of media-only communications (Flay, 1987).

Community prevention programs can be organized as supporting units for local public health services or grass-roots agencies that lack staff or expertise beyond their primary mandates to serve clients in need of clinic-based services. One approach to working within communities is the "lead agency" model, in which a single powerful organization is given responsibility for action, including whatever coalition-building or coordination of others' work is needed to meet objectives. This may also be termed an "inside" approach, in that the origination of the work within the community requires that the selected lead organization change from within. Large-scale community programs require a great deal of planning and coordination among several organizations. However, as experience with coordinating efforts of several agencies increases, the amount of energy and resources required of a "lead" agency to coordinate the additional, incoming organizations decreases. The infrastructure for coordination is in place, reducing the per-organization resource effort, which leads to efficient inter-agency collaboration.

ALCOHOL USE BEHAVIOR OF ADULTS: A CASE STUDY

The city of Eagle Pass, Texas—on the Mexican border west of San Antonio—has been the site of a health promotion pilot study conducted by the Center for Health Promotion Research and Development of the University of Texas School of Public Health at the Health Science Center in Houston. The study investigated how multifactor (integrated) efforts can be most efficiently conducted. From 1985 through 1989, Eagle Pass served as a treatment community, with the nearby city of Del Rio serving as a control site. Baseline surveys in 1985 and 1986 found that, among the Mexican-Americans who made up more than 90 percent of the study populations, alcohol use was comparable in the two sites.

The details and results of the social modeling, community organization, and mass media efforts implemented in this study have been reported (McAlister et al., 1992). The results of the case study demonstrated that it is feasible to combine efforts to influence alcohol use with programs to promote cessation of smoking and other changes in risk factors for cancer and cardiovascular disease. Smoking concerns were the primary focus of the study, not alcohol, and the results seemed to reflect this emphasis. For example, an analysis of the relationship between heavy alcohol use (more than six drinks on a single recent occasion) and other variables found modest associations with tobacco use, lower participation in preventive screening, and dietary practices of fat avoidance. Additionally, heavier drinkers reported more sick days and more perception of financial stress. They were also less educated and younger than their lighter drinking counterparts.

There was no difference between the treatment and control groups in changes in drinking behavior over the course of the program. Both communities had a reduction in the proportion of respondents who reported more than six drinks on a single occasion during the past month.

Although the topics of alcohol and drug abuse received 30 percent of the media campaign exposure, fewer than half of those episodes concerned reduction in drinking among adults. Thus it can be argued that the program was too diluted to produce an effect.

A significant program effect may require environmental changes related to marketing alcohol, taxation, criminal policy, and treatment of alcoholism. These were not implemented in the first phase of study, although a process to select appropriate objectives for small-town action has since been organized in Eagle Pass.

LIMITS TO INCLUDING ALCOHOL ABUSE IN AN INTEGRATED PROGRAM

From a methodological perspective, there are limits on the inclusion of alcohol use and abuse in a broader community study. Measurement instruments for alcohol use and abuse are available and well-standardized, and a variety of physical and social indicators can be used to supplement self-reports. Yet, the number of questions that can be included in an interview tend to discourage the expansion of instruments necessary to include multiple factors into a single interview.

The dilution of treatment intensity is of greater concern, particularly for community experimenters with limited access to media channels and networks of communication. To the extent that experimental programs are constrained in opportunity, a community researcher must be cautious in attempting too much. A purely pragmatic concern further limits integration. Fragmented, disease-oriented federal agencies avoid funding efforts that cross bureaucratic lines of control. For the latter reasons, reduction of alcohol use/abuse has tended not to be included in objectives of community studies of health promotion in the United States.

Active participation of the target audience in the identification of needs, goal-setting, and program planning is a common ingredient of several theoretical approaches necessary for success among large-scale and smaller, institutional-based interventions. Yet, community-wide programs tend to limit local input, particularly in the planning and evaluation stages of the intervention. Large-scale public health interventions would be more efficacious if the planning and evaluation procedures were mostly determined at the local level, whereas resources for implementation would be provided by the central or nationally-focused aspect of the intervention (Green and McAlister, 1984).

The inclusion of youth (ages 12-17) in a study presents an additional difficulty because of the parental consent required for home or telephone interviews of minors, especially when sensitive issues such as alcohol abuse are included. Successive cross-sectional surveys of persons at or above the age of eighteen can be of use to estimate the delayed effects of prevention at earlier ages.

The expansion of prevention objectives within an established community program, as described here, can raise methodological concerns about effects of prior treatment and the generalizability of programs that are built on unique local structures. The issue of contamination is not serious if comprehensive baseline data are collected before the first phase of treatment begins and if the prior treatment was originally documented.

The experience in Texas supports the idea that existing community studies with a focus on other health topics can be usefully expanded to include the prevention and control of alcohol abuse. Community leaders and volunteers, who themselves see alcohol and drug abuse as the largest current threat to health, have been helpful in the expansion of organizational sponsorship to support new activities. The only objections experienced in Texas arose early in the discussion of high-risk counseling, when local treatment providers needed to be assured that reimbursable treatment services were not being provided. Young people see connections between alcohol, tobacco, and other drugs and, in the community events, rapidly transfer skills-training and norm-setting exercises among the different substances.

CONCLUSION

More research is needed on how programs that address multiple health problems, including alcohol abuse, can be best integrated in schools, mass media campaigns, community organization, and policy advocacy. With many different health programs and agencies already competing for the attention of subpopulations at risk, any new initiatives to modify behaviors such as alcohol abuse must be carefully interfaced with existing community organizations serving cultural and geopolitical constituencies. From an attributable risk estimate of lost years of life, alcohol abuse is by far the greatest health threat in South Texas. Access to health services is a concern that includes treatment of alcohol abuse and cuts across other disease categories. Concentrations of risk-taking behaviors are found among some marginal groups that are currently being involved in community studies of AIDS prevention. A major challenge for future research and analysis will be the integration of health-related community programs with actions to influence social problems.

8

Prevention Experiments in the Context of Ongoing Community Processes: Opportunities or Obstacles for Research

Robert L. Stout

INTRODUCTION

The scientific study of alcohol problem prevention is fraught with difficulties. Prevention trials are costly, lengthy, and rarely unambiguous in their findings. The costs of such trials, however, are dwarfed by the social costs of alcohol abuse and its consequences (Secretary of Health and Human Services, 1990: Chapter VII). The costs of prevention trials are even small in relation to the money and effort expended for ongoing prevention efforts, about whose effectiveness little is known (Secretary of Health and Human Services, 1990: Chapter IX; Institute of Medicine, 1989: Chapters 5-6). Better know-ledge about the relative effectiveness of different approaches to prevention should enable us to make optimal use of the limited resources available for prevention.

To learn the most we can from prevention trials, we have to examine their limitations and seek ways to overcome them. One of these limitations is that, since we lack realistic laboratory analogs of communities, we must do our research in real communities. Such research is rather like doing clinical case studies—the number of "subjects" is small, and the focus is typically on within-case change over time more than on comparisons of groups of cases receiving differing treatments. There are, however, several aspects unique to community-based research: for example, the diversity within each community

The research described in this chapter was supported by the project "Rhode Island Alcohol-Related Health Problems Study: A Community-Based Alcohol Abuse Prevention Project," which was funded under CDC-NIAAA Cooperative Agreement Number U50/CCU100832. The project's Principal Investigator was William J. Waters, Jr., Ph.D. of the Rhode Island Department of Health.

and the historical context of events in and around each community. This chapter is an attempt to grapple with the significance of salient events in community history—to understand how these events affect prevention efforts and the evaluation of prevention findings.

The case study that provides the context for this chapter is the Rhode Island Community Alcohol Abuse/Injury Prevention Project. The project interventions and results are described in detail elsewhere (Rhode Island Department of Health, 1989a, 1989b); an overview of the project and its initial results are given below.

THE RHODE ISLAND ALCOHOL ABUSE/INJURY PREVENTION PROJECT

Three Rhode Island communities were selected for the project, based on size, incidence of alcohol-related health problems, sociodemographic characteristics, and community resources. The demonstration community, Woonsocket, was selected at random; the comparison communities were Newport and Westerly.

The intervention strategy was directed at changing the knowledge, attitudes, and behavior of gatekeepers in their roles as regulators of community drinking practices. Two important groups of gatekeepers are servers (i.e., people who sell or serve alcoholic beverages in licensed liquor establishments) and law enforcement officers. The three main intervention efforts were community mobilization, training in responsible service of alcoholic beverages, and increased and improved liquor law enforcement.

Community Mobilization and Publicity

The first intervention was to mobilize the influence of civic and political leaders in behalf of the program and to encourage broad media coverage of project activities. The purpose was to gain credibility and support for the project, to encourage gatekeepers to participate in the project, and to educate the public about the dangers of drinking in situations of high injury risk.

Responsible Alcohol Service/Training

The second intervention effort was designed to secure the cooperation of owners and managers of package stores, bars, restaurants, and private clubs in a training program to increase responsible alcohol service in Woonsocket. Owners and managers of liquor establishments were asked to adopt a written policy statement endorsing principles of responsible alcohol service. Owners and managers were asked to have their sales and service personnel participate in a training program developed and tested by the National Highway Traffic Safety Administration (NHTSA). This program taught servers techniques for identifying minors and intoxicated patrons and for denying, slowing down, or cutting off service. The training program also informed them of their legal liability if they failed to obey dram shop laws and taught them ways to protect customers' safety.

More Intensive and Visible Law Enforcement

The third intervention was to secure the cooperation of law enforcement personnel in Woonsocket to increase arrest rates for driving while intoxicated (DWI) and other liquor law violations and to reduce levels of drunken driving. Police officers were trained (using NHTSA materials) to recognize intoxication in drivers, to operate breathalyzer equipment, and to conduct sobriety checkpoints. The officers were encouraged to increase radar patrols, sobriety checkpoints, and selective enforcement visits to liquor establishments.

Project Evaluation

By the end of the demonstration project, after 18 months of baseline study and 30 months of intervention, the following objectives were achieved:

1. 100% of off-premise establishments and 79% of on-premise establishments had adopted written policies for responsible alcohol service.
2. 388 sales and service personnel had been trained in the techniques for responsible alcohol service. This represents nearly 61% of servers estimated to be employed in the community.
3. All members of the Woonsocket police force had received training in recognizing and measuring intoxication, the role of alcohol in police work, police liability in dealing with intoxicated citizens, and on-scene investigation of motor vehicle crashes.
4. The police department had initiated 73 sobriety checkpoints, 47 additional radar patrols, and 11 selective enforcement patrols covering 300 visits to liquor establishments.

Evaluation Results

Several process indicators suggest that the gatekeepers responded appropriately to the interventions. A posttest of servers done 12 to 18 months after the training shows enduring changes in attitudes and behavior. The police carried out a vigorous enforcement campaign; arrest data show that alcohol-related arrests increased in Woonsocket, while the other two communities showed level or decreasing rates.

The impact of the project on health outcomes is less easy to document. Accident rates in Woonsocket increased, but rates in the comparison communities remained stable. In 1987, the first year major interventions were begun, the number of alcohol-related accidents increased sharply, followed by a modest drop in 1988 (see Table 8.1). The 1988 level, however, was still above the 1985-86 baseline. On a population basis, the Woonsocket rates for 1987-88 were the highest values seen in the study, suggesting enforcement and/or reporting effects.

It is impossible to disentangle fully the effects of improved reporting of alcohol-relatedness (due to the increased sensitivity of investigating officers to alcohol issues) from changes due to prevention effects. As a percentage of total accidents, alcohol-related accidents peaked in 1987 and then showed a substantial drop in 1988 to levels below the baseline years (see Table 8.2).

One possible interpretation of the peak in 1987 and drop in 1988 is that the peak represents a reporting improvement and the drop a genuine prevention effect whose size may be somewhat attenuated by improved reporting. If the reduction in the proportion of accidents reported as alcohol related is interpreted as a prevention effect, it corresponds to the prevention of 11 accidents with injury per year.

TABLE 8.1
Alcohol-Related Motor Vehicle Crashes

	1985	1986	1987	1988
Woonsocket				
Number	80	79	96	86
Rate*	177	176	211	189
Newport				
Number	49	54	49	46
Rate*	164	184	165	155
Westerly				
Number	17	29	32	25
Rate*	88	148	162	126

*Note: The rate figures refer to events per 100,000 persons per year.

TABLE 8.2
Alcohol-Related Crashes as a Percentage of all Crashes in Woonsocket

	1985	1986	1987	1988
Ratio of alcohol-related crashes to all crashes	6.6%	6.4%	7.2%	6.0%
Ratio of alcohol-related crashes with injury to all crashes with injury	11.0%	12.5%	13.1%	9.0%

The pattern of a peak in 1987 followed by a drop in 1988 can be seen in several of the more specific alcohol-related motor vehicle crash (MVC) rates, including MVCs with DWI, alcohol-related MVCs with injury, with transportation to the ER, with severe or fatal injury, or with high risk (high risk being defined as crashes involving a single vehicle with a male driver under 30 occurring late at night [10 p.m.-2:59 a.m.] or on a weekend). The reduction in alcohol-related crashes with severe or fatal injury is especially noteworthy because of its magnitude—a 50% drop. However, the number of events involved is so small (14 versus 7) that it is difficult to assess its significance.

The conclusions we can draw from these data are of necessity modest and provisional. The power of the study to detect differences is limited by the rates of the events of interest. The reporting of alcohol relatedness is also a major area of concern; there are many reasons for believing that the proportion of accidents in which alcohol is involved is substantially higher than the above data would indicate. There are, unfortunately, many obstacles to accurate reporting of alcohol involvement. Another drawback is the lack of data for 1989. Additional funding has been obtained to gather 1989 data, so we will be able to assess the durability of the changes seen in Woonsocket and obtain a better perspective on their significance.

UNEXPECTED EVENTS IN THE RHODE ISLAND PROJECT

The course of the Rhode Island project was affected by many unplanned events and circumstances, prominent among which was a young man's death and its consequences. This man, who was under the legal age of 21, was served in a Woonsocket bar some time before he lost control of his vehicle and was killed upon crashing into a tree. This event became of increased significance to the project when the man's mother filed a $2,000,000 lawsuit against the bar where he had been served and the server who had waited on him. The events connected with the death received considerable publicity in the local press. The death and lawsuit happened to coincide with the beginning of server training by project staff (see Figure 8.1). Prior to this event, liquor licensees and servers had shown limited enthusiasm for the training program; afterwards, the level of interest increased markedly. Woonsocket licensees formed an association and became much more active.

The effect of the death and lawsuit on the licensees and servers should not, however, be overestimated. There were still many uncooperative licensees, and more than one-third of the servers never took part in the training. It still took considerable effort on the part of our Community Coordinator to schedule the trainings and get servers to appear. Nonetheless, there is no doubt that the server intervention was much more readily accepted; the lawsuit was a constant topic of conversation in the server-training sessions.

What happened in Woonsocket also affected the rest of the state. A state legislator introduced a bill that would have mandated statewide server training.

FIGURE 8.1
Rate of Server Training in Woonsocket

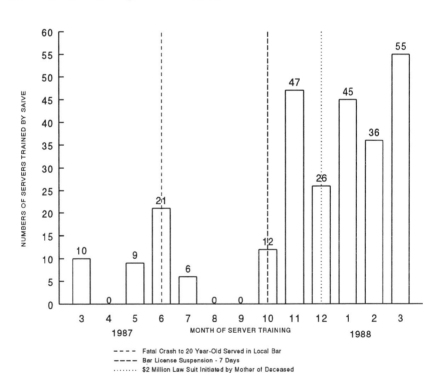

The bill passed the legislature but was ultimately vetoed by the governor. This effort would probably have happened without the Woonsocket incident, but it was given a boost by that event.

RAMIFICATIONS OF CRITICAL EVENTS

What effect do events like the Woonsocket incident have on the community and on prevention efforts and outcomes? In this particular instance there was some synergy between the events and project efforts, but other kinds of events such as changes in key personnel (e.g., mayor, chief of police) could also have deleterious effects. One's perspective on such events depends on the priority one places on different aspects of prevention studies. For example, Table 8.3 contrasts the perspective of a classical experimental scientist, whose sole concern is gaining knowledge, with the more practical perspective of an organizer whose main goal is to make progress toward preventing harm.

Though these two roles are somewhat caricaturized, they illustrate the contrast of perspectives. Classical science calls for simplicity and control; lack of these can weaken a study to the point of meaninglessness. Simplicity and control, however, are often not easy to obtain in modern American communities. In any study with significant community involvement, there will be tensions between building a firm knowledge base that will in a possibly distant future lead to saving more lives, versus doing everything possible to save lives in the here and now, versus maintaining a comfortable if possibly dysfunctional status quo in the community. The community organizer is at the focal point of these tensions and has to reconcile them as best he or she can if anything is to be accomplished. Scientists have a tendency to treat unexpected events or community resistance to and/or deviations from the protocol as potentially threatening at best; however, researchers must learn to see these situations through the community's eyes as well as from their own point of view. Intervention approaches that make allowances for local variations and chance events will fit more naturally into communities, and may be more effective, than rigid protocols.

It is, however, still important to have quantitative information about how much and how often unexpected changes affect prevention outcomes. If outcome levels are routinely subject to major fluctuations due to unusual historical events, then that fact must be taken into account in the design and planning of prevention studies. If, on the other hand, outcome levels only rarely undergo major transitions in the absence of an intervention, then less concern is needed. The only way to find out if outcome levels undergo frequent major shifts is to examine the data.

TABLE 8.3
Ideal Prevention Study Characteristics

Scientist's Perspective	Community Organizer's Perspective
Implementation: The study intervention is implemented instantaneously. Before the target date, there is no prevention activity; after the target date the interventions are working full throttle—they should not be delayed or interrupted by complications.	**Implementation:** Components of the effort are gradually phased in as the leaders and members of the community are ready and the necessary groundwork is laid. Rushing the implementation is likely to backfire.
Design: The interventions are a tightly specified package worked out in advance. Changing plans in midstream, or having somewhat different intervention plans in different sites, complicates the evaluation by muddying the waters. Losing control of the intervention means losing the ability to replicate.	**Design:** Any outside researcher who comes in and starts trying to give orders to the locals should be shot. The success of a project depends in large part on participation by community members who always have their own ideas, sometimes good ones, about how things should be done. The research intervention plan is a starting point, a foundation on which to add improvements.
Isolation: The sites should be independent; outside events should not affect the target communities, and conversely events within the communities should not leak outside and potentially affect other sites.	**Isolation:** No community is isolated; local people are interested in taking advantage of new ideas from outside they think might stop the damage they see being done. The program at one site may seem to be so successful that outside communities spontaneously adopt it.
Events: Events add noise to the outcome data even if they work in favor of the intervention. While minor events are to be expected, major ones threaten replicability. This can be a critical problem since prevention studies so often are single-case or few-case designs.	**Events:** A community in which unexpected events never happen would be grossly anomalous. The most likely events are related to the mortality/morbidity we are trying to prevent. These events, though regrettable, represent opportunities for education and motivation; the intervention team should be ready to take advantage of these incidents.

EXPLORATORY STUDY OF OUTCOME TRENDS

If events such as those described above do influence mortality and morbidity, then under at least some conditions we should be able to see evidence of this in the data. Detecting the effects of any single historical event is difficult for the same reasons that determining the effect of a deliberate effort at prevention can be troublesome: Effects may be gradual, delayed, transient, and difficult to see against a noisy background. For example, the fatality described was just the beginning of an extended chain of events, including the bar license suspension, the filing of the lawsuit, and subsequent developments in the suit. At each point in this chain there was publicity and community reaction, which conceivably could affect outcome rates either immediately or after a delay. Of course, while one chain plays out, other events can occur to complicate the picture further. Any potential effects we see looking forward in time from any one historical event are very difficult to link directly to the event, and we cannot replicate a unique event at another time in another community to see if the effects are similar. Nonetheless, we may be able to attack the problem from another angle—we can examine trends in accident rates for evidence of naturally occurring major shifts in outcome levels and see if we can work backward from any to ascertain their possible causes.

Such an exploration of outcome trends is of more than technical interest. If we can discover why, for example, accident rates abruptly increase or decrease, that knowledge might suggest new approaches to prevention. What we are looking for in the Woonsocket accident data are changes in accident rates long enough and large enough to be of substantive interest, taking into account known sources of variation in accident rates (e.g., seasonal trends) and secular (very long-term) drift in the rates.

Modern exploratory data-analysis techniques allowed us to undertake such a search. Briefly, our procedure involved the following steps:

1. For a given data set (the accident rates for a single city over time) a time-series model was formulated that took into account seasonal and secular variation.
2. From this model, we calculated 80% confidence bands around the predicted values for each time point.
3. An observed value that lay outside the confidence interval was considered a potential outlying point—a point at which the rate of accidents was unusually high or unusually low given the time of year and the general rate of accidents. Since we are interested primarily in prevention, the main concern was with events where the accident rate was below normal. We already know of many

factors that can temporarily inflate the rate of accidents (weather, heavily attended sporting events, and so on).

4. Since some points will be outside the confidence bands by chance, we took an additional step to protect against chasing after random noise. We did this by looking for runs of below-normal accident rates. While all "natural" prevention events are of some interest, the longer-lived ones are of the most interest. A single low reading has a high likelihood of being due to chance, but a run of successive low readings may well be of some significance.

Six outcome series were studied: overall accident rates and alcohol-related accident rates for each of the three communities. In each analysis, the dependent measure was the mean number of accidents per day. The accident data were aggregated over 2-week periods, providing 26 time points per year. The rates of events were sufficiently low that the data, especially for Westerly, were strongly affected by random noise; however, a coarser time resolution would have made it difficult to see shifts lasting less than several months.

In general, the time-series models fit these data relatively well.[1] There are few runs of points above or below the confidence bands. Possible exceptions include a dip in Woonsocket in overall accidents during mid-1987 (see Figure 8.2). The fatal accident discussed above occurred in June 1987 near the beginning of the low period; that is also a time when stepped-up traffic enforcement, including a new series of radar patrols, was being done. There is less evidence of a dip in the alcohol-related accident series at that time; the alcohol-related accidents data are more noisy because of the smaller number of events. Another possible rate shift occurred in Newport in late 1985 through early 1986 (Figure 8.3). In both Woonsocket and Newport, the effects seem transient, with the accident rates returning to established long-run patterns. The data for Westerly are very noisy, and no firm conclusions can be drawn about the presence or absence of runs. Runs tests show no statistically significant clumping of points above or below trend in any of the series; however, these tests are not powerful and it would be premature to conclude that the shifts seen are only noise.

The statistical properties of the accident rates from the different cities are distinct. For example, the overall accident rate for Woonsocket shows a strong upward trend not seen in the other cities or in the alcohol-related accidents in Woonsocket. The amount and pattern of seasonal variation differs substantially. Holiday effects differ, and at a more detailed level accident patterns by day of week are also unique. The kinds of accidents also differ, although this information has yet to be explored fully.

CONCLUSIONS

It appears on the basis of these 12 city-years of data that events that cause major, enduring shifts in accident rates are relatively rare.   The threat to evaluation studies posed by such events thus seems to be modest; however, the sample of communities studied is decidedly unrepresentative.   Also, indicators other than accident rates might show a very different pattern.   For example, some critical events might strongly affect community attitudes about drinking practices, but these major changes in attitudes might have only slow, delayed effects on accident rates which would be difficult to detect with these techniques.

Even if the threat to research validity posed by major unexpected events is low, we should still take what actions we can to minimize the threat still more.   One important step would be always to have at least two intervention sites and two comparison sites.   Though expensive, this approach would avoid the hazards of putting all one's eggs in one basket.   As another step, intervention planners should anticipate that major events might occur in the intervention or the comparison sites and give thought in advance to ways to respond to some of the more likely ones.   The kinds of events that happen

FIGURE 8.2
Motor Vehicle Crash Rate in Woonsocket over Time

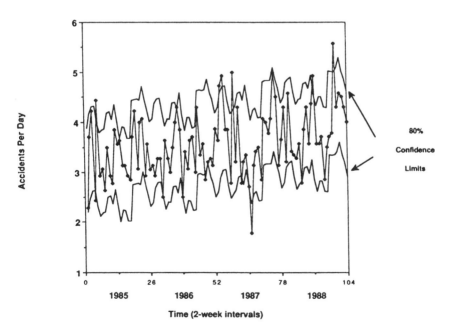

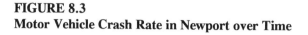

FIGURE 8.3
Motor Vehicle Crash Rate in Newport over Time

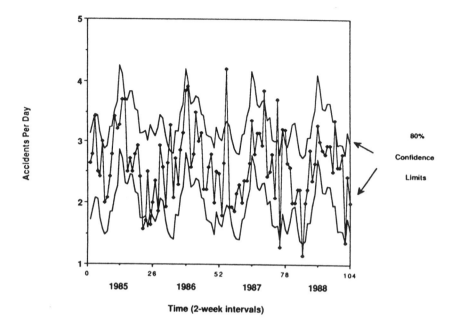

often enough for contingency planning include traffic deaths from drunken driving, involvement of community figures in addictions-related problems, changes in key community personnel, community growth and economic development, turnover in licensed establishments, and major structural changes related to the intervention (e.g., in traffic patterns, treatment services, or liquor regulations). One obviously cannot have detailed plans for all contingencies, but contingency plans could include preparation of publicity to be used when major addictions-related events occur, plans to enlist the cooperation of new civic and/or business leaders who might affect interventions, plans to make prompt contact with new liquor licensees (if they are a target for intervention), and avoidance of too much dependence on specific individual contacts.

A longer-term response to how to deal with unexpected events is to build a data base to support research into the effects of these events. Funding agencies should insist on careful monitoring of intervention and comparison communities, including descriptions of potentially important events and circumstances, especially obstacles to or aids in implementing the interventions. While such histories are useful within a single study, they would be even more valuable if they could be compared across studies at a variety of sites.

Agencies that support prevention research should give consideration to maintaining archives of such histories, with the corresponding outcome data bases, for secondary research. Modern information technology makes such secondary research a feasible and cost-effective way of improving research productivity.

Prevention, like engineering, is an applied science. Like other applied sciences, it relies on a mixture of basic scientific knowledge and practical experience. Our basic scientific knowledge base is quite weak. We have no knowledge, for example, about how different patterns of accident rates in two cities might be expected to affect the impact of a given preventive intervention. A city with many hazardous curves and intersections might have a higher alcohol-related MVC rate than another otherwise comparable town, and an intervention in the more hazardous city might have a larger impact than in the less hazardous one But such a relationship has not even been tested, much less established. We can still do prevention—people built successful bridges long before there was any solid scientific understanding of the strengths and weakness of different materials and designs—but our efforts are likely to be inefficient. We need to know how and why communities change in their drinking-related attitudes and practices in the absence of major interventions as much as we need to know the effects of planned interventions. We should continue to do studies aimed at gaining "engineering" knowledge—e.g., how to work with different segments of a community, or the best ways to stage the phases of an intervention—but basic science should be a priority. Major projects should be expected to produce basic science information even if the primary goals are more practical and immediate.

NOTES

Many people contributed to the Rhode Island prevention trial; however, special recognition is due to the original Project Director, Sandra Putnam, Ph.D., her successor Catherine Harrington, and Research Analyst Mary C. Speare.

1. SAS procedure AUTOREG was used for the timeseries modeling (SAS Institute, Inc., 1984). The time-series model fit to each of these series used twelve degrees of freedom for seasonal effects, a linear (secular) trend term, a term for holidays, and a first-order autoregression term. Tests indicated that further autoregression terms were not needed. A confidence limit of 80% was used so that approximately 10% of points would be expected to be high and 10% low.

Part V

Research Designs, Methods, and Analytic Models

9

Estimating the Effects of Community Prevention Trials: Alternative Designs and Methods

Charles S. Reichardt

INTRODUCTION

Designing a study to estimate the effects of a community-based prevention program is not easy. Many options are available for estimating effects of interventions, but each is fraught with potential difficulties and uncertainties. The purpose of this chapter is to outline four of the most promising design options: the interrupted time-series design, the randomized experiment, the nonequivalent group design, and the regression-discontinuity design. The strengths and weaknesses of each of these design types are discussed.

Before that discussion begins, however, it must be acknowledged that even well-conceived and well-funded intervention plans can be difficult to implement. As a result, it is important to document the intervention carefully as it is delivered, so that effects can be properly attributed. For example, the lack of an effect might be attributed incorrectly to the intervention as planned when, in fact, it was due only to implementation failures (McLaughlin, 1985); in that case, the source of impotence would be misidentified. In addition, because an intervention can change over time, it is important to document the intervention over the entire length of the study.

Further, it can be important to assess differences both in effects among participants and in the effectiveness of different treatment components, so that individuals and treatment regimens can be matched (Finney and Moos, 1986). To assess the potential benefits of matching treatment components to individuals, the researcher must document the quality and quantity of the treatments that are received by different individuals as well as the characteristics of the individuals. It also can be valuable to document differences in contexts and to incorporate a wide variety of outcome measures in the research design.

THE INTERRUPTED TIME-SERIES DESIGN

An interrupted time-series design can be implemented with a single individual or with a group of individuals such as a community. Throughout this chapter, I shall use the term "unit" to refer either to an individual or to a group of individuals.

In an interrupted time-series design, the unit or units under study are measured on the same variable on several different occasions. Then the treatment is implemented, and the unit or units are again measured repeatedly on the same variable. Finally, the effect of the treatment is estimated by comparing the observations made before and after treatment. Specifically, the "before" observations are used to predict what the "after" observations would have been if the intervention had not been implemented. The difference between the actual outcomes and the predicted outcomes is the estimate of the treatment effect.

An example of an interrupted time-series design is provided by a study of the effect of Outward Bound on self-confidence (Smith et al., 1976). The Outward Bound program consists of a wilderness expedition designed to teach both intra- and inter-personal skills. To assess the effects of the program, the self-confidence of the Outward Bound participants was measured for several weeks before the program began. Figure 9.1 plots the mean of these self-confidence ratings over time. The respondents then participated in the wilderness expedition, as indicated by the vertical line between weeks 15 and 20 in Figure 9.1. Finally, the participants' self-confidence was assessed for several more weeks after the wilderness expedition. As Figure 9.1 reveals, there is a sharp jump in the mean self-confidence ratings coincident with the Outward Bound experience. Projecting forward the trend in mean self-confidence ratings from before the Outward Bound experience produces a gap between the predicted and actual mean ratings observed after the Outward Bound experience. Unless threats to validity are present, this gap is due to the effect of the Outward Bound program.

Design Options

The interrupted time-series design can be implemented with data from a single individual. Or the design can be implemented using N (>1) individuals where each individual supplies a separate time series of observations. Similarly, the design can be implemented with data from a single community or with data from N communities where, in each case, each community supplies a separate time series of observations.

FIGURE 9.1

Mean Self-Confidence Ratings before and after an Outward Bound
Program

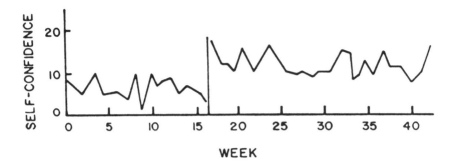

Source: Smith et al., 1976; Glass, 1988.   Copyright © 1988 by the American Educational
           Research Association.   Reprinted by permission.   Also reprinted with permission of
           Sage Publications, Inc.

When N is greater than 1, the differential effects of the treatment might be studied across the N units. When the units are individuals, this means the researcher might study differences in the effects of the treatment across the different individuals. When the units are communities, the researcher might study differences in the effects of the treatment across the different communities.

It is also possible to use the interrupted time-series design to study the effects of two or more interventions in sequence. For example, the participants in the study of Outward Bound could have been given a seminar on self-confidence during week 30. In this case, the interrupted time-series design could have been used to assess the effect of both the wilderness expedition and the later seminar. The ability to assess the effects of multiple interventions can be especially useful if the intervention changes over time, even if the changes are not planned. However, one drawback is that the size of the effects of later interventions may be contingent on the size of the effects of prior interventions. Further, if there are diminishing returns for later interventions, the power of the analysis to detect these differences can be reduced. On the other hand, demonstrating repeated effects over time for the same or similar interventions can increase the credibility of the results because it can reduce the plausibility of alternative explanations.

Statistical Analysis of the Data

The logic of the analysis of data from an interrupted time-series design is to fit a regression line to the pre-intervention data, project this regression line forward, and compare this projection to a regression line that fits the post-intervention data. Unfortunately, ordinary regression techniques usually are not appropriate for fitting these two regression lines; observations collected on the same units over time tend to be correlated, which violates the assumptions of traditional regression techniques. Autoregressive integrated moving average (ARIMA) models are the classic procedures for taking account of the effects of these overtime (i.e., auto) correlations (Box and Jenkins, 1970; Glass, Willson and Gottman, 1975; McCleary and Hay, 1980). These ARIMA models can be used by themselves or in combination with ordinary regression techniques.

Using the ARIMA methodology, a researcher can specify that the time course of the intervention effect takes any one of a wide variety of shapes, as illustrated in Figure 9.2 (Box and Tiao, 1975; Campbell and Stanley, 1966; Glass, 1988). The effect of an intervention might shift the mean level of the observations, it might change the direction or slope of the observations, or it might do both. In addition, the effect of an intervention might be immediate or delayed, permanent or temporary. That it allows a researcher to study how the treatment effect changes over time is one of the great strengths of the interrupted time-series design.

Although the effect of the intervention might take many shapes, an analysis will not have equal precision and credibility in estimating all of the potential shapes. Estimates of effects that produce gradual changes will have the least precision and credibility, while estimates of effects that produce abrupt and dramatic effects will have the most precision and credibility. This difference is because the projection of the pre-intervention regression line becomes less accurate and certain the farther it is projected into the post-intervention time period. In other words, it is more difficult to be confident that a small and gradual change is due to the treatment than it is to be confident that a large and abrupt change is due to the treatment.

When N is greater than 1, each of the N individual time series of observations can be analyzed separately using the ARIMA methodology. Alternatively, the N separate time series can be analyzed jointly (Bryk and Raudenbush, 1987; Dielman, 1989; Simonton, 1977; Swaminathan and Algina, 1977). Either approach enables the researcher to study individual differences in effects across units. Which approach is preferred usually depends both on the number of time points of observations and on the quality of the data.

FIGURE 9.2
Different Shapes of Effects that can be Studied with the Interrupted-Time Series Design

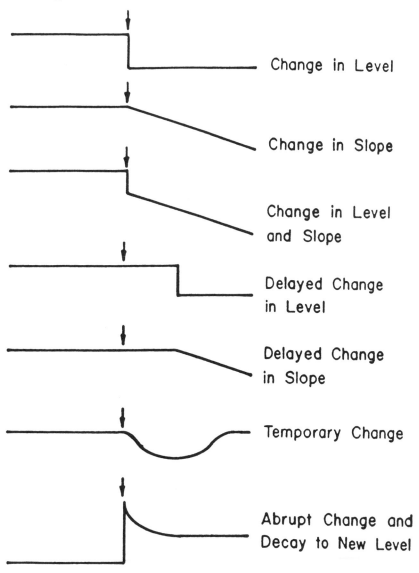

Change in Level

Change in Slope

Change in Level and Slope

Delayed Change in Level

Delayed Change in Slope

Temporary Change

Abrupt Change and Decay to New Level

Time flows from left to right. The arrow marks the point of the intervention.

When N equals 1, the most widely accepted rule of thumb is that an analysis using the ARIMA methodology requires at least 50 observations (time points). In fact, what constitutes an adequate number of observations (i.e., what is an adequate length for the time series) depends on the variability in the data. Variability usually depends on the units and on the outcome measure. For example, a time series of observations from an individual often is far more variable than a time series of observations from a community. When there is relatively little variation, useful estimates can be obtained from a time series that is substantially shorter than 50 time points.

In addition, when N is greater than 1 and the N time series are analyzed jointly, the length of each time series often can be much shorter than if each time series were analyzed separately. The reason is that a joint analysis can use estimates of variability across individuals in place of estimates of variability within individuals. However, the joint analyses do not tend to offer as much flexibility in modeling the shape of the treatment effect over time as does the $N=1$ methodology.

Threats To Validity

One of the most obvious threats to internal validity is the effect of history. History means any event other than the intervention that takes place at the same time as the intervention. For example, if the respondents in Smith et al.'s (1976) study had chosen to participate in Outward Bound upon graduation from college, the change in self-confidence might have been due to graduation rather than to the Outward Bound program. In this case, the effect of graduation would be an effect of history.

One way to take account of the effects of history is to add a control time series to the research design. Data from the control series would be collected at the same points in time as data on the experimental series. Further, the control series would be chosen so that the control observations were susceptible to the same effects of history as the experimental time series but did not receive the intervention under study. For example, the Outward Bound study could include a control series of observations on similar individuals who graduated from college but did not participate in the Outward Bound experience. In this way, the effects of history, if any, could be estimated from the control series and this estimate could be used to distinguish between the effects of history and the effects of the intervention in the experimental series (Reichardt and Gollob, 1989).

Instrumentation is another potential threat to validity. This happens when the way in which the dependent variable is measured changes at the same time as the intervention is introduced. Such a change might occur because of the intervention itself. For example, the number of crimes that were officially recorded increased sharply when Orlando Wilson was appointed Police Chief in Chicago in the 1960s (Cook and Campbell, 1979). However, the increase did not reflect a true increase in crime, only an increase in officially-recorded crimes because of reforms in the recording system that were imposed by Wilson. If an intervention to decrease crime had been implemented at the same time (or if Wilson's appointment were taken to be an intervention), the change in the recording system would have biased the estimate of the effect of the intervention. Similarly, an instrumentation effect might occur in an alcohol abuse prevention program if, for example, methods used to assess drunkenness were changed at the same time as an intervention were introduced to reduce drunk driving, perhaps because of the publicity surrounding the intervention.

Instrumentation often can be ruled out as a threat to validity by direct observation of the measurement process or by adding a control time series. In addition, this threat to validity is often reduced when the time-series observations are obtained after-the-fact from archival records. Indeed, one of the advantages of time-series methodology is that it often can be implemented with archival data. The disadvantage is that archival data is not always relevant to the questions that social and behavioral researchers want to ask. This is because archival data is more frequently collected on economic rather than on social variables.

Another potential threat to internal validity is the effect of testing. Testing is a threat when the act of measuring a variable changes the later measurement of that variable. For example, asking for a person's opinion on a topic might cause that person to think about the issue under question, which in turn might cause a change in the person's opinion at a later time, which would not have occurred if the initial question had not been asked. One way to avoid testing effects is to assess different individuals at each different time interval. This was done, for example, in the Smith et al. (1976) study of Outward Bound. Several hundred individuals participated in the Outward Bound program, but at each time period only a small random sample of the respondents was asked to fill out a questionnaire on self-confidence. However, such precautions often are unnecessary in time-series designs. Testing usually is a serious threat to validity only in short time series because the effects of testing tend to decrease as the number of repeated measurements increases.

One last limitation that may seem obvious, but is nonetheless worth mentioning, is that the simple interrupted time-series design assumes that the intervention will bring about changes compared to previous behavior. However, with some prevention efforts *no* change over time is the preferred outcome. For example, in attempting to *prevent* (rather than reduce) abusive drinking, the researcher hopes that individuals are not abusing alcohol before the intervention and that these individuals continue not to abuse alcohol after the intervention. In this case, the researcher would need to use a control time series to demonstrate that abusive drinking would have increased in the absence of the intervention.

Summary

The interrupted time-series design is relatively easy to implement and is applicable under a wide range of circumstances. However, the design may have low power to detect treatment effects if there is substantial variability in the observations over time and if the effect of the intervention is gradual rather than abrupt. A time-series design often can be strengthened by adding control or comparison time-series.

THE RANDOMIZED EXPERIMENT

In a randomized experiment, units are assigned to different treatment conditions at random. Usually one of the treatment conditions is a control or comparison condition that consists of the absence of any special treatment. After the units are assigned to conditions, the different treatments are applied (or not applied in the case of a control or comparison condition), and one or more outcome variables are measured. Then the differences in the outcomes between the treatment groups are used to estimate the differential effects of the treatments.

The simplest randomized experiment consists of a single treatment condition and a single control condition. More complex experiments may consist of many different treatment conditions, including conditions where more than one treatment is applied simultaneously (e.g., factorial designs). Such complex designs enable the researcher to study interactions between the treatments. Multiple dependent measures are also possible, and each measure could be repeated over time so as to track the time course of the effects of the treatments.

Units

The units that are randomly assigned to the treatment conditions could be individuals or groups of individuals such as communities. For example, in the COMMIT cancer study (Pechacek, 1987), 22 communities were assigned randomly to either an intervention or control condition. However, most randomized experiments use individuals as the units.

Whether the units are communities or individuals, randomized experiments require that more than one unit be assigned to each treatment condition; the more units that are assigned to each condition the better. The power of the design to detect treatment effects increases with the number of units. The greater the variability that exists among the units on the outcome measure, the greater is the number of units needed to have adequate power to detect treatment effects. The number of units that is required for adequate power can be estimated before the design is implemented based on knowledge of the likely variability in the data and the effect size (Kraemer and Thiemann, 1987; Lipsey, 1990).

Note that if two or more communities are randomly assigned to treatment conditions, and individuals are randomly sampled from the communities, the design is a randomized experiment using communities as the units, but the design is *not* a randomized experiment using individuals as the units. Rather it is a nonequivalent group design (as described below) because individuals have self-selected, rather than randomly assigned, themselves into the different communities. If a randomized experiment is to use individuals as the units, the individuals must be *directly* assigned to the treatment conditions at random. Without such random assignment, a statistical analysis of the data using individuals as the units would have to grapple with the difficulties that are described in the later section of this chapter on the nonequivalent group design.

When the researcher seeks to study *community-based* prevention programs, the above restriction makes it difficult to create a randomized experiment where the individuals are the units. All members of the community tend to be exposed to the same treatments, so it may not be possible to assign individuals randomly within a community to a control condition. Nonetheless, even if a community-based program can not be studied as a whole using individuals as the units in a randomized experiment, subcomponents of the intervention might be assessed using individuals as the units in a randomized experiment. For example, if a school-based educational component were part of the intervention, individuals might be assigned at random to receive or not receive this one component of the treatment.

The Value of a Pretest

A randomized experiment does not require a pretest (i.e., baseline) measure. That is, the units in a randomized experiment need not be measured (or pretested) before the treatments are administered. The only required observation is the measurement of the dependent (outcome) variable, or posttest. Nonetheless, pretests offer two potential advantages (though researchers also should recognize the possible disadvantage of introducing testing effects when using pretests).

First, pretests can be used to increase the power of the analysis. Power can be increased with a pretest either by matching or by an analysis of covariance. In matching, units are matched on the basis of the pretest score and then randomly assigned to treatment conditions from within each matched group. For example, if there are three treatment conditions, units are matched in blocks of threes based on the pretest score. Then one member of each block is randomly assigned to each of the three treatment conditions. The membership of the blocks is then taken into account in the analysis in a way that can increase power. In the analysis of covariance, the pretest is used as a covariate to reduce the residual error variance and thereby increase power. Whether matching or analysis of covariance is more powerful depends largely on the size of the correlation between the pretest and the posttest. In particular, the power of the analysis of covariance increases relative to the power of the matching strategy as the correlation increases (Cox, 1957; Feldt, 1958; Reichardt, 1979).

With both matching and the analysis of covariance, more than one pretest can be used. Pretests that are most highly correlated with the posttest increase power the most, for both matching and analysis of covariance. Often the pretest that is most highly correlated with the posttest is a pretest that is operationally identical to the posttest. However, this may not be the case in prevention research, for example, when the posttest assesses behavior such as alcoholic consumption if such consumption is rare at the time of the pretest (Cronbach, 1982).

Second, pretests enable the researcher to study individual differences in the treatment effects. This task is accomplished by looking for interactions between pretest characteristics and treatment conditions (Cronbach and Snow, 1981). Again multiple pretests can be used to study individual differences in treatment effects on multiple dimensions.

Advantages and Disadvantages

Without random assignment, units would be self-selected into the different treatment conditions. Under these circumstances, different types of units generally will select different types of treatment. As a result, initial selection differences can bias the estimates of the treatment effects. The primary advantage of random assignment to treatment conditions is that biases due to initial selection differences are avoided at the start.

Because of this advantage, many methodologists and practitioners believe that, when randomized experiments can be implemented, they are virtually always preferable to the nonequivalent group design in which units are not randomly assigned (Berk et al., 1985). Nonetheless, there are relative disadvantages to the randomized experiment. Some methodologists and practitioners believe that these disadvantages often outweigh the advantages of the randomized experiment in practice (Cronbach, 1982).

Randomized experiments usually are far more difficult to implement than nonequivalent group designs. It usually is more difficult to convince units to accept random assignment to treatments than to accept assignment by self-selection. Further, studying only those units that agree to random assignment can reduce the generalizability of the results.

In addition, various threats to the internal validity of a randomized experiment can arise, such as the diffusion or imitation of treatments, compensatory rivalry, and resentful demoralization, as described by Cook and Campbell (1979). These threats to validity fall under the rubric of contamination. While these rival hypotheses can arise with nonequivalent group designs, they will often create greater problems for randomized experiments. For example, resentful demoralization is more likely to arise in a randomized experiment than in a nonequivalent group design because random assignment to treatments is likely to be more frustrating (for those who do not receive their choice of treatments) than self-selection to treatments (Fetterman, 1982).

Instrumentation is also a potential threat to internal validity, though it may be equally likely to pose a problem in randomized experiments as in nonequivalent group designs. Instrumentation is a threat to validity in between-group comparisons when the way the outcome measure is assessed differs across treatment conditions. For example, the police in different communities might use different protocols to detect the alcohol level in the bloodstream of drivers involved in automobile accidents. Such instrumentation differences might arise because the intervention raises awareness, for example, of the need for improving the protocols that are used to detect alcohol levels.

Further, even though random assignment avoids biases due to initial selection differences, this advantage can be vitiated if there is differential attrition from the treatment groups. Some attrition is almost certain to occur in any field study, and the differential attractiveness of the treatments will tend to make the attrition greater in some treatment conditions than in others. Adding incentives for continuing to participate in the study can help minimize attrition. Another suggestion for reducing attrition due to the differential attractiveness of the treatments is to require that participants agree to participate in the study regardless of the treatment condition to which they are assigned or to institute a trial period of compliance before randomization. But limiting the study population either to those who agree to participate regardless of treatment assignment or to those who fulfill compliance criteria can reduce external validity.

When differential attrition occurs, researchers should try to take account of its potentially biasing effects. One procedure is to examine the pretest differences between those who drop out and those who do not, then to try to adjust for these differences analytically, perhaps with analysis of covariance (Bracht and Glass, 1968; Yeaton, Wortman, and Langberg, 1983). It is also recommended that, when posttest measures are available on those who failed to complete the treatment, researchers analyze the complete set of data according to treatment assignment (rather than according to treatment realization). This procedure tends to produce an underestimate of the effect of the treatment, but at least the direction of the bias is known, and the size of the bias often can be estimated as well (Bloom, 1984). However, one common suggestion that does *not* work is to match units before random assignment and then discard the entire matched group whenever any member of a group drops out. This procedure does not avoid attrition bias as it might appear to do, and researchers are just as well off *not* discarding units and, instead, trying to adjust for biases using analysis of covariance. In any case, differential attrition can reduce greatly the relative advantages of the randomized experiment compared to the nonequivalent group design.

Finally, it should be noted that the randomized experiment offers little, if any, advantage over the nonequivalent group design for studying naturally occurring variations in the treatments. The effects of such variations may well prove to be more noteworthy than the effects of the planned variations (Cronbach, 1982). Nor does the randomized experiment offer much, if any, advantage over the nonequivalent group design in studying the process by which the intervention operates.

Summary

A randomized experiment can be a very credible and powerful procedure both for estimating the effects of treatments on average and for studying individual differences in treatment effects. Unfortunately, randomized experiments are difficult to implement, and, because of differential attrition, a randomized experiment can easily degenerate into a nonequivalent group design. A well-implemented randomized experiment often will be superior to any other design for estimating effects; but a poorly implemented randomized experiment may be no better, or may even be worse, than other types of designs.

THE NONEQUIVALENT GROUP DESIGN

The nonequivalent group design (or observational study) is similar to the randomized experiment, so much of the prior discussion applies. The prominent difference between the two designs is that, in the nonequivalent group design, units are not assigned to treatment conditions at random. Instead units are self-selected into the treatment conditions or are selected on some other nonrandom basis.

If enough communities could be studied, communities could be assigned to the treatments nonrandomly and could be the unit of analysis. However, a more common way to design a nonequivalent group study is to choose a single community in which to implement the intervention and to use a similar community as a control. Then data are collected on either a randomly or nonrandomly selected sample of individuals within each of these two communities. In this case, individuals could be the units. But do not be misled; even if the treatment conditions had been assigned to the two communities at random, using individuals as the units would make the study a nonequivalent group design.

The Need for a Pretest

A pretest usually is critical in the nonequivalent group design. Without random assignment, selection differences can severely bias the estimate of the treatment effect, and a pretest usually is necessary to adjust for the effects of this bias, as described below. The pretest need not be operationally identical to the posttest, but this approach typically will be best.

Unfortunately, even with an operationally identical pretest, none of the procedures for taking account of selection differences are infallible. As Lord (1967:305) stated, "With the data usually available for such studies, there simply is no logical or statistical procedure that can be counted on to make proper allowances for uncontrolled preexisting differences between groups." Therefore, it is advisable to make biases due to selection differences as small as possible by selecting control or comparison groups that are as similar to the treatment groups as possible.

It also can be useful to have the pretest repeated at several different times before the treatment is implemented. This repetition enables the researcher to test alternative analysis strategies. Specifically, the researcher would analyze the data from two pretests that were collected at two different times as if these data had been a pretest and a posttest (Wortman, Reichardt, and St. Pierre, 1978). In such a "dry run" nonequivalent group design, the treatment is known to have no effect because it was not implemented between the time of the pretest and the pseudo-posttest.

Just as in the randomized experiment, the pretest observations are also necessary if the researcher is to assess individual differences in treatment effectiveness. However, in the nonequivalent group design, the estimates of individual differences in effectiveness are subject to the same types of biases due to selection differences as are the estimates of average effectiveness.

Statistical Analyses for the Longitudinal Design

In the prototypic nonequivalent group design, individuals are the units, and a pretest and a posttest are measured on each individual (Campbell and Stanley, 1966). Let us call this the "longitudinal" nonequivalent group design.

There are at least three common ways to take account of the biasing effects of selection differences in this design.

The first approach is the analysis of gain scores (i.e., before-after differences). In this analysis, the researcher estimates the treatment effect as the mean difference between the treatment conditions in pretest/posttest gains. For the pretest/posttest gain to be meaningful, the pretest and posttest usually have to be operationally identical measures. The null hypothesis in such an analysis is that, in the absence of a treatment effect, the difference or gap between the treatment groups will remain unchanged from the pretest to the posttest. Such a null hypothesis may or may not be correct. Some gaps tend to increase; the rich get richer. Other gaps tend to decrease. This change can occur, for example, when groups have been selected into treatments based on extreme scores, which produces regression to the mean. The trick with this analysis strategy is choosing to use it only in those situations where it is reasonable to assume that the gap will remain constant in the absence of a treatment effect.

The second analysis strategy encompasses both matching and the analysis of covariance (Reichardt, 1979). In matching, individuals from the different treatment groups are matched on the pretest scores, and an analysis of variance is used to examine the posttest differences of the matched individuals. With the analysis of covariance, the only difference is that units are matched on the pretest via statistical, rather than physical, means before differences on the posttest are assessed. In this way, both matching and the analysis of covariance attempt to remove any biasing effects of differences on the pretest. The two potential difficulties with these strategies are measurement error in the pretest and omitted variables.

When the pretest is measured with error, as is virtually always the case, neither matching nor the analysis of covariance makes proper adjustments for pretest differences between the groups. Statistical techniques such as LISREL (Joreskog and Sorbom, 1988) can be used to try to model and remove the effects of measurement error, but they require multiple measures of the fallible pretests.

"Omitted variables" refers to the problem that pretest differences may not be the only initial differences that need to be taken into account to produce an unbiased estimate of the treatment effect. A pretest that is operationally identical to the posttest is probably the single best covariate to use to take account of initial differences, but using such a pretest still does not guarantee success in removing all selection differences (Campbell and Reichardt, 1991). Substantive research is the only way to discover the covariates that need to be included in the analysis (Cordray, 1986).

The third procedure is called selection modeling (Heckman and Robb, 1985; Rindskopf, 1986; Stromsdorfer and Farkas, 1980). As the name suggests, the logic of the procedure is to model the way in which units are

selected into the different treatment conditions.   In essence, modeling the
selection process creates a variable representing the probability of assignment
into the different conditions, which is then used in a regression analysis to
predict the posttest (Barnow, Cain, and Goldberger, 1980).   Although this
procedure is relatively new, it shows promise, even though it may not prove to
be as useful as the other analysis strategies when individuals are the units and
treatment conditions are assigned to communities.

Other Design Options

The alternative to the longitudinal design with individuals as the units is a
"cross-sectional" design in which different individuals are assessed on the
pretest and posttest.   Such a nonequivalent group design arises, for example,
when the intervention is implemented in one community, another community
is used as a control or comparison group, a random sample of individuals from
each community is assessed on the pretest, and a different random sample of
individuals from each community is assessed on the posttest.   That the same
individuals are not assessed on both the pretest and posttest avoids both testing
effects that can threaten internal validity and problems of attrition that can
threaten external as well as internal validity.   However, having different individuals assessed on the pretest and posttest also reduces the analytical options
available for removing the effects of selection differences.   Of the three strategies described above, the only one available for the cross-sectional design is
the gain score analysis.   If testing effects and attrition are thought to be serious
problems, perhaps the best compromise is to combine the longitudinal and
cross-sectional designs.   That is, chose samples of individuals so that some
individuals are assessed on both the pretest and posttest, and some individuals
are assessed on only one or the other.

If communities are the units of analysis and if there are a good number of
communities in each treatment condition, the analysis options described above
can be used.   However, when communities are the units and there are very few
communities per treatment condition, these strategies can not always be
applied effectively.

Threats to Validity

As described above, the nonequivalent group design must contend with
potential biases due to selection differences that, under ideal conditions, can be
avoided in the randomized experiment.   In addition, all the threats to the
internal validity of the randomized experiment are also potential threats to the
validity of the nonequivalent group design.   However, in the nonequivalent

group design the biases caused by these threats tend not to be as severe. For example, resentful demoralization will often be less pronounced in the nonequivalent group design than in the randomized experiment because units are allowed to choose their own treatments rather than being randomly assigned (Fetterman, 1982). However, one exception is worth noting.

The exception is the rival hypothesis of local history. Local history refers to any event that occurs in the control condition but not in the experimental condition (or vice versa), where the event is not part of the intervention and where the event biases the comparison between the treatment conditions. Often local history is likely to pose more of a threat in the nonequivalent group design than in the randomized experiment, especially in nonequivalent group designs where there is only a single experimental and a single control community. For example, if the mayor of the control community is killed in an alcohol-related automobile accident, the publicity surrounding that event might be as effective a deterrent to drunken driving as the intervention that was planned in the experimental community. So if this effect of history went unrecognized, an incorrect conclusion would likely be drawn about the effectiveness of the intervention. This outcome is less likely to occur in a randomized experiment, only because a randomized design could not be implemented with only a single experimental and single control community. A randomized experiment requires many communities in each treatment condition. The number of communities, along with random assignment, would increase the likelihood that history effects were more evenly distributed across the treatment conditions.

Summary

Nonequivalent group designs typically are easier to implement than the other three design types considered in this chapter. But researchers get what they pay for: Inferences about the effects of the intervention that can be drawn using the nonequivalent group design are often far weaker than the inferences that can be drawn using the other three design types, if these other designs are well implemented.

THE REGRESSION-DISCONTINUITY DESIGN

The regression-discontinuity design is a very special subclass of the nonequivalent group design. In the prototypic and simplest regression-discontinuity design, each unit is assessed on a pretest. In addition, a cut-off score on the pretest is selected and units are assigned to treatment conditions depending upon where their pretest score falls relative to the cut-off.

Specifically, units with pretest scores below the cut-off are assigned to one treatment condition, while units with pretest scores above the cut-off are assigned to the other treatment condition. All the units are then assessed on a posttest measure.

The treatment effect is estimated by regressing the posttest scores on the pretest scores separately in the two treatment conditions and then comparing these two regression lines. The null hypothesis is that, in the absence of a treatment effect, the two regressions would fall on the same line. A treatment effect is evidenced by a shift in one of the regression lines relative to the other (Cain, 1975; Campbell, 1969b; Thistlethwaite and Campbell, 1960; Trochim, 1984).

A hypothetical example of data from a regression-discontinuity design is given in Figure 9.3, which provides a plot of posttest versus pretest scores. The vertical line at the score of 80 on the horizontal axis is the cut-off score used to assign units to treatment conditions based on the pretest scores. The Xs are data points for the units in the treatment condition, the Os are data points for the units in the control condition. The differences between the separate regression lines for the X and O data are used to estimate the effect of the treatment. In this case, the treatment has lowered the scores on the posttest because the regression line for the X data is lower than the regression line for the O data.

The pretest that is used to set the cut-off score can be any quantitative measure; it need not be related to the posttest. This means that the regression-discontinuity design is particularly relevant whenever eligibility for a treatment can be quantified in some fashion. Examples might be welfare payments that are conditioned on income levels or entrance into educational programs based on test scores.

Limitations

The prototypic regression-discontinuity design involves only two treatment conditions. Even if the prototypic design is expanded by adding more treatments and, therefore, more cut-off scores, it still can be used in practice to compare only a limited number of treatments.

The units in a regression-discontinuity design can be individuals or communities, but in either case a large number of units usually is required to produce precise estimates of the separate regression lines and therefore provide a precise estimate of the treatment effect. Further, given the same number of units, the estimate of a treatment effect obtained from a regression-discontinuity design is not as precise as the estimate obtained from a randomized experiment. For example, even under ideal conditions, 2.7 times as many

FIGURE 9.3
Hypothetical Data from a Regression-Discontinuity Design

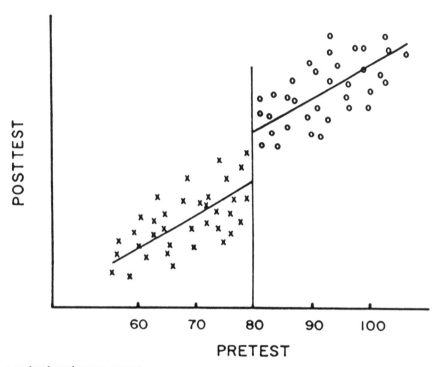

x = treatment group scores
0 = control group scores

units are required for the regression-discontinuity design to produce as precise an estimate of the treatment effect as for the randomized experiment (Goldberger, 1972). The same relationship holds for power as well.

The regression-discontinuity design does not allow for the study of individual differences in treatment effectiveness except along the dimension of the pretest used to establish the cut-off score. (Such individual differences are estimated by projecting the regression line from the treatment group into the region of the scores from the control group or vice versa.) That is, except for individual differences along the pretest dimension, the design enables the researcher to estimate only the effect of the treatment averaged across the individuals in the study.

If the researcher does not fit the proper regression line to the data, the estimate of the treatment effect can be biased. For example, if the true regression line is curvilinear, but straight lines are fit to the data, an effective treatment can be made to look ineffective or even harmful, and vice versa.

Summary

The regression-discontinuity design requires a large number of units, is relatively difficult to implement, and provides limited information about the effects of a very limited number of treatment conditions. But when the regression-discontinuity design is well implemented, it can provide far more valid estimates of treatment effects than the prototypic nonequivalent group design; by using a cut-off score to control the assignment to treatments, the regression-discontinuity design controls for the effects of *all* selection differences (not just those along the dimension of the pretest that is used for assignment) far better than does the typical nonequivalent group design (Rubin, 1977). In other words, the researcher is better able to remove the effects of selection differences by controlling how the units are assigned to treatment conditions (with the regression-discontinuity design) than by not controlling how the units are assigned to treatment conditions (with the nonequivalent group design).

THE ROLE OF IMAGINATION AND CREATIVITY IN RESEARCH DESIGN AND ANALYSIS

This chapter has described four types of designs that are among the most useful for estimating the effects of community prevention trials. Although any one design is fallible, combining designs often can greatly improve the credibility of the results (Cook, 1985). For example, an evaluation of a criminal justice program by Lipsey, Cordray and Berger (1981) masterfully combined all four design types to produce far stronger conclusions than would have been possible with any one design by itself.

Similarly, Blose and Holder (1987a) used multiple comparisons to assess the influence of changes in liquor-by-the-drink laws on alcohol-related traffic accidents. Up until 1978, legislation forbade restaurants to sell liquor-by-the-drink in North Carolina. In 1978, several counties in North Carolina voted to allow liquor-by-the-drink, and Blose and Holder used an interrupted time-series design with monthly data to demonstrate that this change increased police-reported alcohol-related accidents by 16% to 24%. This effect was replicated using a second set of counties that voted to allow liquor-by-the-drink in 1979. In performing this replication, the first set of counties was used as a control for the effects of history in the second set of counties, and vice versa. The threat of history was also assessed using control time-series from counties that were matched to the experimental counties but did not authorize liquor-by-the-drink. The conclusions were then further replicated using a different dependent variable: single-vehicle nighttime accidents involving male drivers. This measure was partitioned into accidents involving male drivers over 21 years old and male drivers under 21 years old. The effect of liquor-by-the-drink was found only for the older age drivers, as expected, because the drinking age for liquor was 21. Taken together, these multiple analyses allow credible inferences to be drawn about the effects of the intervention.

Glass (1988) also reveals how a research design can be strengthened by adding additional comparisons. Figure 9.4 plots enrollment in the Denver Public Schools from 1928 to 1975. In 1969, a Federal District court forced racial integration in the public schools in Denver and, as the figure shows, enrollment declined thereafter. The question of interest is whether this decline represents "white flight" due to the court's decision, or whether the decline would have occurred even if racial integration had not been mandated. The data in Figure 9.4 are equivocal, but Glass argues that the question,

> could be resolved fairly conclusively by breaking down and plotting in several alternative ways the total enrollment series in Figure [9.4]. Breaking the enrollment data down by grade might cast a little light on things. If it's really white flight that is causing the decline, one might expect a larger decline at the elementary grades than at the secondary grades, particularly grades 11 and 12 where parents would likely decide to stick it out for the short run. If enrollment data existed separately for different ethnic groups, these time series would provide a revealing test. If they showed roughly equal declines across all ethnic groups, the "white flight" hypothesis would suffer a major setback. Data on enrollment that could be separated by individual school, neighborhood, or census tract would be exceptionally valuable. These various units could be ranked prior to looking at the data on their susceptibility to white flight. Such a ranking could be based on variables like "pre-1969 ethnic mixture," or "mobility of families based on percentage of housing values mortgaged or amount of disposable income." If the large enrollment declines fell in the highly susceptible regions, the pattern would constitute some degree of support for the white flight hypothesis. (Glass, 1988:460)

Finally, consider the British Road Safety Act of 1967, which instituted crackdowns on drunken driving. The effects of the British Road Safety Act became most evident only when the data were disaggregated to show fatalities separately for different hours of the day and for different days of the week (Glass, 1988; Ross, Campbell, and Glass, 1970). An effect is evident only for certain times because drunken driving in Britain occurs much more heavily on weekend nights when the pubs are open than during commuting hours when pubs are closed. For this reason, an examination of the disaggregated data revealed effects that would have been dramatically underestimated by an investigation of the aggregated data alone.

FIGURE 9.4
Enrollment in Denver Public Schools

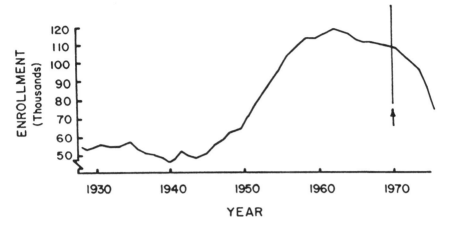

The arrow marks the beginning of the court-mandated desegregation.

Source: Glass, 1988. Copyright © 1988 by the American Educational Research Association.
           Reprinted by permission.

These examples illustrate that it is useful to think through the implications both of the intervention and of threats to validity that might arise in studying the intervention and then to investigate as many of these implications as possible. Such research calls for creativity and imagination, and it is usually well rewarded in the credibility of the results.

STUDYING THE PROCESS BY WHICH EFFECTS ARE PRODUCED

In addition to estimating the effects of an intervention, it can be valuable to study the process by which the effects are produced. Understanding the process can help improve the effectiveness of the intervention.

One difference between estimating the effect of an intervention and studying the process that produces an effect lies in choosing which cause and effect to study. In estimating the effects of an intervention, the intervention itself is the cause under study. However, in studying the process by which an effect is produced, intermediate effects become causes. For example, to estimate the effects of a change in variable A on variable C, the change in variable A is the cause. However, to determine if a change in A brings about a change in C because A first changes variable B, a researcher also would want to study the effect of B on C. Therefore, in studying the process by which A has an effect on *C*, many of the same issues about design that have been discussed in this chapter are relevant. All that differs is the variable that represents the cause under study. Of course, to study process in this way, the researcher must first have some idea of the causal chain by which an intervention has its effects and then be able to measure the intermediate steps in the causal chain (Mohr, 1988; Mark, 1990).

CONCLUSIONS

There are many different types of prevention programs (many of which are multifaceted), many different types of individuals served by these programs, many different contexts in which the programs might operate, and many different variables upon which to assess the effects. Almost certainly, effects will vary with all of these features. It is difficult to know which types of programs, which types of individuals or communities, which types of contexts in which to implement the intervention programs, and which types of outcome measures should be the focus of attention. Therefore, it is difficult to know which are the best questions to ask about the effects of alcohol-abuse prevention programs.

It is also difficult to know how to assess the effects of an alcohol-abuse prevention program. Each of the design types that has been considered in this chapter has its strengths and its weaknesses. Which design and analysis options will work best depend on the circumstances (also see Cook and Campbell, 1979; Judd and Kenny, 1981).

Because of the uncertainties that surround both the asking and answering of questions about the effects of interventions, researchers should not become over-committed to any one question or to any one research method (Reichardt and Gollob, 1987; Stoto, 1988). Rather, researchers must be prepared to shift their attention to promising new questions and to adapt their methods accordingly.

10

Case-Control Studies: Can They Evaluate Preventive Measures for Reducing Alcohol Problems?

Cornelia J. Baines

INTRODUCTION

Should case-control methodology be applied to research in the prevention of alcohol-related problems? Many of the fundamental questions in alcohol problem prevention remain unanswered. One reason may be the study designs that have been used. Although the randomized controlled trial is extolled as the "gold standard" for arriving at scientific "truth," alternative methods such as case-control studies can be used to answer research questions, especially those on causation, in chronic disease epidemiology. The reason is straight-forward: Compared to randomized controlled trials, case-control studies are supposed to be easy to implement, relatively quickly completed, and less costly. Furthermore, case-control studies require relatively few subjects and confer no risk to the subjects.

For those who are unfamiliar with case-control studies, a cardinal characteristic is that they are retrospective, analyzing events that occurred in the past. *Thus, they depend on the exploitation of groups of people who have been or become identified as cases and controls, both having had equal opportunities to be exposed in the past to the intervention or exposure that is being studied.*

Unfortunately, case-control methodology is not simple. It has given rise to "terminological tiffs" (Spitzer, 1985) that have resulted in suggestions for changes in nomenclature such as case-referent and case-compeer (Breslow and Day, 1980) and trohoc (Feinstein, 1973). These suggestions illustrate the continuing attempts to re-define and understand the concepts underlying case-control studies. More challenging issues are the appropriate selection of controls (Feinstein, 1985; Linet and Brookmeyer, 1987; Weiss, 1983), matching, and analytic approaches.

To answer the question this chapter poses, a brief outline of the evolution of case-control studies is presented, followed by a summary of problems associated with them, examples of case-control methodology used to evaluate preventive strategies, and, finally, an overview of alcohol prevention initiatives that may stimulate new applications for case-control methodology.

THE EVOLUTION OF CASE-CONTROL STUDIES

In case-control studies, the underlying concept was based on going back-wards in time from effect (disease) to cause (the exposure being studied). People with disease were compared to people without disease with respect to that exposure. The goal was to understand causation. This approach seems first to have been applied in 1920 (Broders, 1920), in a study comparing 537 cases and 500 controls, which concluded that pipe-smoking was associated with cancer of the lip. Although used in sociology in the 1920s and 1930s, epidemiological case-control studies only began to be used substantially in the 1950s and accelerated in the 1970s. With accelerated use came greater complexity. For example, nested case-control studies (Lubin, 1986) draw from cohort data, incorporating time to event and allowing direct estimation of the relative hazard. Over time, the goal has also changed. Thus case-control studies not only examine exposures that *cause* disease but also interventions that *prevent disease* or, if the interventions do not prevent disease, may at least *prevent death* from the disease. The broadening scope of case-control studies from an etiological focus to an evaluation of a preventive intervention and the change from being grounded in prevalence to being grounded in incidence are, however, much easier to grasp than are the ever more complicated processes of choosing who will be controls and of avoiding bias and confounding, which will be discussed later.

The manner in which case-control study findings are presented is based on the frequency of the effect being studied in those who were exposed, compared to the frequency of the effect in those who were not exposed. This comparison is expressed as the odds ratio (Schlesselman, 1982) but is approximated by and frequently referred to as a relative risk (Breslow and Day, 1980) when the disease is rare. More recently, the term relative hazard is encountered, paralleling the shift from prevalence to incidence cases (Lubin, 1986). While the subtle implications in the varieties of advocated terms are not easily grasped, they all convey the same message: the exposure increased, decreased, or had no impact on whatever effect is being studied.

Two illustrations may be helpful. First, in a case-control study designed to reveal etiology, namely the link between smoking (exposure) and lung cancer (outcome), the relative risk is basically the risk of lung cancer in those exposed to smoking divided by the risk of lung cancer in those not exposed to smoking. The risk might be 10:1. Put in words, the risk of smokers getting lung cancer might be 10 times the risk that it is in nonsmokers. Second, in a case-control study designed to evaluate a preventive intervention, namely the link between screening and death from breast cancer, the relative risk is basically the risk of breast cancer death in those exposed to screening divided by the risk of breast cancer death in those not exposed to screening. The risk might be 7:10. A relative risk of 10:1 is usually expressed simply as 10, implying a tenfold increase. A relative risk of 7:10 is expressed as 0.7, implying diminished risk vis-à-vis the comparison group.

Clearly a major change has occurred in the concepts underlying case-control methodology: from hospital-based prevalent case-control comparisons to population-based incidence studies and those nested in existing cohort studies; and from an examination of exposures associated with an increased risk of disease to exposures associated with a decreased risk of disease or its worst outcomes. However, the basic elements of a case-control study remain the cases, the controls, and the exposure/intervention of interest. It seems useful to review briefly current ideas about their appropriate selection.

Cases

Cases may be prevalent, incident, or deceased. They are designated "cases" because they display the effect that is being studied. In the same way that it is important in etiological studies to specify the criteria by which an objective diagnosis is made of the disease, which will define those eligible to be cases, so is it essential in prevention-evaluation studies to be very specific about the outcome that is being assessed. In a sense the two kinds of studies are inversely related. In the etiological study, exposures are studied that are likely to increase risk of disease and, therefore, the odds ratio/relative risk will be in excess of unity. In prevention evaluation studies, the outcome/effect tends to be desired, for example, reduced mortality from disease X, and the preventive intervention is expected to have a beneficial effect. Then the odds ratio/relative risk will be less than unity and indicates a lower risk of an adverse outcome in those exposed to the preventive intervention. The specification of an outcome that is a disease or death, although not without possibilities for ambiguity and misclassification, will often be more straightforward than choosing outcomes for evaluating some preventive maneuvers.

In both etiological and prevention studies, the exposure/prevention must occur not only before the effect occurred, but sufficiently before, in that there was a period of time long enough for the intervention to have effect. In simple terms, a history of smoking beginning one month before the diagnosis of lung cancer could not be considered a relevant etiological exposure. Thus, in a well-designed case-control study, eligibility criteria should specify the time frame within which exposure did or could have occurred.

Next, cases, like controls, probably should have had a reasonable probability of experiencing the exposure being studied. Yet Rothman (1986) considers exposure opportunity to be irrelevant in case-control studies, arguing that the fact of exposure, not opportunity for exposure, is of interest. While this is certainly a minority opinion among authorities on case-control studies, it may become accepted in the future.

Finally, cases should be newly diagnosed or incident cases of the disease in etiological studies, not only for investigators to be assured that there have been no changes in diagnostic classification but also because the cases' recall of past events should be exercised close to the time of diagnosis, avoiding the influence of post-diagnosis events on the recall of pre-diagnosis experiences. This criterion is easily applied to prevention studies if the effect being assessed is a discrete event for which ascertainment of cases is complete or almost complete. The more important problem associated with prevalent cases, namely, that the exposure studied should be associated with disease incidence and *not* with survival, is examined in detail elsewhere (Schlesselman, 1982; Rothman, 1986) under the label of "prevalence/incidence bias," which is discussed below.

Controls

According to Spitzer (1985), the most difficult decision in case-control research theoretically and practically is the choice of controls. It is generally accepted that controls, like cases, must have been potentially at risk of experiencing the exposure/ intervention and developing the effect. For example, in an etiological study of the relationship between post-menopausal estrogen supplements and endometrial cancer, one would not choose hysterectomized women for controls. It is also reasonable that controls should be representative of the same population from which the cases were drawn, not necessarily of the general population (Rothman, 1986). Traditionally in etiological studies, controls have been drawn from hospitals, disease or tumor registries, Vital Statistics, physicians' practices, neighborhoods, or geographically defined areas. It seems to have been generally accepted that in hospital-based case-control studies, controls who have been admitted for exposure-related disease should be excluded (Breslow and Day, 1980), while those with only a history of exposure-related disease should not (Lubin and Hartge, 1984).

Some have recommended caution in using a nonhealthy control group (Linet and Brookmeyer, 1987) for cancer case-control studies, not only because it alters the interpretation of relative risk (which usually is comparing the risk of becoming a case relative to remaining healthy) but also because, among the nonhealthy, experience of the exposure may be different from among the healthy. Others disagree, concluding that the advantages of using "other cancers" as controls outweigh the disadvantages, but suggesting that controls from two sources (e.g., hospitals and the general population) may provide reassurance if results from the two sources are similar (Smith, Pearce, and Callas, 1988).

As well as unhealthy controls, some investigators have chosen dead controls in studies where cases were deceased; the appropriateness of dead controls depends on the exposure studied. Exposure variables associated with an increased risk of premature death tend to be overrepresented in dead controls compared with living controls, while exposure variables not associated with increased premature death tend to be more or less similar (McLaughlin et al., 1985).

Also to be considered is whether controls will be matched or unmatched to cases. Matching is a strategy to control confounding variables. In etiological case-control studies, confounding is the distortion of a disease/exposure association brought about by the association of other factors with both disease and exposure, the latter association with the disease being causal (Breslow and Day, 1980). Put another way, confounding variables distort the apparent magnitude of the effect of a study factor on risk; they are determinants of the outcome of interest; and they are unequally distributed among those exposed and not exposed to the study factor (Last, 1983).

Confounding can occur in preventive studies. Confounders may inflate or hide true associations. Strategies to avoid confounding include individual matching of one case to one or more controls. Another option is frequency or category matching by age group, sex, or race. Matching is most advantageous when a confounding variable has very different distributions comparing controls to cases, when the exposure is only weakly related to the disease, and when the exposure has a low prevalence in the population. Matching is supposed to improve the precision of the odds ratio, where precision is the inverse of the variance of the estimate (Last, 1983). But if one matches for a variable that is not a confounder, precision will be sacrificed. Matching requires an appropriately matched analysis. If the costs associated with matching greatly reduce the size of the study, an unmatched design may be preferred.

Exposure/Intervention

Much more is written about selection of controls than choice of the exposure/intervention. Since case-control studies are retrospective, the exposure/intervention has already occurred; the researcher has probably neither controlled nor applied it. The exception to this would be a nested case-control study in a cohort study with which the investigator was associated. To carry out a case-control study, the researcher usually depends on the accuracy of the study subjects in their reporting of the type, date, duration, and dose of exposure or on the availability, completeness, and accuracy of appropriate records. In preventive studies, there can be an advantage. The nature or structure of the intervention, the "dose," and who received it may be well documented, as in population breast cancer screening programs that were evaluated with case-control studies (Collette et al., 1984; Verbeek et al., 1984). In both types of studies, whether etiology-based or prevention-based, an unbiased method of collecting data about exposure is essential.

It is discouraging that an extremely well-designed and well-implemented case-control study may yield a null result because there is little variability in the distribution of the exposure. Thus, some case-control studies have failed to find significant associations between food and disease—for example, dietary fat and breast cancer risks—because diets (i.e., the exposure) were too uniform in the communities studied (McKeown-Eyssen and Thomas, 1985).

PROBLEMS IN CASE-CONTROL STUDIES

This topic can be dealt with here in only a superficial fashion. Some problems associated with the selection of controls have already been mentioned. Interaction has not been discussed, but it is an issue in the analysis. The overriding concern in case-control study design is to avoid bias. No description of case-control methodology would be complete without acknowledging the catalogue of biases that, even with the most careful study design, can undermine confidence in the conclusions reached by many studies. Although Sackett (1979) has described literally dozens of possible biases, only a few are mentioned here.

Very important to avoid in case-control studies is detection bias, which Feinstein and Horwitz (1978) describe as the fallacy obtained when the rate of occurrence of disease (outcome) in one group of people is compared with its rate of occurrence in another group in circumstances where the two groups have received a different intensity and frequency of the procedures used to detect the disease. This bias corresponds to Sackett's diagnostic access bias, a term little used but attractively descriptive.

Also of concern in case-control studies is recall bias (Sackett's rumination/anamnestic bias) when it is theorized that, by virtue of being cases, cases may recall previous exposures in a way that is consistently different to the controls' recall of previous exposures. Other biases include: "prevalence-incidence bias" when "a late look at those exposed (or affected) early will miss fatal and short episodes" (Sackett, 1979), also known as length bias (Last, 1983); response bias when those who agree to enter a study (as cases or controls) systematically differ from those who refuse to participate; and biases in the measurement, collection, and interpretation of data. All are pitfalls in the execution of case-control studies as they are in other study designs. Nevertheless, even more formidable than any potential bias is the lack of consensus on the basic principles of case and control selection, matching, and, although not discussed, analysis. It becomes important for the investigator to choose the principles that appear appropriate in the context of the proposed study, which are feasible and which are justifiable.

CASE CONTROL STUDIES: APPLICATION TO PREVENTIVE INTERVENTIONS

Standard textbooks of epidemiology (Mausner and Kramer, 1985) offer straightforward definitions for three kinds of prevention. Primary prevention prevents the disease (or other outcome) from occurring. In disease, primary prevention may be achieved by health promotion interventions or by specific measures such as immunization. Secondary prevention is early detection of asymptomatic disease permitting prompt treatment in the hope of "curing" the disease. Tertiary prevention attempts to limit disability and rehabilitate, or to offer palliative care to the diseased person. In the final section, an attempt will be made to superimpose these three levels of prevention, as defined by epidemiologists, on alcohol prevention research. In this section, examples will be drawn primarily from cancer epidemiology where case-control methodology has been used as an evaluation procedure for prevention programs in progress.

Case-control studies have been used to evaluate primary prevention, for example, a screening program designed to detect individuals in a precancer state, thus preventing incident cancers at a later date. (Screening is generally regarded as secondary prevention. However, screening can be either for the detection of predisease states with the goal of preventing disease, or for early disease states with the goal of curing the disease. These different goals have different implications for the selection of cases and controls.) Clarke and Anderson (1979) evaluated the screening efficacy of cervical cytology to detect dysplasia or carcinoma-in-situ of the cervix and to prevent invasive carcinoma. Other investigators (Aristizabal et al., 1984; La Vecchia et al., 1984; Macgregor et al., 1985) also evaluated cervical screening with case-control studies. A different kind of example was a case-control study evaluating the effectiveness of mass neonatal Bacille Calmette-Guérin (BCG) vaccination among Canadian Indians (Young and Hershfield, 1986) to achieve primary prevention of tuberculosis. Case-control methodology has also been applied to evaluate "primary prevention" of benign breast disease as a result of oral contraceptive use, although, obviously, oral contraceptives are administered with other purposes in mind (Berkowitz et al., 1984).

Examples of secondary prevention can be drawn from cancer screening programs other than those for cervical cancer. Here the goal of screening is to detect early disease, thereby increasing the likelihood of cure and decreasing the probability of death. A case-control design has been used to evaluate screening for stomach cancer in Japan (Oshima et al., 1986) and lung cancer (Ebeling and Nischan, 1987). The most frequent case-control evaluations have focused on breast cancer screening, one form of which is breast self-examination (BSE), where the preventive exposure was the reported performance of BSE and the outcome was earlier stage of cancer at diagnosis. Weiss (1983) cites six studies in which cases were women with advanced breast cancer and controls were women with less advanced breast cancer (Foster et al., 1978; Greenwald et al., 1978; Smith et al., 1980; Huguley and Brown, 1981; Senie et al., 1981; Feldman et al., 1981). However, none of the six studies were reported explicitly as case-control studies. Smith, one of his cited authors, subsequently did publish an explicit case-control study of BSE (Smith and Burns, 1985). Weiss counsels against using as controls women with early disease, since such controls will be likely to have had greater exposure to screening than cases with advanced or fatal disease, and the comparison would lead to spuriously concluding that screening had been efficacious. The comparison should be between late-stage cases and persons who are representative of the population of *disease-free* persons from whom the cases arose.

Screening programs for breast cancer employing mammography with or without physical examination of the breasts have also been evaluated with the case-control design (Collette et al., 1984; Verbeek et al., 1984). In these studies, the overall approach was to select dead breast cancer cases and living controls (who might or might not have breast cancer themselves), both having received invitations to be screened in the past. Both studies concluded that ever being screened was protective against death from breast cancer. One bias of potential concern, respondent bias, was ruled out since it was determined that there were no apparent differences between controls who consented to be part of the study and those who refused.

Even though the case-control design could be applied to tertiary prevention, looking at a potential exposure, such as palliative care, and an outcome such as the quality of life during a terminal illness, no references relevant to tertiary prevention were found. In any case, tertiary prevention, although important, probably occurs too late in the natural history of human afflictions to attract the attention that primary and secondary prevention deserve and receive.

Indisputably, there are precedents for applying case-control methodology to prevention research. Before exploring its potential in alcohol prevention research, an examination of the special characteristics of cases and controls in the context of prevention may be helpful.

Sasco, Day, and Walter (1986) offer an extremely detailed description of the characteristics of cases and controls to be selected for the evaluation of screening programs. Their conclusions may offer insights in addressing the problems of evaluating alcohol prevention programs and may provide a template for case-control studies of alcohol problem prevention. They specify a "Type A" situation that corresponds to secondary prevention. Here, cases must have "advanced disease" or even be dead, and their screening history up to the time of diagnosis must be known. The screening history of the matched control must correspond to the time during which screening was available to the case. In addition, the control must be free of the disease up to the time the case was diagnosed. This guideline implies that the control could develop the disease at a later date and remain a control. Sasco and associates state that, with such criteria for choosing cases and controls, one can estimate the relative risk of dying from the disease, comparing groups with different screening histories.

The analogy for this Type A situation in studies of alcohol prevention may be strained. Alcohol problems can potentially lead to two kinds of death: accidental and violent death associated with alcohol impairment, and death due to the chronic diseases associated with alcohol abuse, such as cirrhosis, hemorrhage due to portal hypertension, or even some neoplasms. But the questions arise: What corresponds to early stage asymptomatic disease in alcohol-prevention studies and what are the appropriate exposures? If the cases are alcohol-impaired teenagers who have died in motor-vehicle accidents, early asymptomatic disease might have been behavioral problems in high schools, and the exposure might be a screening test to identify an association of particular behavior problems with specific alcohol habits, followed-up by appropriate therapy/counseling. If the cases are adults who have died of cirrhosis, the exposure might have been a screening test to identify alcohol problems or dependence in patients registered with a health-care facility such as a health maintenance organization.

Sasco and associates go on to describe a "Type B" situation that corresponds to primary prevention, namely, to detect with cervical cytology a precancerous state such as dysplasia in order to reduce the risk of invasive cervical cancer. Drawing an analogy here for alcohol prevention reveals how arbitrarily "definitions" can be created. What has been called "early stage asymptomatic disease" above could equally well be considered a "preproblem/predisease" state. Thus, intermittent excessive alcohol use in teenagers, alcohol dependence in adults before major morbidity has occurred in target organs, fatty livers before cirrhosis has developed—all seem eligible for the two different classifications (primary or secondary prevention)—depending on one's point of view. Probably the single most appropriate situation for the detection of predisease would be identifying children with a genetic predisposition for alcohol problems. But in order for a case-control study of these children to be implemented, one would first have to find an established program where high-risk children were invited to receive such screening.

Sasco and associates have different eligibility criteria for cases and controls according to whether a Type A or Type B study is being carried out; they further differentiate Type B criteria according to the mode of disease detection. The Type B case-control study begins by requiring cases to have the disease or problem that one wishes to prevent. These cases may be detected in two different ways: by clinical diagnosis when symptoms are present or by screening when there are no symptoms. When the exposure of interest is the screening history, the relevant history for clinically diagnosed cases must have occurred prior to diagnosis, and it is suggested that screening tests performed less than six months to a year prior to diagnosis be excluded from the screening history. Appropriate controls for clinically diagnosed cases are those who are alive at the time of diagnosis of the case, with no previous diagnosis of the disease, but who are at risk of the disease. In contrast, screen-detected cases should be matched with controls who were screened at the same time as cases but were free of disease, the relevant screening history being screening that occurred prior to the case's diagnosis. Such a study would estimate the odds ratio of prevalence rates of disease among individuals with different screening histories.

A potential problem in the alcohol prevention context may well be that the interval between the premorbid and morbid state may be very long or quite unpredictable. The lead time between preclinical and clinical detection of breast cancer may be one to three years. If the lead time is many years, or if the premorbid condition frequently regresses to normal, case-control studies will not flourish.

For both Type A and B studies, controls should be subjects at risk of disease. This feature has very different implications for alcohol prevention research than for cancer research. Any woman with breasts is at risk for breast cancer, but it is doubtful that all women are at similarly high risk for alcohol problems. But there are other definable groups in whom alcohol problems are prevalent, such as young males or native Americans.

POTENTIAL FOR APPLICATION OF CASE-CONTROL METHOD-OLOGY IN THE EVALUATION OF THE EFFICACY OF ALCOHOL PREVENTION ACTIVITIES

Perusal of three general reviews of alcohol and health (Secretary of Health and Human Services, 1987; U.S. Preventive Services Task Force, 1989; Rankin and Ashley, 1986) has led to an attempt to categorize current alcohol prevention activities into three tiers, namely primary, secondary, and tertiary prevention and to further categorize these tiers by applying to them the epidemiological triangle of host, agent, and environment (Table 10.1). It was hoped that this approach would enable one to ascertain more easily which prevention activities lent themselves to case-control studies and, further, that case-control studies in other fields would assist in the definition of criteria of eligibility for cases and controls. Scientists already involved with alcohol research are likely to perceive omissions and opportunities that are not obvious to a cancer epidemiologist. (It should be noted that this conception is based on conventional epidemiological thinking, and readers based primarily in alcohol research will have to keep in mind that this approach differs from their own.)

TABLE 10.1
Alcohol Prevention Restructured

The Epidemiological Triangle	The Intervention (Exposure)	The Outcome (Effect)
I. Primary Prevention		
A. *The "Person" (Host)*		
The general population	Measures to reduce per capita consumption, e.g., programs to increase awareness of hazards or alcohol; delay legal age for drinking	Reduced per capita consumption
Youth - public school students - adolescents - college students	Health promotion in schools and workplace Driver education programs	Reduced incidence of alcohol dependence, morbidity, and mortality Changes in knowledge, attitude, and behavior of individuals
High risk groups - ethnic groups - pregnant women - the elderly - children of alcoholics - native peoples - genetically predisposed	Mass media campaigns (similar to those promoting cholesterol and breast screening) Driver surveillance programs Disincentives/punishment	
B. *The "Agent"*		
Alcoholic beverages	Increase prices for all alcoholic beverages	Reduced per capita consumption
	Differential pricing to favor low alcohol content	Reduced alcohol-related morbidity and mortality
	Restrict availability of alcohol - decrease time for sales - decrease number of outlets - discourage self-service - alter milieu where sales occur to decrease time spent	Reduced overall individual consumption as well as high volume per occasion consumption
	Promote alternative beverages	Reduce acute alcohol-related morbidity and mortality
	Server intervention programs	Reduced high volume per occasion consumption and thus alcohol-related trauma

TABLE 10.1
Alcohol Prevention Restructured (Continued)

The Epidemiological Triangle	The Intervention (Exposure)	The Outcome (Effect)
I. Primary Prevention (Continued)		
C. *The "Environment"*		
The family	Reduce direct and indirect promotion of alcohol in the media	Decreased promotion/endorsement of alcohol use in the media
The school		
	Alter social norms so that alcohol abuse is discouraged	Changes in knowledge, attitude, and behavior of communities
The media		
The workplace	Provide role models to discourage alcohol abuse	
The community		
	Health promotion programs directed at influencing specific groups in the community	
II. Secondary Prevention		
A. *"The Person"*		
Those at high risk for serious alcohol morbidity and mortality	Screening by health professionals followed by effective "therapy"	Altered drinking habits, either moderation or abstinence
Potential risk markers include: - Binge drinking - Chronic heavy drinking with or without dependence - Children with alcoholic parents - Pregnancy in heavy drinkers - Social, job, or family problems related to alcohol abuse - Involvement in accidents or violence while alcohol impaired	Punishment and disincentives - withdrawal of car license - imprisonment - fines Educational programs	Reduced incidence of alcohol-related morbidity and mortality Reduced frequency of impaired driving
B. *"The Agent"*		
Alcoholic beverages	Reduce palatability (Antabuse?)	Reduced consumption by people at high risk
	Reduce accessability	Reduced alcohol morbidity and mortality
	Server intervention programs	
C. *"The Environment"*		
Health Care System	Alcohol training for health professions at undergraduate level and in continuing professional education programs	Increased detection of high risk individuals Increased delivery of appropriate remedial interventions
	Routine screening for problems with alcohol using CAGE or MAST questionnaires	
	Availability of appropriate therapeutic facilities	
The Workplace	Employee assistance programs for those with alcohol-related problems	Reduced absenteeism, accidents, and employee turnover
		Increased productivity
Volunteer Agencies	Alcoholics Anonymous, self-help programs	Altered lifestyle in individuals
		Reduced morbidity and mortality

TABLE 10.1
Alcohol Prevention Restructured (Continued)

The Epidemiological Triangle	The Intervention (Exposure)	The Outcome (Effect)
C. *"The Environment"* (Continued)		
The Educational System	Systematic identification and appropriate referral of alcohol-related problems	Improved social and academic performance
		Decreased vandalism
		Decreased morbidity
III. Tertiary Prevention		
A. *"The Person"*		
Individuals with severe or life-threatening alcohol-related problems	Appropriate diagnostic, therapeutic and supportive programs, the latter extending to family members	Improved quality of life
	Improved nutrition	
B. *"The Agent"*		
Alcoholic beverages	Decreased availability of toxic substitutes for conventional forms of alcohol	Decreased consumption by the individual or a less harmful manner of consumption
	Total withdrawal from alcohol during custodial care	
C. *"The Environment"*		
Shelter	Provision of acceptable lodging for the destitute	Improved quality of life
Health care facilities	Appropriate number and accessability of facilities providing expert care	

The application of case-control design will always be restricted by the investigator's particular circumstances. Is there some form of "registry" available from which he or she can draw a representative sample of cases displaying the outcome that the preventive measure of interest was supposed to influence? Will he or she be able to randomly sample controls who come from the population from which the cases emerged? How accurately will he or she be able to determine the history of the exposure? Are there cohorts in progress or completed in which a case-control study can be nested?

In Table 10.1, section I, an outcome such as reduced per capita alcohol consumption does not seem amenable to case-control evaluation; however, specific interventions to achieve this outcome might be eligible, were subsidiary outcomes available. For example, do programs to increase awareness of the hazards of alcohol lead to a decreased risk of alcohol problems? To apply a case-control study to this very unspecific question would require that an awareness program had been carried out (or was in progress), and that the people to whom it was offered were identifiable. However, the program would have to have been optional and not obligatory. Were it obligatory, the controls would have equal exposure to the cases.

Furthermore, in alcohol prevention programs, an appropriate outcome (which should be less prevalent in those exposed to the program than in those unexposed and which can be reliably and completely ascertained) may be elusive. Also the longer the time between a health-promotion exposure and the outcome occurrence, the more difficult it will be to find the appropriate controls. Compared to a screening intervention (as in breast cancer screening where acceptance of the screen-examination enhances follow-up of those exposed to the intervention), health-promotion interventions may be less suitable for case-control evaluations. Still with reference to Section I, nothing described in B seems to lend itself to case-control design, and only health-promotion programs in C offer some potential for this type of evaluation.

From an outside perspective, no opportunity is perceived in Section I to define an indisputable outcome (e.g., chronic alcohol dependence or alcohol-related death) that might reasonably have been prevented by a specific intervention.

The situation changes in Section II. If you have a high-risk group, in which everyone has had a potential exposure to some preventive intervention, and if a reliably ascertainable outcome is available, case-control studies should be applicable. Unfortunately, if you consider how one would evaluate a policy of routine screening for alcohol problems by health professionals in an HMO, it probably would be best accomplished by a cohort study or randomized controlled trial. The problem is that for the exposure to be evaluatable, not everyone should receive it, although everyone should be offered it. Thus, in any situation where the "whole population" that is theoretically eligible to become cases or controls receives the health promotion or the screening intervention, the possibility for case-control evaluation is effectively ruled out. As was true in Section I, preventive strategies involving the "Agent" will be more easily evaluated using cohort designs, randomized controlled trials, or before/after comparisons.

Environment-related interventions in Section II at least satisfy the criterion that the exposure be offered to the population at risk of becoming cases, without being accepted by everyone. This is true for the services of Alcoholics Anonymous or voluntary employee-assistance programs in the workplace. But then the problem of "volunteer" bias arises. Entering into such programs is perhaps a favorable prognostic factor in isolation from, and separate from, the program itself. Certainly, in breast screening it has been observed that women who refuse to be screened have a lower incidence but a higher mortality from breast cancer than those who accept screening. The advantages of randomized controlled trials become immediately apparent. They permit one to recruit a cohort, all members of which are susceptible to volunteer bias and then to randomize them to one or more preventive interventions, permitting unbiased evaluation of the program.

If it is correct to assume that many alcohol-prevention intervention initiatives focus globally on a relatively small group—students at a high school, pregnant women at an obstetrical clinic, clients at a detoxification center—it may also be correct to conclude that before/after studies or cohort studies are preferable to case-control studies.

Although it is disappointing to conclude that case-control studies may have a relatively minor role to play in evaluating alcohol prevention initiatives, it is quite possible that researchers in the alcohol field will disagree and demonstrate that there are many opportunities awaiting imaginative investigators. In Rothman's (1986) opinion, case-control studies are "the most outstanding methodological development of modern epidemiology"; however, he also warns that "a casual approach to their conduct and interpretation invites misconception and possibly serious error." The challenges are to identify the opportunities for case-control study design and then to design and conduct them meticulously.

NOTE

Both Professor M. J. Ashley and Professor G. Eyssen are thanked for critiquing this chapter and making very helpful suggestions.

11

Some Alternative Models Based on Relative Risk Regression for the Analysis of Community-Based Intervention Studies

Steven G. Self

INTRODUCTION

This chapter describes how relative risk regression models can be used to analyze the results of community-based intervention studies when the endpoint is the occurrence of events associated with individuals residing in the community. We focus on methods that characterize the change in rates of endpoint occurrence over time within a single community, with particular attention to the timing and magnitude of this change relative to the timing and intensity of the intervention activities. This approach requires that sufficient data be collected to characterize fluctuations in the endpoint event rates both before and after implementation of the intervention. We believe that characterization of changes within a single community over time is the appropriate focus of detailed modeling activities, even when there is more than a single community participating in the study. Such attention to characterizing changes in each community considerably enhances the internal validity of the inferences. Because of the difficulties in characterizing differences between communities, and because there are typically few communities participating in any such study, we believe that less formal comparisons across communities, conducted after detailed analysis of each community, are most appropriate.

The problem of modeling trends in event rates over time is also encountered in epidemiologic cohort studies. Considerable development of models and statistical methods for the analysis of epidemiologic studies has occurred during the last four decades, and this work has resulted in an arsenal of statistical methods based primarily on relative risk regression models and their grouped-data analogs, Poisson regression models. In some circumstances these standard epidemiologic methods can be applied to community intervention studies; however, in other circumstances these methods would be inappropriate.   For example, the underlying assumptions in a Poisson regression analysis are that the variance of an observed count of endpoint events is proportional to its expectation and that event counts observed during nonoverlapping intervals of time are uncorrelated. It will be shown that these assumptions obtain under fairly mild conditions, provided that the underlying event rate fluctuates slowly over time.   This is typically the situation in epidemiologic cohort studies in which incidence rates of chronic diseases are stable over time.   However, noisy endpoint rates that fluctuate more rapidly over time will induce a correlation structure among the observed event counts, thereby violating the assumptions of the Poisson regression approach.   We believe this is the more common situation in the context of community intervention studies.

In this chapter, the connection between relative risk regression models and Poisson regression models is reviewed.   Particular emphasis is placed on identifying regression parameters associated with individual-level covariates in the relative risk regression models with parameters in the models for grouped data.   An additional component to the model is also developed that attempts to accommodate underlying endpoint rates that are noisy.   This corresponds to an extension of the standard Poisson regression analysis to incorporate a model for correlation structure among the observed endpoint counts.   We believe that this shift in emphasis and generalization of the standard methods used in epidemiologic cohort studies will be useful for community-based intervention trials.

STRATEGIES FOR DESIGN AND ANALYSIS

Any interpretation of changes in endpoint rates in a single community over time as being caused by the intervention can only be supported by a characterization of the changes that is sufficiently thorough to rule out any competing hypotheses and threats to internal validity.   Thus, "the analysis" of changes in a community over time ideally consists of a suite of statistical analyses.   These attend to the timing and magnitude of changes in primary endpoint rates relative to the timing and intensity of the intervention, the statistical adjustment for other processes in the community that affect endpoint rates but are independent of the intervention, the changes in intermediate endpoints or process variables through which the intervention is thought to affect primary endpoint rates, and the changes in rates of secondary or alternative endpoints.

Practical considerations preclude the possibility of collecting data from every individual in the community for use in each of the different analyses mentioned above.   It is most likely that data will be collected from different individuals in the community at different levels of intensity.   At the first level, only information regarding the number of endpoints occurring during each of a series of intervals in calendar time would be obtained. Ideally, these counts represent the total numbers of endpoints occurring among all community residents. These data can be quite inexpensive to obtain and may often be available from administrative data bases already existing in the community. Some methods for the analysis of such a time-series of endpoint counts and issues surrounding the interpretation of these analyses are given later in this chapter.

A second level of data collection involves obtaining both endpoint and follow-up data from individuals in the community. In this context, "endpoint data" refers to a record of times at which an endpoint event occurs for an individual and "follow-up data" refers to a record of the times during which the individual could theoretically undergo an endpoint event that would be recorded. Conceptually, these data correspond to the contributions of an individual to the numerator and denominator of an observed rate of endpoint occurrence. They represent the minimum amount of data that is logically required in order to make inferences about changes in the rates of endpoint occurrence. Thus, these endpoint/follow-up data are the basis of the most important analysis of change in the community. Ideally, these data would be obtained from every individual in the community, but this is rarely possible. Such data may be collected from a representative subset or cohort of individuals within the community. Statistical methods for the analysis of endpoint/follow-up data from such a cohort are also described in a later section of this chapter.

A third level of data collection involves obtaining information from individuals in the community about intermediate or process variables in addition to endpoint/follow-up data. The intermediate or process variables are assumed to reflect characteristics of either individuals within the community or aspects of the community structure itself through which the intervention will theoretically affect rates of the endpoint events. By monitoring changes in these processes over time, a measure of intervention effect is obtained, which is more proximal than endpoint rates and is tied to the theory of how the intervention will ultimately affect endpoint rates. Modeling these changes provides information that is useful in explaining the observed changes in rates of endpoint events and strengthens the argument for causal inference. These measurements also form the basis for a "structural" analysis that models the effect of these variables on endpoint rates and the possible changes in these effects over time. Estimates of the structural model can be combined with information about the change in the distribution of intermediate variables over time to construct an estimate of the magnitude of change in endpoint rates due to the effect of the intervention on the intermediate variables. This estimate can then be compared to the total change in endpoint rates actually observed. Methods for estimating parameters in these structural models and the use of different strategies for collecting data to use in these analyses have been well developed in the context of epidemiologic cohort and case-control studies. These methods are developed in considerable detail by Breslow and Day (1980, 1987) and Kalbfleisch and Prentice (1980) and will not be described in this chapter.

Although the models and statistical methods described here are quite general, it is useful to describe them in the context of a specific example. For this purpose, we will use Blose and Holder's (1987a) study of the effect of legalization of the sale of liquor-by-the-drink (LBD) on alcohol-related traffic crashes in North Carolina. In this study monthly time-series data on the number of alcohol-related traffic crashes during the 10-year period 1973-1982 were assembled for four groups of counties in North Carolina. For two of the groups of counties, permits for LBD were first issued during the end of 1978 and the beginning of 1979. LBD was not available in the other two groups of counties during the study period. The latter two groups of counties were matched to the first two groups on two indicators of socioeconomic change occurring during the study period: percentage of population change and percentage change in per capita income. Two different measures of alcohol-related traffic crashes were used: police-reported, alcohol-involved "had been drinking" (HBD) crashes; and single-vehicle nighttime crashes involving male drivers (SVNM). SVNM was also partitioned into SVNM crashes involving male drivers age 21 or older (SVNMO) and SVNM crashes involving male drivers younger than 21 (SVNMY). Blose and Holder use time-series and Box and Tiao's (1975) intervention analysis modeling techniques applied to log-transformed event counts to examine pre- versus postintervention contrasts within counties and intervention versus nonintervention contrasts between counties for each endpoint.

RELATIVE RISK REGRESSION MODELS

We begin by describing the history of endpoint events for individuals in the community as a multivariate counting process. Let $N_i(t)$ represent a stochastic process the value of which represents the number of endpoint events occuring for individual i in the community at time t or before. For a group of k individuals, the multivariate counting process $N = (N_1,...,N_k)$ is the collection of k (univariate) counting process that may be dependent on each other but for which there are no simultaneous jumps. Thus, in the context of the LBD study, if the time variable is chosen to represent calendar time measured in months then $N_i(t+1)-N_i(t)$ would represent the number of SVNM that individual i was involved in during the tth month of the study. If there are k individuals residing in the community during the tth month, $\Sigma_i[N_i(t+1)-N_i(t)]$

would represent the tth observation in the time series of SVNM counts analyzed by Blose and Holder.

Under mild regularity conditions, the multivariate counting process N has an intensity process denoted by $g = (g_1,...g_k)$ where $g_i(t)dt$ is defined as the probability that N_i jumps in the time interval $[t,t+dt)$ conditional on the history of the entire process, N, prior to time t. Thus g has the interpretation of the instantaneous rate of occurrence of endpoint events, and characterization of the dependence of g on the intervention is the object of the statistical analyses.

Let $dN_i(t)$ denote the number of events occuring for individual i during the time interval $[t,t+dt)$ and let F_t denote the history of the process prior to time t used in the definition of the intensity process, g. Then certain useful properties of the conditional moments of $dN_i(t)$ obtain from the theory of martingales. In particular,

$$E[dN_i(t) \mid F_t] = g_i(t)dt,$$

$$\mathrm{Var}[dN_i(t) \mid F_t] = g_i(t)dt,$$

$$\mathrm{Cov}[dM_i(t),dM_j(s)] = 0 \text{ for all } s,\ t \text{ and}$$

$$\mathrm{Cov}[dM_i(t),dM_i(s)] = 0 \text{ for all } s \neq t$$

where $dM_i(t) = dN_i(t) - g_i(t)dt$.

The definition of the history of the process at time t, F_t, that is used in the specification of the intensity process g includes a complete specification of the path of the counting process N prior to time t, as well as all other events that will be included implicitly or explicitly in a model for g, which can be thought of as having occurred before time t. For example, some individuals might move out of the community during the course of the study, in which case their rate of endpoint event occurrence would drop to zero. This follow-up information should be incorporated into a model for g. Define a stochastic process $Y = (Y_1,...Y_k)$ such that $Y_i(t) = 1$ if individual i is under observation just prior to time t and $Y_i(t) = 0$ otherwise, and include the path of the process Y prior to time t in F_t. We can now specify a statistical model for g that is written

$$g_i(t) = Y_i(t)\,\lambda_i(t).$$

This is a special case of the multiplicative intensity model described by Aalen (1978). Under certain independence assumptions (Kalbfleisch and Prentice,

1980), λ_i has the interpretation of the intensity of endpoint occurrence in the absence of any censoring or loss to follow-up.

Relative risk regression models specify a multiplicative form for $\lambda_i(t)$

$$\lambda_0(t) \, r\{(Z_i^T(t)\beta)\}$$

where λ_0 is an arbitrary, unspecified background intensity function, $Z_i(t)$ is a data-analyst defined vector of numerically coded covariate information calculated from information obtained prior to time t (i.e., $Z_i(t)$ is in F_t), β is a vector of regression coefficients to be estimated from the data and $r(\cdot)$ is a monotone function of specified form standardized so that $r(0) = 1$. Typically $r(\cdot)$ is taken to be the exponential function $e^{(\cdot)}$ although there are certain applications in which the linear function $1 + (\cdot)$ may be preferred (Prentice et al., 1988). This model can be further generalized by allowing the baseline intensity, λ_0, to vary arbitrarily over levels of stratification variables that may also be time-dependent, provided they are contained in F_t.

The multiplicative model for $\lambda_0(t)$ represents the structure for the end-point event rate in the absence of an intervention that we will assume in this chapter. When calendar time is taken to be the time variable in the model, general time trends in the rates such as cyclical seasonal fluctuations can be included in specifications of the baseline intensity function λ_0. Effects on the rates of factors such as age that vary from individual to individual are modeled via the time-dependent covariate vector $Z_i(t)$. Alternatively, some individual risk factors such as age can be accommodated in the model by time-dependent stratification. With this approach, the event rate at calendar time t for individual i in the jth age stratum is given by

$$\lambda_{0j}(t) r\{(Z_i^T(t)\beta_j)\}$$

where, in this formulation, the parameter β can also vary across age strata. If age is taken as the time variable in the model, then general time trends in the rates may be modeled by covariates that are functions of age and year of birth or can be accommodated by time-dependent strata.

We will assume throughout that the intervention affects the endpoint event rates via a term of the form $\exp\{(X_i^T(t)\gamma)\}$, which multiplies the basic model for the rates given above. Thus, regardless of the choice of the time variable, the basic model assumed for endpoint event rates is given by

$$Y_i(t) G \lambda_{0j}(t) r\{(Z_i^T(t)\beta_j\}\exp\{X_i^T(t)\gamma_j\}$$

where the intervention effect is also allowed to depend on age. We note that any components of β and γ that vary over age strata can be represented by a model with stratum-independent parameters and appropriately defined age-dependent covariates. For notational simplicity, we will use this representation and suppress subscripts on the parameters β and γ.

The covariate $X_i(t)$ is a data-analyst defined function of calendar time and possibly other variables such as age. It will typically take a value of zero prior to the start of the intervention. After implementation of the intervention it will take values that reflect prior beliefs regarding the timing and magnitude of the intervention's putative effect on rates relative to the timing and intensity of the realized implementation of the intervention. The associated unknown regression coefficient, γ, represents the magnitude of intervention effects; tests of the hypothesis, $\gamma=0$, are the formal significance tests of whether or not the intervention affects endpoint event rates. The covariate $X_i(t)$ serves exactly the same purpose as the "transfer function" used by Blose and Holder (1987a). See Box and Tiao (1975) for a discussion of specific forms that incorporate the possibilities of a time lag between the start of intervention and the start of its effect on endpoint rates, a gradual change in endpoint rates over time to a maximum change which subsequently maintained, and the decay of intervention effects over time. We also note that, technically, a modeling term representing intervention effects that is intrinsically nonlinear in its parameters can be used in place of term $\exp\{X_i(t)\gamma\}$. However, we believe that the log-linear form provides sufficient flexibility in modeling so this generalization would rarely be warranted.

AN ANALYSIS OF ENDPOINT COUNT DATA

In this section we will develop a model and describe a method for the analysis of intervention effects on endpoint event rates when the only data available are a time series of endpoint event counts. We begin with the age-stratified model for the intensity and calendar time as the time variable. The intensity of the counting process, $\bar{N}_j(t)$, which represents the total number of events in age stratum j at time t, is given by the sum of the individual intensity processes over all individuals in that age stratum. This intensity is given by

$$\Sigma_i[Y_i(t)r\{Z_i^T(t)\beta\}] \; \lambda_{0j}(t)\exp\{X_j^T(t)\gamma\},$$

which, after multiplying and dividing by $E[\Sigma_i Y_i(t)r\{Z_i^T(t)\beta\}]$, may be written

$$\lambda_{0j}(t)E[\Sigma_i Y_i(t)r\{Z_i^T(t)\beta\}]\exp\{X_j^T(t)\gamma\} \; \eta_j(t)$$

where $\eta_j(t)$ is a random variable with mean 1. The term $\eta_j(t)$ has the form of an average taken over the entire population. Provided the population base for the study is fairly large, the variance of $\eta_j(t)$ will be negligible relative to other sources of variation in the data. At this point, we will assume that $\eta_j(t)$ is identically one.

The term $E[\Sigma_i Y_i(t)r(Z_i^T(t)\beta]$ represents trends in the numbers of individuals at risk and fluctuations in the average levels of risk factors. Using a log-linear form, $\exp\{W_{1j}^T(t)\xi_1\}$, one can model these trends with community-level covariates, $W_{1j}(t)$, derived from census or survey data collected across time. For example, in the analysis of alcohol-related traffic crashes, time trends in the number of vehicle miles traveled (VMT) would provide credible surrogate information for the numbers of individuals at risk. Inclusion of such covariates into the model should be carefully considered in the context of the mechanism through which the intervention is thought to operate and the goals of the analysis. For example, suppose the goal of an analysis is to test the efficacy of an intervention designed to reduce alcohol-related traffic crash rates by reducing the overall per capita consumption of alcohol in the community. The inclusion of a covariate in such an analysis that is a survey-based estimate of per capita alcohol consumption would drastically reduce the power of the test. However, such a model could be quite informative in secondary analyses to characterize the mechanism through which the intervention actually operates.

Modeling of the baseline event rate function, $\lambda_{0j}(t)$, is problematic. This function includes systematic long-term and cyclical fluctuations in the baseline rate of endpoint events over time as well as short-term fluctuations that may not be able to be characterized from the available data as being systematic. These two aspects of $\lambda_{0j}(t)$ can be modeled by a parametric form representing the systematic component and a random term with a specified covariance structure representing the nonsystematic component. A log-linear form, $\exp\{W_{2j}^T(t)\xi_2\}$, can be used for the systematic component where the covariate $W_{2j}(t)$ is composed of functions of calendar time designed to capture any long-term or cyclical trends. The nonsystematic component can be modeled by a mean-stationary latent process, $\epsilon_j(t)$, with covariance function $\sigma_{ij}(s,t)$. Writing $W_j^T(t) = (W_{1j}^T(t), W_{2j}^T(t))$ and $\xi = (\xi_1, \xi_2)$ we have a model for the intensity of the age-stratified event counting process, $N_j(t)$, conditional on the latent process, $\epsilon_j(t)$,

$$\exp\{W_j^T(t)\xi + X_j^T(t)\gamma\}\ \epsilon_j(t).$$

Let $O_j(t)$ denote the number of events occurring in age stratum j during the time period $[t,t+1)$ (i.e, $O_j(t) = N_j(t+1)-N_j(t)$). Then an obvious discrete-time approximation to the continuous-time model described above leads to a specification of the mean of $O_j(t)$ conditional on the latent process, ϵ, given by $\mu_j(t)\epsilon_j(t)$ where

$$\mu_j(t) = \exp\{\alpha + W_j^T(t)\xi + X_j^T(t)\gamma\}$$

with $\exp\{\alpha\}$ representing $E[\epsilon_j(t)]$. Assuming that the discrete-time approximation also inherits the covariance properties of the continuous-time model, the
conditional variance of $O_j(t)$ is approximately equal to the conditional mean,
and the conditional covariance between different increments of O_j and between
increments of O_j and O_i is approximately zero.

The first two marginal moments of $O_j(t)$ are given by

$$E[O_j(t)] = \mu_j(t),$$

$$\text{Var}[O_j(t)] = \mu_j(t) + \sigma_j(t)\mu_j^2(t)$$

$$\text{Corr}[O_j(t),O_i(s)] = \text{Corr}[\epsilon_j(t),\epsilon_i(s)]/A$$

where Corr denotes correlation, $A^2 = \{1+[\sigma_j(t)\mu_j(t)]^{-1}\}\{1+[\sigma_i(s)\mu_i(s)]^{-1}\}$ and
$\sigma_j(t)$ denotes $\sigma_{jj}(t,t)$. Specification of the covariance structure of the latent
process, $\epsilon_j(t)$, in terms of a few unknown parameters results in a complete
parametric specification of the first two moments of the data, which allows
efficient procedures for the estimation and testing of parameters in the model
to be derived.

Note that in the special case when the baseline event rate $\lambda_{0j}(t)$ fluctuates
only slowly over time, then an adequate description of λ_{0j} could be obtained
using the systematic component $\exp\{W_{2j}^T(t)\xi_2\}$. This would imply that both
the mean and variance of $O_j(t)$ equal $\mu_j(t)$ and that the correlation between $O_j(t)$
and $O_i(s)$ is zero. These are the conditions required for the use of standard
Poisson regression techniques and, with the exponential form of $\mu_j(t)$ described
here, the statistical models correspond to the class of log-linear models.

Zeger (1988) describes an approach for efficient estimation and testing of
parameters for the general model described above in which the latent process is
assumed to have a homoscedastic, autoregressive covariance structure. This
approach is an extension of the generalized estimating equation approach
(Liang and Zeger, 1986) and is analogous to the method of quasi-likelihood
(Wedderburn, 1974; McCullagh, 1983). Zeger proposes that estimates of ξ
and γ be defined as solutions to the system of equations

$$U(\xi,\gamma) = D^T V^{-1}(O\text{-}\mu) = 0$$

where O represents the vector of observed endpoint counts during each time
period, μ represents the marginal mean of O, D represents the derivative of μ
with respect to ξ and γ, and V represents the variance-covariance matrix of O
evaluated at ξ, γ, and $\hat{\theta}(\xi,\gamma)$ where $\hat{\theta}$ is a consistent estimator of the parameters, θ, in the model for $\sigma_{ij}(s,t)$. The method of moments estimator of θ given
the parameter values ξ and γ would be a reasonable choice for $\hat{\theta}$. The matrix
$D^T V^{-1} D$ provides a large sample estimator of the covariance matrix of the

proposed estimators of ξ and γ upon which hypothesis tests and confidence intervals can be based. Zeger describes a simple computational strategy for solving the estimating equations that involves an iteratively weighted and filtered least-squares algorithm. These estimators of ξ and γ enjoy a robustness, in that they are consistent even if the covariance structure is misspecified. However, misspecification of the covariance structure invalidates the variance estimator so that if the covariance structure was not modeled appropriately, confidence interval widths and p-values would not be reliable.

The modeling and statistical analysis of a time series of event counts described above has certain features in common with the standard time-series analysis of log-transformed event counts that is described by Blose and Holder (1987a). In both approaches the following occurs:

1. A multiplicative form is used in the modeling process.
2. An attempt is made to explain as much of the variability in event counts as possible on the basis of past trends and patterns before introducing terms that characterize intervention effects, and valid inference about intervention effects relies on the assumption that the modeling of such past trends and patterns is complete and that these trends and patterns persist after the intervention is implemented.
3. Terms that characterize intervention effects are crafted in such a way as to acknowledge the timing and intensity of the actual implementation of the intervention as well as the relative timing and magnitude of intervention effects.
4. Careful modeling of the covariance structure of the series is required in order for valid inferences about intervention effects to be made.

With both approaches, the art in the data analysis lies in decisions made to partition fluctuations in the event rates into three components: a systematic component based on preintervention data that is assumed to persist after the intervention is implemented, a systematic component representing intervention effects, and a nonsystematic component modeled through the covariance structure of the process.

There are some differences that are worth noting between the approach described here and the standard time-series approach. First, in this approach the multiplicative model is derived from a more detailed structural model of event rates for individuals in the community so that under the modeling assumptions, the parameter γ has a direct interpretation in terms of these event rates. As a consequence of this feature, results can potentially be related to results from other, more detailed analyses of individual-level data by virtue of the parameters that the two types of analyses share. This difference is particularly important when attempting to integrate results from a variety of analyses of a single, carefully studied community.

Second, the multiplicative model applies to the structure of the mean rather than to the data itself. The data are not log-transformed, and normality assumptions about the transformed data are not required. In particular, these methods are appropriate for endpoints that are relatively infrequent, which is a situation that causes problems with the log-transform time-series approach. It is interesting to note that Blose and Holder mention that they were unable to analyze fatal crashes and nighttime fatal crashes because these endpoints were too infrequent, even though these endpoints have been suggested as more reliable measures of alcohol-related traffic crashes than SVNM crashes.

A third difference between the time-series approach and the approach described here is that finite sample inference procedures based on the t- and F-distributions are available under the assumption of Gaussian distributions with the time-series approach, but only large sample inference procedures are available with the methods described above. This difference is likely to be of minor importance in most cases because the simple log-linear form of the model and the weighted least-squares type estimators for the approach described suggest that the large sample normality of the estimators would be attained rather quickly. Also, strict normality of the log-transformed counts is a dubious assumption, particularly with counts that are relatively small so that, in practice, the inference procedures used in the time-series approach also depend on a large sample approximation. Nevertheless, careful attention to the finite sample properties of both methods is warranted in any particular application and additional methodologic work to characterize the small sample properties of the method described above would be most useful.

A last difference between the two approaches is the relative maturity of the statistical methods. Statistical methods for the analysis of Gaussian time-series data have a long and illustrious history with many different types of models described and their statistical properties characterized. In contrast, the ideas of quasi-likelihood and generalized estimating equations are only 15 years old. The application of these methods to time-series of count data is even more recent. Although there is no reason why classes of models that are rich in possible covariance structures and associated statistical methods cannot be developed, they are not available to date. Zeger's (1988) work with a covariance structure induced by an autoregressive latent process provides some useful initial results. However, this is an area of methodological research that would be most profitable to pursue.

AN ANALYSIS OF ENDPOINT COUNT DATA USING A PROPORTIONAL RATE MODEL

In this section, we describe an approach for the analysis of a time series of event counts in which data from a second endpoint are assumed to be available. The observed counts for the second endpoint are used to adjust for fluctuations in the primary endpoint rates and in the unobserved follow-up data via a proportionality assumption in order to obtain valid inferences about intervention effects.

We start with the model developed in the previous section for the primary endpoint event rate in age stratum j during the time period $[t,t+1)$ given by $\mu_j(t)\epsilon_j(t)$ where

$$\mu_j(t) = \exp\{\alpha + W_j^T(t)\xi + X_j^T(t)\gamma\}.$$

As before, $O_j(t)$ will represent the observed number of endpoint events occurring in age stratum j during the time period $[t,t+1)$. Now assume that event count data are available for a secondary endpoint and that, through the same modeling exercise, the form of the event rate for this endpoint in age stratum j during the time period $[t,t+1)$ is given by $v_j(t)\epsilon_j(t)$ where

$$v_j(t) = \exp\{\alpha^* + W_j^T(t)\xi^* + X_j^T(t)\gamma^*\}.$$

A key assumption is that the same random term $\epsilon_j(t)$ that appears in the rate for the primary endpoint also appears in the rate for the secondary endpoint. This implies that the rate of the secondary endpoint must be subject to the same nonsystematic fluctuations over time as the primary endpoint.

Let $\tilde{O}_j(t)$ denote the observed number of secondary endpoint events occurring in age stratum j during the time period $[t,t+1)$. It follows that the conditional probability $p_j(t)$ that an event in the jth age stratum and t^{th} time interval is a primary endpoint, given that an event occurred at all, is given by

$$p_j(t) = \mu_j(t) / \{\mu_j(t) + v_j(t)\}$$

$$= [1 + \exp\{-(\alpha-\alpha^*) - W_j^T(t)(\xi-\xi^*) - X_j^T(t)(\gamma-\gamma^*)\}]^{-1}.$$

Thus, a logistic regression model for the conditional probabilities, $p_j(t)$, is induced with parameters $(\alpha-\alpha^*)$, $(\xi-\xi^*)$, and $(\gamma-\gamma^*)$. These parameters can be estimated using standard likelihood-based inference techniques for logistic regression models by treating the $O_j(t)$ as independent binomial random variables with denominators $\tilde{O}_j(t) + O_j(t)$ and probability parameters $p_j(t)$. Details of this technique are described in Breslow and Day (1980).

From the form of the parameters in the logistic regression model for $p_j(t)$, it is clear that an unbiased estimate of the intervention effect on the primary endpoint rates is possible only if the intervention has no effect on the selected secondary endpoint (i.e., $\gamma^*=0$). Thus, the art in this approach to the analysis of event count data is the selection of a secondary endpoint that is similar enough to the primary endpoint so that its rates are subject to the same nonsystematic fluctuations over time as the rates of the primary endpoint but, at the same time, is different enough from the primary endpoint that its rates are not affected by the intervention. If such a secondary endpoint is available, this approach enjoys a great advantage over the methods described in the section "Relative Risk Regression Models" in that a detailed modeling of the covariance structure is not required.

In the field of cancer epidemiology, considerable caution has been used in the interpretation of results from proportional incidence or mortality studies. This caution is because of difficulty in interpretation due to the fact that a proportional excess can reflect either an increase in the absolute rate of the primary endpoint or a decrease in the absolute rate of the secondary endpoint. For this reason the approach has typically been relegated to descriptive or hypothesis-generating studies. However, in the context of community-based intervention studies, the proportional rate analysis has the potential to provide stronger inferences. In intervention studies, the theoretical basis for the intervention can provide specific information useful in the selection of an appropriate secondary endpoint, and the effects on the proportional rates that are being examined are quite specific in terms of their timing and form.

In their analysis of alcohol-related traffic crashes, Blose and Holder examined the event rates for single vehicle nighttime crashes involving males under the age of 21 (SVNMY) and those involving males age 21 or older (SVNMO) using separate time-series analyses. They found no effect of the change in liquor-by-the-drink (LBD) laws on SVNMY, but they did find an effect on SVNMO. The choice of SVNMY as a secondary endpoint by Blose and Holder was motivated by the fact that the minimum drinking age in North Carolina for distilled spirits was 21 throughout the study period. They state that "the impact of LBD on younger drivers should be less than for older drivers, if it exists at all." Since both the younger and older drivers are subject to the same local road, weather, and traffic conditions, the assumption that the rates of both events share the same nonsystematic component is also plausible. If so, the method of analysis described above would provide a more formal framework for Blose and Holder's comparison of SVNMY and SVNMO. This method would also generate formal estimates of intervention effects.

ANALYSIS OF ENDPOINT COUNT AND FOLLOW-UP DATA

In this section we describe some models for event rates that are useful when endpoint and follow-up data are available for all individuals in a cohort which comprises a representative subset of individuals in the community. Ideally this cohort comprises all individuals in the community. Technically, we define endpoint and follow-up data to be individual-level counting process, $N_i(t)$, which identifies the times of all endpoints occurring for individual i and the individual-level "at risk" process, $Y_i(t)$, which is an indicator for whether individual i is under observation at time t. Both of these processes were described in the section "Relative Risk Regression Models."

There are two approaches to modeling these data. The first approach uses continuous-time models for event rates and statistical methods based on the theory of partial likelihood (Cox, 1975) in order to nonparametrically estimate the effect of the time variable, and simultaneously estimate the effect of individual-level covariates, on the event rates. The second approach is based on grouped data and uses modeling and statistical methods that are quite similar to those described in the section "An Analysis of Endpoint Count Data." We will first discuss some of the problems with using the continuous-time models; we will not describe the partial likelihood-based methods for inference in these models. For details of these statistical methods, the reader is referred to Kalbfleisch and Prentice (1980) and Breslow and Day (1987) and the many references contained therein. We will then describe models and statistical methods for grouped data.

We begin by recalling the assumed form of the intensity function for individual i

$$Y_i(t)\lambda_{0j}(t)r\{Z_i^T(t)\beta\}\exp\{X_i^T(t)\gamma\}.$$

As mentioned above, the partial likelihood-based methods for inference with this continuous-time model provides a nonparametric estimate of the baseline rate, $\lambda_{0j}(t)$, and simultaneously estimates regression parameters associated with individual-level covariates. Recall that $X_i(t)$ in this model is a covariate that represents the effect of the intervention. If the time variable in this model is taken to be calendar time, then $X_i(t)$ is the same for all individuals in the cohort. In this case, the model reduces to

$$Y_i(t)\lambda_{0j}^*(t)r\{Z_i^T(t)\beta\}$$

where the new baseline event rate, $\lambda_{0j}^*(t)$, equals $\lambda_{0j}(t)\exp\{X_j(t)\gamma\}$ with $X_j(t)$ denoting the common value of $X_i(t)$ for all individuals in age stratum j. Because $\lambda_{0j}^*(t)$ is estimated nonparametrically, there is no opportunity to separate the effects of the intervention from other fluctuations in the baseline event rate over calendar time.

The other obvious choice for the time variable in continuous-time models for event rates is age. With age as the time variable, functions of calendar-time vary over individuals of equal ages, so regression coefficients associated with covariates summarizing intervention effects and covariates summarizing trends and cyclical patterns in rates over calendar time can be estimated. Any fluctuations in the event rates as a function of age will be accommodated nonparametrically. The main advantage with this approach is that the non-parametric estimation of age effects potentially reduces the total number of parameters that are required to be estimated. This can have potentially important implications for validity of the large sample approximations to the distribution of test statistics.

Although there is some advantage to using continuous-time models with age taken as the time variable, the validity of the model should be carefully considered. One potential problem with this model is the possibility of nonsystematic fluctuations in the event rate as a function of calendar time. These fluctuations can be accommodated in models for the analysis of grouped data through a latent process whose covariance structure must be modeled. However, if such a random term is included in the continuous-time model, then the partial likelihood-based methods can no longer be applied. Of course, random fluctuations in the event rates that occur as a function of age cause no problems at all with the partial likelihood technique. Thus, a reasonable approach to model selection might be first to consider age-stratified models for grouped data that include a latent process that generates fluctuations in event rates over calendar time. If there is no evidence for such a latent process on the basis of these analyses and if many age strata are required to accommodate fluctuations in the event rates across age groups, then continuous-time models should be considered.

Incorporation of follow-up data into the analysis of grouped event counts requires only a slight modification of the models and methods described in the section "An Analysis of Endpoint Count Data." In that section a model for the rate of the total number of events in age stratum j at time t was described with the form

$$\Sigma_i[Y_i(t)r\{Z_i^T(t)\beta\}]\lambda_{0j}(t)\exp\{X_j^T(t)\gamma\}.$$

Multiplying and dividing this expression by the random term

$$\Sigma_i Y_i(t)\ E[(\Sigma_i Y_i(t)r\{Z_i^T(t)\beta\})/\Sigma_i Y_i(t)]$$

yields the model

$$\Sigma_i Y_i(t)\lambda_{0j}(t)E[\Sigma_i Y_i(t)r\{Z_i^T(t)\beta\}/\Sigma_i Y_i(t)]\exp\{X_j^T(t)\gamma\}\eta_j(t)$$

where $\eta_j(t)$ is a random variable with mean 1 and variance proportional to the inverse of the number of individuals in stratum j at time t. As discussed earlier, we assume that the variance of $\eta_j(t)$ is negligible relative to other sources of variation in the data, and so we take $\eta_j(t)$ to be identically one. Now, using a log-linear form to model the term $E[\Sigma_i Y_i(t) r\{Z_i^T(t)\beta\}/\Sigma_i Y_i(t)]$, which represents the average event rate relative to the baseline rates in the absence of intervention effects among all individuals who are under observation in stratum j at time t, and modeling $\lambda_{0j}(t)$ with a systematic and a random part exactly as in the earlier section, yields a event rate model

$$\Sigma_i Y_i(t) \exp\{W_j^T(t)\xi + X_j^T(t)\gamma\} \epsilon_j(t).$$

The only difference between this model and the model derived in "An Analysis of Endpoint Count Data" is the appearance of $\Sigma_i Y_i(t)$ and the interpretation of the first components of the covariate $W_j(t)$.

The simple discrete-time approximation to the continuous-time model leads to an expression for the conditional expected number of events occurring in age stratum j during the time period $[t, t+1)$ of the form $n_j(t)\mu_j(t)\epsilon_j(t)$ where

$$\mu_j(t) = \exp\{\alpha + W_j^T(t)\xi + X_j^T(t)\gamma\}$$

and $n_j(t)$ represents the total number of person-months of follow-up realized in the jth stratum during the time period $\{t, t+1)$. Algorithms for computing $n_j(t)$ from the individual-level follow-up data, Y_i, are described in Breslow and Day (1980). Inference about parameters in this model can proceed using the same statistical methods as described earlier with only minor and obvious modifications to accommodate the known multiplier, $n_j(t)$.

APPLICATION TO AN ANALYSIS OF ALCOHOL-RELATED TRAFFIC CRASHES

To illustrate the use of some of the methods described above, we have applied them to Blose and Holder's (1987a) data on the sale of liquor by the drink and alcohol-related traffic crashes. We present results from a subset of this analysis here and compare it to Blose and Holder's results based on log-transformed time-series methods.

We fit models of the form described in "An Analysis of Endpoint Count Data" to the time-series of numbers of police-reported "had been drinking" (HBD) traffic crashes in the Group I intervention and control counties. A log-linear form for the means of these series was used. Trends in the log-means of these series were modeled by term of the form $\alpha + W^T(t)\xi$ where elements of the covariate vector W evaluated at month t include t, t^2, $\sin(2\pi t/12)$,

$\cos(2\pi t/12)$, $\sin(2\pi t/6)$ and $\cos(2\pi t/6)$. Intervention effects were modeled as a shift in the intercept, linear, and quadratic terms in the preintervention model for trends in event rates where the shift is applied at the time of intervention. If T_I represents the month during which the change in LBD laws went into effect, then the intervention effects enter into the log-mean as the term $\underset{\sim}{X}^T(t)\gamma$ where the vector $\underset{\sim}{X}(t)$ has components given by $I_{T_I}(t)$, $(t-T_I)I_{T_I}(t)$ and $(t-T_I)^2 I(t)$ where $I_{T_I}(t)=1$ if $t \geq T_I$ and $I_{T_I}(t)=0$ if $t < T_I$. A second order autoregression model was used to model the correlation structure of the latent process $\epsilon(t)$. An additional parameter was included in the specification of the variance function to give added flexibility to the model. To be specific, the variance of the event count at time t was assumed to be $\phi\mu(t) + \sigma^2\mu^2(t)$ where ϕ and σ^2 are unknown parameters to be estimated from the data. Zeger's (1988) quasi-likelihood estimation technique was used to provide estimates and standard errors for the regression parameters in the mean.

In Table 11.1 we present estimates and standard errors of the regression parameters. In addition, we present the estimate of the change in risk at the time of intervention, $\exp\{\gamma_1\}$, where γ_1 is the coefficient associated with the intervention effect covariate $I_{T_I}(t)$. This is compared to the intervention effect as estimated by Blose and Holder. Although the two estimates of intervention effect for the Group I intervention counties are quite similar, those for the Group I control counties are not. It seems likely that this discrepancy for the control counties is explained by the more complicated trends observed in the HBD crash rates for the control counties, both before and after implementation of the intervention in the matched counties, as evident from the plots of these series given in Figures 11.1 and 11.2. These figures display the observed time series of counts of traffic crashes and the expected value of these observations as estimated by the model fit. The expected value curves in these figures are plotted after eliminating the periodic terms in the model so as to display the fitted general trends in traffic crash rates without seasonal fluctuations. Note that in both the intervention and comparison counties there are statistically significant changes in the shapes of the trends in event rates at the time of intervention.

DISCUSSION

The variety of models and statistical methods that have been described may be useful in the analysis of community-based intervention studies. The starting point for the derivation of all of the models considered here has been the class of relative risk regression models for the intensity function of counting processes. The focus for the statistical methods described has been the analysis of changes in event rates within a single community over time.

TABLE 11.1
Estimates of Intervention Effects

Parameter	Covariate [+]	Group I, Intervention			Group I, Control		
		Estimate (SE)	Z	p	Estimate (SE)	Z	p
γ_1	$I_{T_I}(t)$	0.12^* (0.04)	3.0	<.01	$0.01^{\pm}$ (0.06)	0.2	.84
γ_2	$(t-T_I)I_{T_I}(t)$	-0.01 (0.35)	-2.6	<.01	-0.61 (0.48)	-1.3	.19
γ_3	$(t-T_I)^2 I_{T_I}(t)$	-0.48 (0.65)	-0.7	.48	-3.00 (0.85)	-3.5	<.01

$\vdash I_{T_I}(t) - 1$ if $t \geq T_I$ and 0 otherwise T_I is month of implementation of intervention.

* Estimated % change in risk of HBD traffic crash at time of intervention is 12%; Blose and Holder estimate is 17%.

$\pm$ Estimated % change in risk of HBD traffic crash at time of intervention in matched counties is 1%; Blose and Holder estimate is 9%.

FIGURE 11.1
Numbers of Monthly Police-Reported "Had Been Drinking" (HBD) Traffic Crashes in Group I, Intervention Counties and Estimated Trends

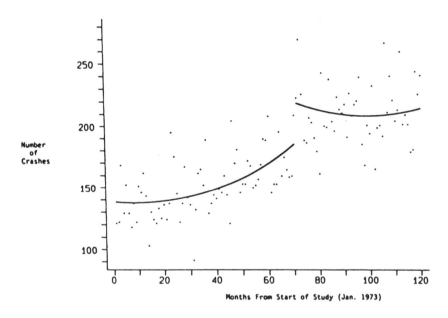

Source: Blose, J. O. & Holder, H. D.   (1987).   Liquor-by-the-drink alcohol-related traffic crashes: A natural experiment using time-series analyses.   *Journal of Studies on Alcohol*, *48*(1), 52-60. Reprinted with permission.

FIGURE 11.2
Numbers of Monthly Police-Reported "Had Been Drinking" (HBD) Traffic
Crashes in Group I, Comparison Counties and Estimated Trends

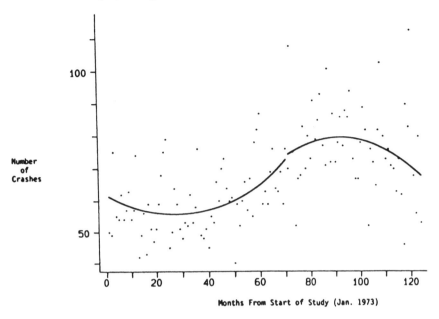

Source: Blose, J. O. & Holder, H. D.   (1987).   Liquor-by-the-drink alcohol-related traffic
           crashes: A natural experiment using time-series analyses.   *Journal of Studies on
           Alcohol, 48*(1), 52-60. Reprinted with permission.

These same two perspectives have been central and unifying themes in the
development of models and statistical methods in the context of epidemiologic
cohort studies.   It is useful to characterize the similarities and differences
between these two types of studies in order to identify how much of the
methodology developed for epidemiologic cohort studies can be directly
carried over to intervention studies.

The major difference between the two types of studies is the nature
and importance of fluctuations of event rates over calendar time.   In
epidemiologic studies of cancer incidence, for example, fluctuations in
incidence rates over calendar time tend to occur slowly.   This reflects the
relatively long time required for cells to be initiated and promoted to a
cancerous lesion and for the lesion to become clinically detectable.   In
addition, effects of individual-level covariate information tend to be the focus
of such studies, with fluctuations in rates over calendar time of secondary
importance.   In intervention studies, however, the endpoint event rates may be
subject to considerably more rapid fluctuations over calendar time.   In some

respects, endpoints with more labile event rates may be the most likely candidates for effective intervention. Also, in intervention studies, the effect of calendar time is of primary importance. Only through careful modeling of the effect of calendar time can the intervention effects be disentangled from other trends and fluctuations in the event rate.

This difference in the nature and importance of calendar time between the two types of studies identifies the major dilemma in directly applying epidemiologic methods to intervention studies. The great strength of the epidemiologic methods is the ability to avoid complicated modeling of a fluctuating baseline event rate by estimating it nonparametrically. Typically the choice between age and calendar time for the time variable in models used in epidemiologic studies is based on which variable exerts the more profound effect on event rates (Breslow and Day, 1987). Unfortunately, in intervention studies, complicated modeling of the baseline event rate cannot be avoided by this device because the intervention effect is entangled with the fluctuations in the baseline rate, and modeling is the only way to disentangle them.

Another difference between the two types of studies is that the timing and form of the effect that is being examined is much more precisely specified in intervention studies than in epidemiologic studies. This information can be used to tailor specific terms in the model, which increases the power to detect an effect.

Finally, the opportunity to build a case for causal inference is much greater in intervention studies because the mechanism of action of the intervention is typically better understood than the mechanisms under investigation in epidemiologic studies. This information about mechanism can be used to identify intermediate variables in an intervention study, which can then be used in a variety of secondary analyses that are typically not possible in epidemiologic studies. Results from these analyses can considerably strengthen the case for causal inference.

12

Community Prevention Programs as Natural Experiments

H. Laurence Ross

INTRODUCTION

Community-based programs of alcohol countermeasures can be treated as natural experiments for producing directed social change. Looking at them in this way permits their evaluation for effectiveness and efficiency. Evaluation can lead to directing resources into the better programs and to improve the poorer ones. In this chapter, I illustrate this potential, concentrating on my own studies of interventions designed to reduce drunk driving. The discussion here is based on the classical methodology handbook of Campbell and Stanley (1966), and on my work with Richard McCleary concerning ways to evaluate drunk-driving laws (Ross and McCleary, 1983).

A social intervention such as an alcohol-problem prevention program becomes a natural experiment because of the way it is looked at for purposes of evaluation, not because of its content. A natural experiment is accomplished by defining an intervention as a purported "cause" and the desired outcome as a change in an "effect." Investigators seek to link the intervention to the change in the effect in a way we speak of conventionally as cause-and-effect.

A prima facie case can be made that causality is present when there is confirmation of a prediction, based on a theory, that a change in the purported causal variable—the intervention, such as a prevention program—will be followed by a change in the purported effect variable—for instance, cirrhosis rates or nighttime highway crash fatalities. However, the mere finding that the prediction is fulfilled is not sufficient to establish causality. The social world is full of influential causes, and any given change might conceivably be the result of numerous changes other than the purported cause. The task of the evaluator of a natural experiment is to look at the situation in such a way as to decrease the number and plausibility of causes other than the one proposed by his or her theory. Although certainty is never achieved for causal explanations in science, our confidence in the correctness of a theoretically based explanation is a rough function of the degree to which alternative explanations have been ruled out by the study design.

THE CLASSICAL EXPERIMENT

In the world of physical science, things are sometimes so simple that the necessity to exclude alternative possible explanations of a theoretically predicted effect does not even occur to us. If a bar of iron is dropped into acid and its weight changes, we feel safe in concluding that the acid alone was the cause of the weight loss. However, social science is characterized by a multiplicity of plausible alternative explanations for nearly all theoretically specified cause-and-effect relationships. Social scientists have had to devise research methods that rule out as many alternatives as possible. The paradigm of research methods is the classical experiment as used in psychology.

The classical experiment compares an experimental group, which experiences the theoretically causal intervention, with an equivalent group termed the control. The equivalence is accomplished either through matching or randomization. Matching is a technique that equalizes the groups on specific variables within the limits of measurement and other error. Randomization *tends* to equalize on all variables, including those not even imagined at the time, within the limits of random variability. Sometimes both techniques are used to gain maximum comparability between the groups. For instance, experimental and control groups may be formed from a classroom of students, equalizing them for age and sex by matching, and tending to equalize them for everything else—for instance, race, political beliefs, sexual preference, or whatever, by assigning age-sex matched pairs to the experimental or control condition by a random process such as flipping a coin. The experimental group is then exposed to the intervention and the control group is not. Actually, the control group is exposed to something else, and the true contrast is between people experiencing intervention X and those experiencing a different treatment, Y, rather than simply X and not-X. The experimental group may view a film on the horrors of drunk driving and the control group may watch television. It is hoped and assumed that the television program contains nothing that can reasonably be expected to affect the criterion variable, such as numbers of drinks consumed during the following week. Any subsequent differences between the two groups can then with some confidence be attributed to the effect of the experimental intervention.

Of course, the classical experiment has its limitations even in very favorable situations: differential "mortality" or dropping out of the study, for instance, can render initially comparable groups quite incomparable at the crucial time of measurement. More examples of limits could be given, but in many situations the classical experiment is an elegant solution to the problem of determining cause and effect in social situations.

The classical experiment was designed for, and works very well in, situations like classroom-based research. If the groups have been rendered the same on all relevant variables except for the experimental one, any difference beyond that ascribable to random variation must in some sense be due to the intervention. However, the need to match or randomly assign people to groups severely limits the usefulness of this design for much social research. This is particularly true for interventions that are practically and ethically hard to vary randomly among individuals. Criminal laws, such as those threatening drunk drivers with heavy penalties, furnish a good example. Laws are hard to formulate so that they apply differently, not to mention randomly, to different individuals within a jurisdiction. Moreover, a fundamental principle of law, that of equal justice, requires that all similar people be treated similarly. This can be viewed as proscribing randomization of treatments.

However, classical experiments need not be ruled out in all cases of social interventions. Several years ago, a colleague and I were approached by the traffic court in Denver, Colorado, requesting a determination of whether their probation and treatment programs were effective in preventing recidivism of drunk drivers. The judges agreed to assign future defendants to fines, probation only, or some form of treatment, according to an arbitrary schedule devised by the researchers to permit true experimental controls. All of the sanctions to be applied were commonly used in the court; the main constraint to which the judges agreed was to vary them for experimental reasons rather than trying to match each offender with what a judge thought was the most appropriate punishment (Blumenthal and Ross, 1975).

THE NATURAL EXPERIMENT

The natural experiment occurs in situations where an intervention is introduced but the analyst is incapable of controlling its timing and placement. This situation is common when the intervention is a legal one. Matching and randomization are not possible, and a control group cannot be created for scientific purposes. Examples are limitless. A few from my experience include a judge deciding to pronounce unusually severe sentences on people brought to his courtroom for drunk driving (Ross and Voas, 1989), police in a rural county announcing a crackdown on drunk driving or some other behavior (Ross, 1977), and a state legislature mandating certain minimum penalties for convicted drunk drivers (Ross, McCleary, and LaFree, 1990). The judge's community, the rural county, and the innovative state constitute treatment groups or quasi-experimental groups.

The crux of the natural experiment is to find a reasonable control group, inasmuch as one cannot be deliberately created. The role of the control group in a natural experiment is the same as in a classical experiment with random assignment: to experience all relevant factors *except* the purported cause, which is limited to the experimental group. The value of the control is maximized to the extent that it is as equivalent as possible to the experimental group.

I offer here some suggestions for possible sources of control groups for natural experiments. The availability and suitability of such "quasi-experimental" controls are matters that have to be determined in each case. With luck, the intervention to be studied will have taken place in a situation where obvious controls of great similarity are available. For instance, an intervention in North Dakota may seek a South Dakota control. At other times, apparently great differences between experimental and control groups may vitiate the usefulness of the natural experimental model; there would seem to be no obvious control state for an intervention undertaken in Hawaii or, in the matter of alcohol countermeasures, for Utah. However, there are likely to be few if any situations where available comparisons are so limited that the investigator would be better off without a control. In that case it would be necessary to assume arbitrarily that differences in conditions before and after the intervention must be caused in the theoretically indicated way. This approach is not the basis of firm and convincing knowledge.

SEGMENTAL CONTROL: THE PAST FOR THE PRESENT

One common kind of natural experimental control consists of prior experience in the very jurisdiction adopting the intervention. One looks at the state of affairs before the intervention and compares it with that prevailing after the intervention. This kind of comparison sometimes rests on observations at merely one point in time before and after the intervention. Such a comparison produces only a weak control. The reason is that conditions at a single point in time are highly susceptible to the influence of chance factors or quirks of fate, resulting in a possibly misleading impression of change when in fact there is none, or the equally misleading impression of no change when change has occurred. This possibility can be minimized by looking at several points before the intervention as well as several subsequent ones. The several points help the analyst estimate the degree of random variation present in the situation and thus the magnitude of an apparent change necessary to justify the conclusion that it probably was not caused by this factor. Moreover, if the points are arranged in a time series, a change caused by the intervention can be distinguished from several kinds of preexisting changes that take the form of gradual trends in the data, as opposed to interruptions in the trend that more typically indicate intervention effects. This methodological approach is termed the interrupted time series.

The effects of an intervention may vary in the abruptness of their inception and in their duration. Figure 12.1 presents some graphs of these different cause-and-effect relationships as seen in time series. They represent ideal expectations, to which the results of a natural experiment can be compared. Through a theoretical understanding of the situation, the experimenter should be clear in advance about the expected form of the intervention effect, for this will help guide the statistician in evaluating the actual data.

The immediate, permanent change is diagrammed at the lower left. This might occur when the intervention occurs abruptly and completely, and the response is immediate. In the lower right the effect is immediate but temporary. Figure 12.2, dervied from serious crashes during drinking hours surrounding the inception of the British Road Safety Act of 1967 (Ross, 1973), shows an immediate, temporary effect in close to ideal form. The law promised an important increase in the certainty of punishment for drunk drivers, but there proved to be less enforcement than was originally expected. Figure 12.2 furnishes strong evidence that the law produced a major reduction in casualties at its inception, but that this effect wore off as people discovered that enforcement was minimal.

FIGURE 12.1
Models of Intervention Effects

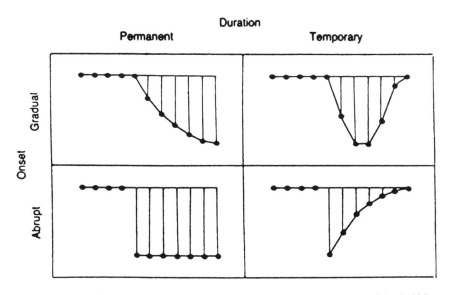

Source: Ross, H. L. & McCleary, R. (1983). Methods for studying the impact of drunk-driving laws. *Accident Analysis and Prevention, 15*, 415-428. Reprinted with permission.

FIGURE 12.2
Crash-Related Fatalities and Serious Injuries in England and Wales during Weekend Nighttime Hours (with corrections for seasonal variation and different numbers of weekends per month)

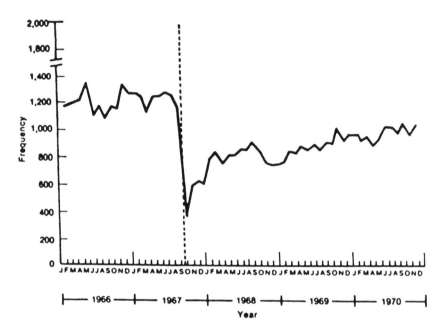

Source: Ross, H. L. (1973). Law, science, and accidents: The British Road Safety Act of
           1967. *Journal of Legal Studies, 2,* 1-78. Reprinted with permission.

The gradual, permanent change graphed at the upper left of Figure 12.1 should occur when adaptation must take place following the intervention. For example, if alcohol interlocks, preventing drunks from starting a car, were mounted on all newly produced vehicles, this model would better describe expectations of the casualty rate than the model of immediate permanent change.

The model at the upper right of Figure 12.1 describes expectations where the gradual change disappears. I include this for logical completeness, but it is hard to think of actual situations where this model would be appropriate.

SIMULTANEOUS CONTROL: NEIGHBOR FOR NEIGHBOR

The interrupted time-series design is a very strong one, perhaps the ideal for analyzing the natural experiment. However, it makes demands of the data that may not be fulfilled in many real-life situations. The interrupted time-series design generally assumes that the theoretical cause is abruptly introduced in a way that produces a large and immediate effect. Modifications of the model can handle incremental effects if these begin promptly following the intervention. However, subtle causes, and ones with long-term effects only, are not easily studied with this method. Moreover, the needed data may not be available, especially from before the intervention. For example, the only available data relevant to the extent of drunk driving in New Philadelphia, Ohio, before Judge Edward O'Farrell introduced 15-day jail sentences for first-offense law violators, were fatalities, but the data base was so small that the effect of even a very successful intervention would have been impossible to detect in time series (Ross and Voas, 1989).

In this situation, a useful comparison may be made between the jurisdiction experiencing the intervention and a similar one lacking the experience. Depending on the similarity found in candidate jurisdictions, the comparison can be revealing.

It proved possible to pair New Philadelphia with the nearby community of Cambridge, Ohio, which could be seen as similar enough to treat as a quasi-experimental control. Table 12.1 presents the kind of data that were reviewed in order for investigators to arrive at the judgment of sufficient similarity. Both impressions from visits and these Census data indicate similarity, but it is also obvious that the communities are not identical. It may suffice to say that among communities close enough to share the geographical and social condi-

TABLE 12.1
Selected Demographic Characteristics of New Philadelphia and Cambridge, Ohio

Characteristic	New Philadelphia	Cambridge
Population, 1980	16,883	13,573
Percent male	67.1	62.7
Percent Black	0.6	3.9
Percent Hispanic	0.2	0.5
Percent 18-64 years old	60.6	56.0
Percent high-school grads	67.5	61.3
Percent college grads	10.6	10.8
Percent unemployed	7.1	7.9
Median household income	$15,612	$12,578

Source: Ross, H. L. & Voas, R. (1989). *The New Philadelphia story: The effects of severe punishment for drunk driving*. Washington, DC: AAA Foundation for Traffic Safety. Reprinted with permission.

tions of New Philadelphia, Cambridge appeared the most similar, and its differences did not appear too large or especially relevant to the issue of the extent of drunk driving.

Surveys were made of drivers on weekend nights in New Philadelphia and Cambridge to determine whether the O'Farrell judicial policy was well known. Figure 12.3 presents the results for the question of whether a jail term was expected. It clearly shows that the policy had an effect on the expectations of these drinking-hour drivers.

In another case (Robertson, Rich, and Ross, 1973), an apparent reduction in traffic casualties in Chicago, at first-glance attributed to a judge-made threat of jail for drunk drivers, was analyzed by comparing Chicago data with those from Milwaukee, selected as a quasi-experimental control jurisdiction. The

FIGURE 12.3
Expectation of a Jail Sentence by Drivers in New Philadelphia and Cambridge, Ohio

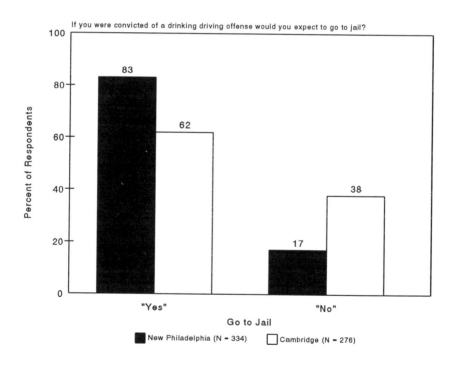

Source: Ross, H. L. & Voas, R. (1989). *The New Philadelphia story: The effects of severe punishment for drunk driving*. Washington, DC: AAA Foundation for Traffic Safety. Reprinted with permission.

evaluators found that Milwaukee, which lacked the intervention, had experienced an even greater casualty reduction than Chicago during the time in question, suggesting that something other than the judicial policy was very likely responsible for the developments in the two cities.

SIMULTANEOUS CONTROL: THE WHOLE FOR THE PART

Sometimes an intervention may be introduced with the expectation that it will affect some part of the population to which it is applied more than other parts. For example, some kinds of personalities might be more attentive to deterrent threats, or the policy might be more effective in certain regions, or at certain times of day. These situations can give rise to natural experiments if the parts most or least likely to be affected are compared with each other or with the whole.

For example, the regions of France differ very much in the extent to which alcoholism is a recognized problem. Paradoxically, alcohol problems are less common in the regions that produce wine, such as the South, and more common in those with less developed production of alcoholic beverages, such as Brittany and the North. In a study evaluating the success of a 1978 law permitting roadblocks for breath testing of drivers, changes in casualties in these regions were compared (Ross, McCleary, and Epperlein, 1981). There was a significant reduction of 15 percent in injury-producing changes in Brittany and the North, whereas the change in the South was only half that amount, and statistically insignificant, reinforcing the interpretation that it was indeed the law that produced the effects in question.

Although the interrupted time-series approach to the effects of the British Road Safety Act of 1976 provides impressive proof of the effect, the data can also be looked at in the framework of simultaneous control. Indeed, two time series can be developed, one (shown in Figure 12.2) graphing casualties during drinking hours, when alcohol is expected to be an important cause, and the other (Figure 12.4) graphing them during commuting hours when pubs are closed, when alcohol use is expected to have been rare at all times. This provides a demonstration of effect for the law that is overwhelmingly convincing, even though no randomization or other experimental manipulation was possible.

CONDITIONS FOR SUCCESSFUL NATURAL EXPERIMENTS

Valid and reliable measurement of the effect variable is necessary for both classical and natural experiments. Where measurement is unreliable, apparent changes can be mistaken for real ones, or changes actually produced

FIGURE 12.4
Crash-Related Fatalities and Serious Injuries in England and Wales during Weekday Commuting Hours (with corrections for seasonal variation and different numbers of weekends per month)

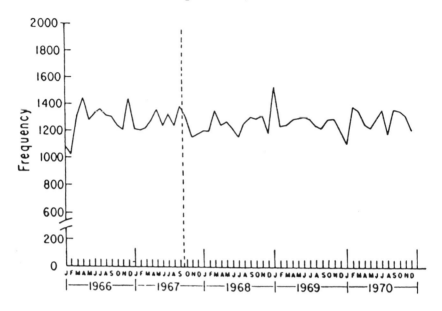

Source: Ross, H. L.   (1973).   Law, science and accidents: The British Road Safety Act of
        1967. *Journal of Legal Studies, 2,* 1-78. Reprinted with permission.

by the intervention can be hidden because countered by misleading changes in the indicators. Where measurement is invalid, i.e., measuring something other than what the researcher thinks it measures, the theoretical understanding of what has happened rests on shaky foundations. The measures used in evaluating alcohol programs vary in the extent to which they typically meet these criteria.

Alcohol consumption, for example, is well measured for most large jurisdictions through tax receipts and similar data, but these can be quite misleading for small jurisdictions. Much of the alcohol sold in Washington, D.C., for example, is consumed in Virginia and Maryland, and much of what is sold in Las Vegas is drunk by visitors from Los Angeles. Self-reports concerning consumption are notoriously biased, seriously understating the amount. This may be tolerable for comparisons over time or with quasi-experimental controls, but where differentials in the completeness of reporting might be expected between the compared groups, the problem can be serious (Ross et al., 1991).

Drunk driving in particular is hard to measure directly, though it can be done through systematic surveys of drivers involving breath tests. However, where refusals are permissible, as is generally the case in the United States, such surveys no doubt underestimate the phenomenon. Arrest rates and police-defined "alcohol-related" crashes are highly unreliable measures. Fatal crashes, especially those at night, which are strongly related to drunk driving, form acceptable indexes since almost all of them are reported. However, fatal crashes are relatively rare events and are likely to be useful for indexing drunk driving only in the largest communities. This is even more true of the best surrogate measure of drunk driving, single-vehicle nighttime fatalities.

Natural experiments are best conducted with interventions that are simple and straightforward, and they are thereby more easily interpreted. Unfortunately, many interventions comprise a complex "market basket" of different measures. If some of these are effective and others not, the net result is likely to be less evident than if only the effective measures were studied. Moreover, if an effect is found, it may be impossible to identify the specific cause from among the potential nominees in the basket. One may conclude that something (or everything) in the basket works, but more detailed studies will then be required for a sophisticated understanding on which policy improvements can be based.

The frequent complexity of interventions to counter alcohol problems is due in part to the urgency of the problems. It is also due to the correct understanding that alcohol problems are complex and probably require complex interventions for maximum control. The best way to manage these legitimate considerations might be for countermeasures to be introduced one at a time, allowing time for evaluation of each before introducing a new one.

It is much harder to recognize small effects than big ones, for the small ones must compete with all the other things that are happening in the world in order to be recognized. Therefore, interventions should ideally be as big as possible, or as big as politically feasible, to avoid the erroneous conclusion that they failed when actually they merely produced small effects. Moreover, some kinds of causes produce effects only in "doses" that exceed a threshold. Deterrent threats with very low probabilities of enforcement probably do little to affect behavior, even though the threatened punishment is quite severe (Ross, 1982).

Immediate effects are also easier to see than those in the long term. The longer the term, the harder it is to distinguish the effects of a specific cause from those of the general causal ferment that characterizes social life. One should not, however, give up on trying to identify long-term causal relationships, but the task is more difficult and the likelihood of erroneous conclusions is greater.

Finally, the search for effects of a given cause should be a broad one, encompassing a variety of measures for expected effects. In addition, the evaluator should be alert to the possibility of unexpected and even unintended effects. Severe punishment, for example, may have the unintended effect of stimulating resistance by alleged offenders to accusations through hiring lawyers and demanding trials rather than pleading guilty to charges. The consequent increase in the burdens on prosecutors and courts can result in a lower likelihood of any punishment at all (Ross, 1976).

Part VI

Implementing Research Designs

13

Protecting the Scientific Integrity of Community Intervention Studies: Confronting Social Realities

Jan M. Howard and Ivan Barofsky

INTRODUCTION

Research of any kind, particularly studies of humans, takes place in a dynamic social context that inherently affects the design, implementation, and interpretation of the research. Moreover, the very social dynamic that inspires and envelops research may compromise its scientific integrity. Community-based health intervention studies (both natural experiments and tests of investigator-controlled interventions) confirm these tenets. The challenge of intervention research in real-world environments is to make social reality a friend rather than a foe of science. Confrontations with reality can stimulate creative applications of available science and generate fundamentally new ways of answering questions.

CLINICAL TRIAL STANDARDS

Randomized controlled trials (RCTs) are posited to be the gold standard for testing interventions in disease prevention and treatment (Friedman, Furberg, and DeMets, 1981). Presumably, they provide the best protection against a biased experiment (Meinert, 1986). Randomization reduces the likelihood that investigators will contaminate the study by assigning the intervention and control phenomena to different sets of persons in terms of known and unknown risk factors. Analogously, concurrent controls reduce the probability that "extraneous" ongoing events will influence study results.

Experienced designers and managers of RCTs recognize that the social milieus of intervention trials are laden with potential threats to their scientific importance and validity. Thus, participants in clinical trials (whether sick or well) tend to be healthier than their counterparts in the world at large (Friedman, Furberg, and DeMets, 1981), which has obvious implications for generalization.   Moreover, participants do not necessarily adhere to study protocols, dropping out of the experimental group or into it in violation of study designs.   Sample size estimates are inflated to take these behaviors into account; and other procedures also lessen the likelihood of drawing false conclusions (e.g., p values that compensate for multiple looks at the data).

More important than *perceived* challenges to the scientific integrity of clinical trials are socially-induced threats that go unrecognized—for example, tendencies by community physicians to prescribe the intervention to control-group patients most at risk of endpoint events.[1]   In spite of elaborate procedures in double-blind trials to protect the identity of assigned therapies, physicians as well as patients have used various means of breaking the blind (Howard et al., 1982), sometimes because patient safety requires it.   These conflicts in priorities may not even be brought to consciousness, outside or inside the study group.

Similarly, investigators may not fully appreciate the differential implications of the two statistical tails of a treatment-effect distribution. Because of proscriptions to "first, do no harm" to patients, policy/data monitoring boards are inclined to stop trials for harm on the basis of less persuasive evidence than they require to stop trials for benefit.   Yet, stopping rules for positive outcomes are undergoing increased scrutiny as patient advocates demand access to drugs that offer reasonable hope of effectiveness.   Thus, the viability of clinical trials depends on ethical principles and their interpretation, which are continually in process of change.

It could be argued that research focused on behavior (or lifestyle) change is more sensitive to demands of the social environment than are traditional drug-efficacy studies. But recent political activity concerning drug testing for AIDS counters this argument. In any event, alcohol focused interventions *are* primarily oriented toward behavioral change, which places alcohol prevention research unequivocally in the social dynamic.   The peculiarities of that dynamic can force decision makers to initiate prevention activity without guidance from research. Even where studies exist, proof of efficacy may be elusive.   And community pressure to curtail alcohol problems can motivate policy makers to act in the absence of certainty. By default, prudence[2] rather than proof may become the yardstick for action.

PRUDENCE VS. PROOF

Ideally, community prevention programs should reflect and build upon the state of the art. Their design and implementation should be guided by existing research findings, and these programs should carry the inquiry further through "evaluation" studies.   Unfortunately, there is a dearth of proven strategies for the prevention of alcohol-related problems, and some approaches that do have track records of effectiveness (such as increased taxes on alcoholic beverages) may be politically unpalatable.   Thus, community decision makers must frequently choose among less-than-preferred options.   In the political arena, these choices may be based on compromise.   But in the world of unknowns, compromise may be irrelevant.

One option is to select an intervention on the basis of a simple hunch, or "common sense." The "Just Say No" campaign may be illustrative. Although hunch approaches can reinforce social norms against problem behavior, untested strategies may also have unanticipated negative consequences (e.g., school curricula that inadvertently encourage experimentation with alcohol [Bruvold and Rundall, 1988; Schaps et al., 1981; Tobler, 1986]).   In contrast to medical interventions (such as prescribed drugs), it seems to be naively assumed that strategies to prevent alcohol problems cannot result in harm.

Leaders wary of making hunch decisions in a climate of uncertainty may pursue alternatives. They can: delay intervention until the evidence for one or another strategy becomes more convincing; undertake expeditious or long-term research in preparation for intervention; select an approach on the basis of promise rather than proof; or conduct a natural experiment, intervening and testing at the same time.[3]   All these options constitute action, but the time frame for implementing prevention strategies (as opposed to research) will vary with the choice.   In the first two cases intervention might be postponed indefinitely.

Selecting Prudent Strategies

Since proof is elusive and rarely closes the door to reasonable doubt, it is appropriate to consider criteria for selecting prudent as distinct from proven prevention strategies.   Given the realities of decision-making environments, the following guidelines appear relevant:

1. Evidence indicating beneficial effects of the proposed intervention needs to be strongly suggestive that the results were more than a function of chance.

Even if tested strategies have not consistently shown statistically significant benefits, the data may clearly point in the positive direction. This is perhaps an operational definition of "promise," which can be objectified through such techniques as systematic data pooling, meta analyses, and consensus conferences. Because the goal of prevention programs is frequently behavioral change, positive placebo effects (from the intervention process itself) might also be considered beneficial.

Additionally, possible spin-off effects of the intervention for the general health of the target population should be taken into account. For example, the curtailment of alcohol abuse may have implications for the abuse of other drugs or for unsafe sexual practices. Even if problems are not directly linked, inferences regarding benefits of particular interventions can be drawn from other areas of research, as long as pertinence can be empirically or theoretically justified.

2. There should be persuasive evidence that the intervention will not cause deleterious behavior or that the possibility of harm pales in comparison to anticipated benefit.

The admonition to "first, do no harm" that applies to physicians should guide community prevention strategists as well. Interventions aimed at reducing alcohol problems can backfire, strengthening the very activities the strategies are designed to curtail (Myers et al., 1991). Moreover, the diversity of prevention goals may permit success and failure to occur simultaneously. It is conceivable, for example, that designated-driver campaigns may reduce drunk driving while legitimizing (enabling) destructive drinking among non-drivers.[4] The pressure to implement stop-gap prevention programs may also have adverse consequences. Premature actions may negate opportunities to introduce more effective strategies later.

Given the predilection of change agents to focus on their positive results, decision makers may have difficulty learning about negative effects of prevention efforts. Yet, reviewers of alcohol prevention research have a propensity for wariness and willingly attack sacred cows (Hochheimer, 1981; Moskowitz, 1989).

3. The longer the perceived waiting time for proof of benefit to be established, the greater the attractiveness of prudent prevention strategies.

Other factors being equal, the value of prompt prudence may outweigh the value of delayed proof. Where immediate administrative action is demanded by the "community," any pause for research might be criticized as irresponsible. The speed with which convincing answers can be obtained from research will depend in part on the endpoint. Changes in knowledge or attitudes may occur sooner than changes in behavior or disease states, but the first set of outcomes need not be predictive of the second. Moreover, financial constraints may require trade-offs and compromises in research approaches that would seriously weaken the quest for proof.

4. Financial costs of the proposed intervention must be evaluated in the context of uncertain outcomes.

The willingness of legislative and administrative bodies to fund prevention programs will undoubtedly reflect the perceived probability of success. Ambiguity is likely to breed caution. Indirect as well as direct costs should be considered, such as the cost of adjudicating alleged violations of new laws to control alcohol abuse. Also important are long-term costs of "booster" strategies to counter the decay of intervention effects.

Particular prevention efforts by a community or government agency may be encouraged or mandated by another public authority with a contribution of targeted funds. Financial aid could make prudent options more appealing. By the same logic, states or municipalities might adopt a prudent strategy because public funds for other programs (e.g., highway construction) were contingent on their doing so.

5. Possible consequences of a potential credibility gap should be considered in implementing prudent strategies.

The more tenuous the evidence supporting prudent actions, the greater the likelihood they will later be ineffective. Public reactions will then depend on factors that may not be known in advance, such as the visibility and price of failure. If no major alcohol-related "incident" occurs, the public may never become aware that the prevention program was flawed. And without intervention *research*, success might simply be defined in terms of action. However, policy makers who base choices on prudence rather than proof might be wise to acknowledge the fallibility of their decisions. The public may later be more accepting of exposed failure if the intervention was initially called an experiment and if contingency plans were put in place.

6. Prevention strategies should be appraised for selection in terms of their intrinsic value.

Preventive interventions carry a message of concern about the problem. Reciprocally, the absence of prevention efforts may legitimize problem-inducing behavior. It may, therefore, be prudent for policy makers to take some action supporting societal norms, to go on record against inertia. At the least, such "statements" heighten the background rhetoric and might facilitate placebo effects—assuming their impact is not deleterious. At best, such actions could have preventive properties in their own right.

7. Where prudent prevention strategies can additionally generate an experiment, their attractiveness should increase.

214   Implementing Research Designs

Strategies that show promise of benefit are not necessarily amenable to further study through experimental designs. It may be deemed unethical to withhold the intervention from the control group, even though proof of effectiveness is still to be established; or its existing use may be so extensive as to profoundly contaminate any randomly selected control group. Breast self-examination (BSE) for early detection of breast cancer is illustrative. Randomized controlled trials of the effectiveness of BSE may be appropriate in certain foreign countries; but in the United States, the opportunity for such studies appears to have passed (Howard, 1984). Similarly, universal interventions like the minimum drinking age may constrain the use of experimental designs.

The potential value of an intervention for reducing alcohol problems may be independent of its value as a catalyst for research. If prudent strategies are selected for the double purpose of implementing and testing a prevention program, the research component may be inordinately vulnerable to co-optation and bias. To protect the study's integrity, evaluators of the intervention-experiment should be devoid of responsibilities or vested interests in the prevention effort. And ideally, funding for the research should come from sources independent of the prevention program.

8. Prudent interventions necessarily reflect objective assessments of political realities.

Alcohol prevention constituencies have multiple concordant and discordant objectives. Moreover, the alcohol beverage industry (also not monolithic) has its own stakes in the prevention dialogue. In choosing viable strategies, decision makers must confront these realities, ultimately translating debate into compromise, consensus, or controllable conflict. To be effective, interventions must be acceptable to the significant populace. Correctly determining who qualifies as significant is an important measure of prudence.

Shaping the Quest for Proof

Social realities that influence the selection of *prudent* prevention strategies in communities also shape the quest for *proven* interventions through rigorous research: risk/benefit ratios, credibility issues, time constraints, financial costs, and political agendas. These factors determine which strategies will be studied, as well as research technologies, target groups, and timing.

It can be argued that successful prevention research in the community requires continuous negotiation (Buka and Speare, 1990) and commitment from all the principal parties (Pentz et al., 1986; Pentz et al., 1989). The best contemporary illustration is drug testing for the prevention and treatment of

AIDS. The quest for proof of efficacy and effectiveness is being shaped through an ever-changing process of combat and negotiation involving researchers, government administrators, and representatives of populations at risk.

POLITICS AND PROOF: THE CASE OF AIDS

The AIDS epidemic has lowered institutional resistance to fundamental changes in the design and implementation of RCTs. These changes are being promoted by AIDS activists (ACT UP, 1989) who have captured the attention of drug development agencies. The activists have questioned the fairness of selection processes for clinical trial participants, the necessity for protocol compliance, the extent to which participants are getting optimal treatment, and the lengthy time for completion of drug development (Palca, 1989).

AIDS activists are also concerned about more basic scientific issues: whether, for example, competent background studies were conducted on the pharmacology of agents to be tested (ACT UP, 1989). And they have challenged research priorities, arguing for greater emphasis on prevention and treatment of opportunistic infections in addition to HIV-focused research.

Some of the activists' concerns stem from features of RCTs that make them appear socially insensitive and impersonal: first, clinical trials (particularly efficacy studies) require adherence to protocol rules independent of the unique circumstances of subjects; second, although investigators try to ensure that clinical trials are "treatment neutral" (and, thus, that randomization is fair), potential participants are often skeptical; third, the structure of an RCT unavoidably reduces participant freedom of choice.

Eligibility criteria for clinical trials include such considerations as sociodemographic attributes, comorbidities, and treatment history. Selection constraints are necessary to protect patients, reduce variance, and maximize the power of inferences from trials. However, rejected subjects may view the selection process as discriminatory, especially in the absence of a viable therapeutic option. AIDS activists also contend that eligibility criteria can be so restrictive they reduce, rather than enhance, chances of demonstrating treatment efficacy.

Numerous factors, including treatment complexities and toxicities, affect patient compliance with trial protocols. Since noncompliance threatens the integrity of the trial, investigators mount major efforts to assure adherence. Patients may well perceive such efforts as a form of coercion that can be hard to resist when their very lives may depend on cooperation.

Additionally, design requirements of an RCT can make potential subjects believe they might receive less than optimal treatment, even though what is considered optimal may be very much in dispute. Concerns may focus on treatment blinding, placebo controls, treatment groups that receive the lower dose of a drug or the more radical surgical procedure, or inclusion of a "standard" therapy of limited value.

Inclusion of placebo controls in an RCT may be the most reasonable way to establish proof of benefit when there is no applicable standard treatment. But faced with certainty of death, AIDS patients want every arm of a clinical trial to include therapies that offer hope of help. The window of opportunity to use placebo-only controls may well have passed, even where standard treatments are inapplicable. However, placebos might be acceptable to patients if they are combined with active drugs in multi-therapy factorial designs or if patients are asymptomatic, particularly if the experimental treatment were known to be highly toxic.

Circumstances under which placebo controls could be scientifically and ethically appropriate are continuously being discussed. Other considerations include whether patients will be concurrently taking an active drug for HIV or the opportunistic infection under study, whether the protocol permits switchovers to the experimental drug in case of disease progression, and how closely patients will be monitored. Some spokespersons for the AIDS community appreciate the value of placebos in drug development and might endorse their inclusion in certain clinical trials.

AIDS activists have attacked the Food and Drug Administration (FDA) for allegedly impeding drug development and evaluation. Many of the complaints about the FDA concern the time it takes to ensure the safety and efficacy of new drugs.[5] In response to the AIDS epidemic, the FDA has implemented new initiatives to expedite the clinical-trial and drug-approval process for patients with life-threatening illnesses.

To address the broader issues, creative approaches have been negotiated by researchers, AIDS activists, and community physicians (Specter, 1989). Strategies include randomized trials without placebo controls, even where patients are intolerant of the standard treatment; "parallel tracking" that permits more widespread access to experimental drugs; and community-based studies that use nontraditional technologies and sanction community control over the design and conduct of certain RCTs (Specter, 1990).

Two trials of the antiviral drug dideoxyinosine (DDI) are comparing its effectiveness with AZT; but a third trial for patients intolerant of AZT is simply comparing low and high doses of DDI. Although a placebo control might be justified scientifically, it was judged unacceptable on ethical grounds. Without a standard control group, demonstrating drug efficacy may be difficult, even with historical controls. Usually, efficacy is determined before tests of optimal dosage.[6]

Pragmatically, AIDS patients have veto power over the design of RCTs containing placebo arms. One drug trial for a serious opportunistic infection failed to accrue sufficient patients when it included placebo controls. As a result, another trial for the same infection was designed to allow patients to state preferences among options that all involve randomization to active therapies. Before being randomized, patients can elect immediate or deferred treatment or to have that decision also be made randomly. In designing the protocol, the investigators solicited input from community physicians, potential subjects, and their representatives (J. Holbrook, personal communication).

Parallel tracking (Secretary of Health and Human Services, 1990), performed concurrently with an RCT, takes advantage of compassionate drug distribution to make promising investigational drugs available to HIV patients who have no therapeutic alternatives and cannot participate in the trial. At a minimum, parallel tracking will help measure side effects (particularly rare toxicities) by expanding the population at risk. The larger, more diverse subject population might also provide clues about the generalizability of RCT results. An approach analogous to parallel tracking, known as "expanded access," already accompanies such studies as the DDI trials. However, researchers have clearly indicated that parallel tracking must not interfere with the viability of concurrent trials. If interference occurs, parallel tracking will be constrained.

The community-based research encourages grass-roots studies. Potential investigations include observations of self-experimentation among AIDS patients (particularly with unapproved drugs and diet), enumeration of opportunistic infections, and systematic assessments of the natural history of the disease. "Low-tech" trials may also be promoted,[7] as well as other nontraditional designs. For example, expanded factorial designs would permit simultaneous assessments of multiple drugs and their combinations.

The program answers community needs at the interface of research and intervention, and thus has implications for alcohol prevention research. Participating institutions include health centers and consortiums not served by the AIDS Clinical Trials Group, whose experienced investigators have access to state-of-the-art resources. Patients represented by the program are "underserved" and undercovered by health insurance, with an emphasis on racial minorities, intravenous drug users, and women. Specific research protocols will come from community-based primary-care physicians rather than referral centers; and clinical rather than sophisticated laboratory outcomes will be stressed, in keeping with "low-tech" resources. In the process of research, physicians will be trained in clinical-trials methodology.

Another issue being discussed in AIDS research is flexibility in protocol compliance. The activists are adamant that subjects who suffer AIDS-related problems during clinical trials receive immediate help with proven or promising therapies, regardless of how the trial might be affected. In response, researchers are attempting to build greater protections for subjects into trial protocols.

Victims of other diseases are beginning to emulate the constructive work of the AIDS activists. Socio-political attempts to influence clinical trials also *predate* the AIDS epidemic. For example, the trial that tested the unconventional drug laetrile for cancer was a direct response to pressure from patients seeking laetrile treatment. The trial demonstrated that laetrile was not effective as a cancer therapy and that it was actually toxic (Moertel et al., 1982). More recently, members of Congress have requested that the Office of Technology Assessment examine the evidence concerning the efficacy of unconventional immuno-augmentative therapy for cancer and develop a protocol to evaluate it (Report, 1990; Holden, 1988).

Another form of socio-political influence in the cancer area is exemplified by those who advocate alternatives to mortality as scientifically justified endpoints for the RCT (e.g., disease-free interval, quality of life, and reduction of symptoms [Criteria, 1989]). These types of outcomes are of particular interest to patients, and in both the cancer and AIDS areas, they are receiving increased attention.

POLITICS AND PROOF: THE ALCOHOL ARENA

The AIDS illustration is a special case of conflict between prudence and proof. The interventions of primary interest are drugs, not behavioral-change strategies; the cost of drug failure is death; only one anti-retroviral drug has officially proven effective in delaying death, and its impact is limited; risk groups are mobilized for political action (Shilts, 1987); and the disease is contagious, which broadens risk. However, the alcohol arena has its own social forces that shape the conduct of science. And some are embodiments and reflections of power structures, ethical principles, health-care practices, and styles of study that have also influenced AIDS research. The following case histories are instructive.

Confronting Vested Interests

For adults ages 21 and older, alcohol is a legal drug that has legitimate recreational, cultural, and medicinal uses in American society. The alcohol beverage industry (including its production and service components) is a powerful political and economic force that spends well over a billion dollars a year on advertising alone (Atkin, 1988; U.S. General Accounting Office, 1989; American Medical Association Board of Trustees, 1986). Although the industry acknowledges that consumption of alcohol can have deleterious consequences, it takes a parochial view of the origin and scope of these problems and the hazards of consumption per se. Thus, industry-initiated prevention campaigns focus on "responsible" drinking by individuals or groups (e.g., the "Know Your Limits" campaign) in preference to environmental interventions that could threaten profits (Paddock, 1989). Server-training programs may be an exception that helps protect the industry from liability suits (McKnight, 1991).

More germane here are attempts by the alcohol industry to influence prevention research and research-based policy making. Segments of the industry actually fund prevention research (e.g., studies of drunk-driving deterrence, but there are clear indications that the industry opposes intervention research that has the potential of reducing alcohol consumption, particularly where whole communities are the targets. It also appears that the industry opposes research-oriented workshops that may generate consumption-reducing policies.

In 1988, representatives of the alcohol beverage industry, in alliance with broadcasters and advertisers, attempted to legally enjoin the Surgeon General's Workshop on Drunk Driving (Surgeon General: Proceedings, 1989).[8] The workshop had been initiated by Congress to explore opportunities for intervention and research on drunk driving (Surgeon General: Proceedings, 1989; Surgeon General: Background Papers, 1989). Although the workshop was allowed to continue, participants were mandated to conduct their dialogue in the presence of industry and media "observers." Predictably, these observers were most concerned about the evolving recommendations regarding advertising, counter advertising, taxation, and constraints on alcohol availability.

It appears that the recommendations were not dramatically affected by pressures of the industry, perhaps because the Surgeon General took a forthright position against contamination of inquiry (Surgeon General: Proceedings, 1989). By contrast, the history of the "Winners Program" in California during the late 1970's suggests that the beverage industry can substantially influence the process of inquiry—shaping and suppressing features of alcohol prevention research.

The "Winners Program" was a three-community demonstration project, sponsored by the California Department of Alcohol and Drug Programs (Wallack and Barrows, 1982-83) and modeled after the Stanford Heart Disease Project (Maccoby et al., 1977). In one community, media and community-action approaches were used; in another, the intervention involved the media alone; and the third community served as a control. Officially, the program had a continuum of goals: changing awareness, knowledge, and attitudes about alcohol problems or use; then changing drinking behavior and per capita consumption; and ultimately reducing indicators of alcohol problems (Wallack and Barrows, 1981). Unofficially, however, there appeared to be some confusion about program goals, especially whether reduction of consumption (even abstinence) or reduction of problems was the primary objective (Room, 1990).

Potential achievement of the official outcomes, particularly reduced consumption, could well be considered a threat to the alcohol industry. And in fact the state wine industry took action against the media messages by involving the Governor of California. According to Robin Room, the project "was born as a political decision and continued to be politicized for as long as it was politically visible" (Room, 1990).

The media campaign was patterned after industry marketing approaches that emphasize immediate gratification from drinking (Wallack and Barrows, 1982-83). Here, however, the theme was gratification by not drinking or by specifically limiting consumption (e.g., to one drink). Airing of the first wave of television spots was suddenly postponed through efforts of the Governor and an influential state assemblyman (Room, 1990), who were concerned about morality aspects of the messages and enunciation of concrete drinking limits (Wallack and Barrows, 1981; Room, 1990). After reviewing the situation, "the Governor ordered that two of the three commercials be replaced and the third one altered" (Wallack and Barrows, 1982-83). The effect of this whole process was to water down the excess drinking message and severely curtail anticipated viewer exposure because of increased cost constraints (Wallack and Barrows, 1982-83; Room, 1990).

Evaluation of program outcomes showed modest increases in knowledge and awareness of alcohol issues but no evidence of changes in attitudes or behavior concerning drinking (Wallack and Barrows, 1982-83; Room, 1990). It might be presumptuous to suggest that the absence of behavioral effects was partially a consequence of industry pressure. Yet, counter advertising in the tobacco arena was apparently an effective strategy for reducing cigarette smoking, at least in the short run (Office on Smoking and Health, 1989); and constraints on the freedom of prevention researchers to test interventions that offer the greatest promise of success clearly weaken and complicate the quest for proof. For example, the smaller the expected effect, the greater the sample size needed to reveal its presence.

Implementation of the most promising "environmental" strategies (e.g., increases in the price of alcohol and decreases in its availability [Secretary of Health and Human Services, 1987]) largely depends on political action. If counter advertising and warning labels are seen as threats to the beverage industry, the prospect of increased taxes on alcohol could stimulate even greater concern (Paddock, 1989).

Those who advocate a public-health approach to alcohol beverage control appreciate the role of "community action" in generating support for environmental interventions, such as curtailing alcohol outlets (Mosher and Colman, 1989). Studying community movements requires qualitative and quantitative methodologies oriented toward analysis of policy planning, organizational dynamics, collective behavior, and conflict resolution. The process by which community objectives are developed, implemented, and achieved or not achieved becomes a research focus in its own right. Thus, analytic methods used by students of technology transfer (including dissemination of change *concepts*) might be adapted to the alcohol area.

Validating Self-Reports

Self-reports of alcohol consumption and problems are commonly used endpoints for epidemiologic and prevention research. However, in treatment research, where respondents tend to be dependent upon alcohol and to have concurrent medical and psychological problems, outcome measures that rely totally on self-report are increasingly suspect. Study sections that review grants for the National Institute on Alcohol Abuse and Alcoholism (NIAAA) are requiring confirmation of the validity of self-reports through blood and urine tests, breathalyzers, and statements of significant others, including therapists.

These approaches are not easily incorporated into large-scale surveys. Hence, epidemiologists who must rely on self-reports may focus on *comparisons* of rates over time rather than their absolute value, implicitly assuming that any biases are essentially constant over time. Unfortunately, self-reports of drinking behavior may be influenced by perceived social expectations. Thus, changes in these reports may simply reflect changing definitions of the normative situation. It may, therefore, be necessary to seek external validation from sources independent of the respondents (e.g., sales data).

In treatment research, *laboratory* validation of self-reports is an established component of clinical trials for alcoholism (Fuller, Lee, and Gordis, 1988) and other diseases. However, a recent experience of NIAAA concerning validation demonstrates that challenging veracity for the purpose of research can seriously threaten "therapeutic communities." This may be particularly true if the quest for proof necessitates testing of "body fluids" (specifically, blood or urine) that must be voluntarily provided by participating subjects.

NIAAA is currently funding a long-term research project that tests an AIDS-oriented primary prevention strategy in an alcohol treatment setting. The subjects are homosexual men undergoing group therapy for alcohol and/or drug abuse in an outpatient clinic. Their baseline incidence of unprotected anal intercourse appears to be significantly higher than the rate for homosexual men in the community, estimated from a randomized survey. This finding is consistent with studies that show positive links between use of alcohol (or other drugs) during homosexual intercourse and high-risk sex (Stall et al., 1986; Valdiserri et al., 1988; Peterson and McKirnan, 1989).

The present study is testing the effectiveness of an educational intervention that encourages in-depth discussion of barriers to and facilitators of safe homosexual sex. The intervention is introduced into half the sessions of a 16-week alcohol treatment program, employing an RCT design with usual-treatment groups as controls. Although alcohol use is not the major endpoint, it is believed to be an important predictor of outcomes of the safe-sex intervention. Moreover, the investigators want to be assured that the safe-sex strategy does not disrupt the alcoholism therapy. They, therefore, measure alcohol consumption patterns during the study.

The investigators initially proposed to assess drinking through questions that measured the consistency of self-reports and through therapist observations. The review committee urged additional validation through urine tests, and the investigators attempted to comply. However, the alcohol clinic directors firmly opposed any collection of urine, inside or outside clinic walls. They felt such procedures would compromise the ethos of trust they regard as essential for the successful treatment of alcoholism. There was also concern that HIV antibody might be discernible in urine and that reporting of persons who are HIV positive might soon be required in that state. Devoid of apparent options, the investigators stood their ground against the urine tests; and the reviewers remained wary of the self-report procedures.

Recognizing the dilemma, NIAAA proposed a compromise, which the clinic accepted: breathalyzer tests. According to the principal investigator, the breathalyzer test was regarded as relatively unobtrusive and not a serious threat to trust or HIV privacy. Furthermore, the NIAAA proposal was viewed as an act of good faith that would enable the research and safe-sex program to be funded.

Challenging Revered Ideologies

Police sobriety checkpoints (roadblocks) on the nation's roads and highways are an established strategy for enforcing laws against drunk driving. The procedure has been judged constitutional by the U.S. Supreme Court, and its randomization features have been sanctioned by several U.S. district courts as a constraint on police discretion. Researchers in drunk driving have taken advantage of roadblocks to study realistically the prevalence of driver intoxication and its risk factors. Without the aid of police, it would be virtually impossible to implement such studies. And self-reports of drunk driving are vulnerable to distortions.

One research approach (the "downstream" procedure) is to piggyback the study on police actions that happen naturally. After a real roadblock occurs, police encourage drivers to help the adjacent researchers by answering questions and voluntarily undergoing breath tests. The second approach uses police for roadblocks entirely dedicated to research. Although the police stop the cars and direct traffic, they do not examine occupants; they simply motion the cars into the study area.

In both situations, researchers try to distinguish themselves from law enforcement, gathering their information confidentially and defining consumption levels according to study objectives. However, they are sensitive to ethical and liability considerations. If drivers who have been drinking are perceived as dangerous, the researchers will drive them home or pay for taxis or a motel. And if the drivers refuse assistance, the police may be notified.

During 1989, a study of "tolerant" drunk drivers[9] that involved police roadblocks encountered unexpected opposition from two ideological extremes: civil libertarians and proponents of law and order. The researchers planned to use the roadblocks to screen prospective volunteer subjects. The police were simply catalysts for the research. Following his usual custom, the principal investigator publicized the roadblocks to inform, reassure, and gain support from potential motorists/subjects. This time, however, the publicity backfired.

Civil libertarians attacked the study for misusing police power and coercing drivers into participating in the research. Law and order enthusiasts voiced opposition because drunk drivers were not being arrested or punished. While public officials debated alternative actions, the study essentially came to a halt. During the pause, the investigators determined that police could legitimately employ roadblocks simply for deterrence, without necessarily arresting anyone. But this theoretical argument did not quell the opposition.

To quiet both sets of critics, the investigators then offered to use the "downstream" approach, allowing the police to arrest obvious drunk drivers while directing "tolerant" (invisible) ones to the researchers. However, it became apparent that this option was no longer tenable, because the police were now using the same sophisticated detection equipment (breathalyzers) as the researchers. Thus, "tolerant" drivers would also be caught in the police net and not be permitted to go "downstream" to the researchers.

The only solution was to use the police simply as research catalysts, but this was now out of the question. So the investigators had to find another site for their research. The moral of the story is in the eye of the beholder. According to the principal investigator, "researchers should not necessarily rely on past written commitments of public officials," which is perhaps another way of saying: Politics has its own momentum, and community research in the alcohol area is by definition political.

CONCLUSION

This chapter had two purposes: First, to describe socio-political constraints on scientific inquiry in domains of community-based prevention research, and second, to identify ways prevention strategists and researchers can deal with these constraints to better serve the goals of science and policy.

The proposed criteria for prudent decision making, in the absence of proof, stress the importance of a research orientation among prevention practitioners. Prudence demands objective assessments of available evidence concerning the success and failure of previous interventions. It also calls for appropriate integration of evaluation research into ongoing prevention activity, to facilitate midstream corrections and to enhance science. The better the scientific foundation underlying the choice and adaptation of prevention strategies, the more effective they will be.

Social, economic, and political realities may force policy makers to move beyond existing knowledge into untested territory or to select options that are less than ideal. Through informed anticipation, decision makers may be able to control future events and to avoid serious disruptions in the momentum of prevention programs. With respect to research, socio-political realities are influencing the armamentarium of scientific inquiry—the design, content, and implementation of community-based research. This effect is most obvious in the AIDS area where fundamental changes are occurring in the choice of comparison groups, the breadth and precision of data collection, the expansion of low-technology trials, and the involvement of community leaders in the development of science.

The relevance of these changes to alcohol prevention research remains to be seen. However, both research milieus involve highly visible emotionally charged problems, articulate political action groups, conflicts of interest between subsections of the community, and demands on policy makers to find solutions that go beyond the state of science.

Clearly, the precepts of science mandate that compromises in research approaches be limited. Yet, freedom of inquiry is bounded by social realities. Through cautious creativity, new styles of research are evolving that do justice to the prerequisites of science and concerns of citizens. Of course, their emer-gence in one field does not guarantee applicability elsewhere. But the universality of the scientific method and fundamental commonalties in human behavior are grounds for optimism that gains in one domain of health science can be exploited by another.

NOTES

Dr. Barofsky had primary responsibility for conceptualizing and writing the section on AIDS, in collaboration with Dr. Howard.

1. E.g., prescribing aspirin to heart attack victims receiving placebo medication, as a means of preventing their subsequent death.

2. Defined in the dictionary as "sound judgment" (Guralnik, 1982).

3.   They might also be falsely convinced through marketing promotions that a particular prevention strategy (e.g., a school curriculum) has proven effective when proof is yet to be established.

4.   Research on this topic is almost nonexistent. However, one study suggests that passengers in drinking groups with designated drivers may consume more alcohol on average than comparable groups without such drivers (Shore, Gregory, and Tatlock, 1991).

5.   Delays in drug development and dissemination are also of concern in the cancer area. High-level debates between representatives of the research establishment are addressing such questions as when and how to share clinical-trial results with physicians and the public (DeVita, 1990).

6.   The effectiveness of an aerosol form of pentamidine for opportunistic infections has already been established by community physicians through a trial that compared three dosage levels of the drug without a placebo control. Because the two higher doses were clearly more effective than the lowest, the drug was judged beneficial. Had there been no difference, the interpretation of findings might have been more problematic.

7.   "Low-tech" trials involve minimal data collection and minimal requirements for expensive or invasive procedures.

8.   In addition, the National Commission Against Drunk Driving (which includes representatives of the beverage industry [Wagenaar, 1990]) tried unsuccessfully to delay release of certain Workshop recommendations for at least 16 months (Surgeon General: Proceedings, 1989).

9.   A high-alcohol "tolerant" driver has a blood alcohol concentration above the legal limit but does not show manifest clinical signs of intoxication.

14

Undertaking a Community Prevention Trial to Reduce Alcohol Problems: Translating Theoretical Models into Action

Harold D. Holder

INTRODUCTION

The previous chapters have identified conceptual and methodological issues for investigators undertaking community prevention trials for alcohol problems. Ways to address those issues have also been suggested. Many of the chapters have been written by professionals who are active participants in ongoing community prevention trials in the areas of heart disease and cancer reduction. There are important lessons that investigators in the alcohol prevention field can learn from these research projects.

This book has also identified important differences between the alcohol field and heart disease and cancer reduction; these differences may suggest unique approaches and strategies. Most likely community-based alcohol-problem prevention trials will represent hybrids, incorporating some of the techniques, approaches, and experiences from other projects in the health area and developing approaches and strategies appropriate to the uniqueness of alcohol problems.

The purpose of this chapter is to build upon the foundation of the previous chapters and suggest some guidelines for undertaking community prevention trials for alcohol problems.

SELECTION OF COMMUNITY PERSPECTIVE IN ALCOHOL-PROBLEM PREVENTION

What perspective should an investigator take in a community prevention trial? As described in the first chapter, it is possible to consider the community as a target population of individuals (or subgroups) who are at risk for specific health problems or other untoward conditions. This perspective most accurately characterizes prevention trials in the area of heart disease, cancer, and alcohol problems resulting from chronic, high-volume use of alcohol, e.g., cirrhosis of the liver.

It is also possible to consider alcohol problems as the product of complex systems, i.e., to take a systems approach to the problem. Thus, systems rather than individuals become targets for intervention in an effort to reduce problems. Each of these two perspectives has important implications for the identification and measurement of target alcohol problem(s) and populations; each perspective affects selection of prevention interventions to reduce the target problem(s).

Catchment Approach

Most of the previous heart disease and cancer community prevention trials have employed a catchment area approach to some degree. There are at least three reasons for using this approach. First, the target of these trials is a well-defined state or condition into which individual residents of the community who fulfill the criteria can be assigned. For example, if heavy smokers are the target group, then individuals who are heavy smokers can be identified, and educational programs for smoking reduction and/or cessation can be developed.

A second reason for employing the catchment approach is that there exists an empirically tested causal model of the condition for individuals. For example, community heart disease projects have made effective use of the link between diet, exercise, smoking, and genetics both to enable individuals who are at risk (due to one or more of these factors) to be identified (including self-identification) and to develop programs to aid these individuals to change behavior. A third reason a catchment approach has been successfully used in previous health prevention trials is that individual behavior can be changed through education. Prior trials have demonstrated that changes in individual knowledge and behavioral skills can result in improved health status.

Within alcohol-problem prevention research, causal models of individual behavior that can be used unequivocally to design prevention trials have not been developed. As will be noted later, such individual-only models are likely to be inadequate. This does not mean that we are without potentially effective prevention tools and approaches; later in this chapter, a number of prevention strategies are summarized.

Alcohol use versus abstinence does not have the same unambivalent status within the community as, say, eating or not eating butter, red meat, and cheese, or not smoking. Norms against smoking in recent years have encouraged nonsmoking as a desired condition but have not encouraged "moderate smoking." However, personal abstinence from alcohol is not a meaningful social or epidemiological community prevention goal (except for alcoholics). Among drinkers, the heavy-dependent users (alcoholics) have the greatest risk for alcohol problems, but they are not the *largest* at-risk group as was documented in the chapter by Saltz et al. in this volume.

Community-level alcohol information and educational programs have been tried in the past. They have typically been one-time investments in education and public awareness, reflecting the belief (or hope) that a "shot" of prevention will render the community safe. Most such educational programs have shown little long-term impact on drinking behavior; their effect has been largely limited to increasing the amount of information people have about alcohol and altering their attitudes (Kinder, 1975; Blane, 1976; Blane and Hewitt, 1977; Cameron, 1979; Wallack, 1983). On the other hand, well-planned intensive community education using the communication approach along with structural changes in alcohol access, particularly in high-risk situations such as driving, has a real potential for success (Hochheimer, 1981; Holder and Blose, 1985). Such programs have not yet been undertaken as part of a large scale prevention trial.

Some environmental strategies have been employed in heart disease and cancer prevention trials. For example, projects have worked to get restaurants to offer low-fat menu alternatives, to make low-salt food products available and prominently displayed in grocery stores, to get warning labels installed about the hazards of smoking at points of sale for cigarettes, and to increase the number of no-smoking areas within public spaces and at the workplace. However, few community health trials have employed public policy alternatives, for example, to mandate the availability of low-fat food alternatives or increase the retail price of cigarettes or legally restrict their availability. Local restrictions on cigarette vending machines as a means to reduce underage smoking have been enacted and "no smoking" areas have been established. There are obviously good reasons for not utilizing such strategies in disease prevention trials, including the avoidance of political issues and debate surrounding the use of law or regulation. In addition, individual education and skill training have been generally accepted by community leaders.

However, alcohol-problem prevention has a long tradition of public policy, e.g., the control and regulation of alcoholic beverages. Every state has some form of state agency for alcoholic beverage control that regulates the licensing of establishments to sell alcohol for consumption on the retail site (on-premise) or for later consumption elsewhere (off-premise). In addition, legal levels of unacceptable alcohol in the bloodstream (Blood Alcohol Concentration—BAC) have been established for operators of motor vehicles, i.e., limits at which point a person is considered too impaired to drive. Even lower levels are set for drivers of commercial vehicles, and a zero level is set for airline pilots.

Systems Approach

One rationale for employing a system strategy is that many alcohol problems are stochastic events, i.e., time dependent and probabilistic. These events are not predictable in terms of individual characteristics only. The probability that any one drinker at any specific time will incur an alcohol-involved trauma or death is usually quite low. For example, the chances of an alcohol-impaired driver being stopped and arrested by the police is estimated to be 1 in 2,000 events on the average, and the chances of an auto crash following drinking are estimated to be even lower (Farris, Malone, and Kirkpatrick, 1977; Fell, 1983a, 1983b; Zobeck, 1986). Thus, one can argue that many alcohol problems are not simply the actions of a set of definable high-risk individuals but, rather, are the accumulative result of the structure and flow of complex social, cultural, and economic factors within the community system.

Most heavily addicted drinkers will continue their drinking pattern throughout their life and never incur an alcohol-involved traffic crash or encounter the police. On the other hand, an 18-year-old with limited driving and drinking experience may cause a serious auto crash with small amounts of alcohol in his or her blood. Physical and cognitive impairment begins as soon as the body begins to metabolize ethanol; impairment increases as more ethanol enters the blood. This means that individuals can become increasingly impaired over time as they continue to drink. The rate of impairment is a function of such factors as alcohol experience and tolerance, body weight, amount of food consumed while drinking, and rate of alcohol intake.

Further, it is not possible to permanently "inoculate" a community population against alcohol-related problems using education and skills training alone. The community is a dynamic system. The system changes as new members enter and others leave; as alcoholic-beverage marketing and promotion evolve; and as social and economic conditions, including employment and disposable income, change. No single educational prevention program, no matter how good, can sustain its impact, particularly if system-level structural changes are not accomplished (Holder and Wallack, 1986; Wallack, 1983).

GUIDELINES FOR THE SELECTION OF COMMUNITIES FOR ALCOHOL-PROBLEM PREVENTION TRIALS

The purpose of a prevention trial is to test or evaluate the ability of a specific set of planned interventions to reduce a targeted set of alcohol-related problems. Therefore, as much as possible, the effects (or lack thereof) of the interventions should not be confounded or confused with other factors such as economic changes (local prices, physical availability of alcohol), social changes (values about alcohol and its appropriate use), demographic changes (in/out migration, age/gender mix of population), and other confounding social processes.

Therefore, the degree of "isolation" of the community from other influences that can affect the dependent variable(s) and thereby obscure the potential effect of the prevention intervention may be important. Examples of exogenous confounding factors include:

1. A prevention effort/program from a physically adjacent or nearby community.
2. Daily commuting to other areas for employment or recreation, including drinking.
3. Regional differences in mass media coverage of alcohol-related matters and/or advertising.

The degree of containment of access to alcohol for members of the target community is also important. For example, if a change in availability of alcohol for consumption at bars and restaurants (on-premise) is part of the intervention, then it is ideal that most on-premise drinking by test community residents be contained within the defined geographical area. A similar observation can be made for off-premise sources of alcohol (liquor stores, etc.). (Note: The author recognizes that it is unrealistic to expect no contagion.)

It should be noted that community alcohol-problem prevention trials within the United States benefit or suffer depending on such matters as:

1. Substantial common exposure of the population to national television programs and thus common portrayals of alcohol use, as well as national beer and wine advertising.
2. The mobility of community residents from their own community to other locations for work and recreation, with associated exposure to alcohol availability and variations in alcohol marketing.
3. A relatively high level of disposable income, thereby the ability to purchase alcohol.
4. Differences in the above factors by subgroups such as racial or ethnic populations and by income groups.

Suggested criteria for selecting a target community for an alcohol-prevention trial include:

1. Geographical boundary of target community closely fits the social/ economic boundary of employment and social/recreational activities, including sources of on-premise and off-premise alcohol.

2. Community residents share a common mass communication exposure in radio, television, local magazines, and newspapers.
3. Population size is such that:
   a. Social networks and community leadership can be efficiently documented and monitored
   b. Number of alcohol outlets is reasonable for potential monitoring and feasible intervention if desired
   c. Overall size of population is manageable for an experimental project and for data collection with the use of sampling procedures where necessary.
4. Interest exists among active community leaders in alcohol issues (drinking and driving) or related matters (e.g., the litter of alcohol beverage containers or noise related to public drinking). There must be sufficient interest in alcohol problems that the community will support specific prevention strategies.
5. Low tourist involvement is desirable in order to remove the confounding factor of alcohol use and misuse by nonresident drinkers. Of course, it is possible for an effective program to be "blind" to the actual residence of persons affected/influenced by the program and for tourists to contribute to total community-level problems sufficiently to be a target themselves for the program. For example, training beverage servers can have beneficial effects on both residents' and nonresidents' high volume drinking and thus related alcohol problems.

ISSUE OF COMPARISON COMMUNITIES

One common research design has been the use of control groups that do not receive a specific stimulus, treatment, or intervention to provide a reference point for a group that does receive such stimulus, treatment, or intervention. The use of this no treatment group provides a reference or comparison to the treatment group. The treatment-no treatment comparison strengthens the inferences that can be drawn about the effect of the treatment, in addition to inferences drawn from pre- and post-comparison of results for the treatment group only.

While such a design may be standard for many types of studies, it is not an absolute protection from threats to validity even in experimental designs. The application of this design to community studies is not without its advantages and its problems. Following are some positive features of comparison communities.

Comparison communities (if equivalent in essential factors to the test or treated community) provide some (not total) control for contemporaneous factors or events that can affect the target dependent variable(s) in both experimental and control communities. Comparison communities can also provide control for trends that can affect the treated and untreated communities as well, e.g., national consumption patterns. (Note: Communities may well have different trends in alcohol problems and, therefore, a comparison community alone is not an absolute protection against differences in time trends, particularly if a pre/post test design is utilized. Thus if the experimental community has a long-term downward trend (prior to the prevention trial) in drinking and driving crashes and the control community had an upward trend in such crashes, one might make incorrect judgments about prevention efforts using only experimental and control comparisons on a pre and post basis.)

A comparison community increases face validity. Given the expectancies of the scientific community, having comparison communities increases the acceptance of the findings and potential funding if the project proposal is peer reviewed. Comparison communities provide additional data to assist in confirmation of statistical analysis of treated communities, i.e., potentially using longitudinal data from other sites as independent controls for national or regional matters, such as traffic crashes.

Problems with use of comparison communities are notable. The cost of collecting data in additional sites increases overall project costs. This is particularly true if household interviews are used. Also, it is difficult to locate a true comparison community that is sufficiently similar to target communities to be useful. A true matched control community does not exist, even if selected via random assignment (perhaps especially if randomly selected). No community is likely to be an unequivocal match for a target community. Community dynamics make selection of true matching control communities unlikely. Furthermore, the use of comparison communities can deflect attention from a careful examination of the target communities. Since all community prevention trials will have limited research funds available, the cost of data collection in a comparison community will reduce funds for indepth study of the experimental community.

Comparison communities are not necessarily blind and, therefore, can initiate their own programs or activities to "show the treatment community" (compensatory rivalry) or could become/assume a defeatist posture and, thus, actually alter the natural processes (resentful demoralization) (Cook and Campbell, 1979). For example, one of the control communities, Greensboro, NC, for the current COMMIT Nationwide Community Smoking Reduction Trials (an effort to reduce heavy smoking), voted to restrict smoking in public places, thereby potentially confounding its status as a true comparison ("no treatment") community (Gallagher, McDonald, and Winbush, 1990).

Communities using long-term time-series data can be used as reasonable controls for themselves. Longitudinal trends and seasonality of community systems can be effectively controlled for only by data from the target communities. For some dependent variables, it is possible to introduce into a time-series analysis of a locality, national or regional data on the same measure as a control, e.g., miles driven, fatal automobile crashes, and beverage rules, as a substitute for a control community.

Suggested criteria for selecting comparison communities include:

1. Similar population size. Though not an essential criterion, it is likely to increase face validity. Also, all things being equal, communities of similar size are more likely to have things in common with each other than with communities of much larger or smaller population.
2. Similar economic and demographic profiles. These factors are likely to be related to changes and differential rates of alcohol problems. Investigators should look at current levels and past rates of change in such variables as:
   a. Per capita or family disposable income
   b. Age and gender mix of community
   c. Previous (and expected) rates of change for in/out migration
   d. Ethnic and minority group size and composition within total population
   e. Rate of economic growth, e.g., retail sales, taxable property, sales tax revenues, etc.
3. Similar cultural tradition and history.
4. Similar regulation of alcoholic beverages and distribution of number and type of alcohol outlets.
5. Similar level of alcohol sales by beverage type.
6. Low tourist involvement. However, a recreational or entertainment-oriented community may develop its own unique prevention program that incorporates nonresidents in its design.
7. No plans to undertake a unique, independent prevention effort—at least one that is dramatically different from other communities in the region or state (e.g., required school-based alcohol/substance abuse education) or even from the normal process of the target communities.

PHASES IN DEVELOPING AND UNDERTAKING COMMUNITY TRIALS

A number of phases and steps have been identified for undertaking community-based prevention trials (see description by Farquhar and Fortmann in this book as well as Greenwald and Caban, 1986 and Flay, 1986). Such discussions share common concepts and approaches. Each highlights and/or separates various phases to emphasize key steps and decision points. They all share some of the following:

1. Prevention trials are research projects and as such are driven by (based upon) prior research, i.e., utilize in a formal and systematic fashion basic research concerning risk factors and potential intervention points to reduce a specific problem.
2. As research projects, community prevention trials are to be subjected to the same scientific rigor as would be expected of basic research projects.
3. Prevention trials are a natural progression from basic research to application, generally aimed at reducing the incidence and prevalence of health problems.
4. While based upon basic research, prevention trials are concerned with the public health and welfare, and their purpose is to develop the means to reduce problems.

The remainder of this chapter suggests a set of steps or phases to develop and undertake a community prevention trial for alcohol problems. These are not intended to be unique or divergent from those phases developed for prevention trials in other health areas. They are suggestive and intended to highlight key steps in the development and implementation of an alcohol-problem prevention trial. Seven steps are described: Problem Identification, Feasibility Assessment, Trial Design, Pre-Implementation Research, Detailed Project Planning, Program Implementation and Evaluation, and Program Effectiveness Assessment and Interpretation.

Step 1: Problem Identification

The rationale for a community prevention trial is the reduction of one or more alcohol problems. Therefore, the first step is an identification of the problem or problems to be reduced. Problem identification has two aspects: epidemiological and political or cultural.

The epidemiological dimension refers to defining or identifying the problem and determining the actual number or extent of the problem in a population (prevalence) and frequency of occurrence over a time period of, say, one year (incidence). Saltz et al. in this volume identify five criteria for selecting a candidate alcohol problem for a community prevention effort. These are community values, relationship to alcohol consumption, reliability of measurement, practical measurement, and potential reduction through purposeful intervention.

The first criterion recognizes that the definition of what is a problem (or implicitly what problems are given priority) reflects community values and beliefs. For example, if large numbers of babies are dying from malnutrition or childhood diseases, then public intoxication may be of lower concern than infant mortality in that community. The community may consider child deaths as the primary problem and judge public drunkenness as acceptable cultural behavior, partially in response to difficult social and economic conditions. On the other hand, in a community dependent on tourists or downtown retail sales, public drunkenness might be considered a serious problem if shoppers are reluctant to come to areas with a high concentration of street intoxication.

Criterion two requires that alcohol consumption be directly or indirectly related to the undesired outcome (e.g., car crashes). This requires a determination of a *causal* link between alcohol and the outcome, not simple association.

Criterion three requires that measures of the condition or outcome be reliable. Low reliability would make it difficult to attribute any changes in the outcome to the prevention intervention, and serious problems with reliability would likely render the measure invalid.

Criterion four emphasizes the practicality of measurement. While it is possible to demonstrate the theoretical value of a particular outcome measure (such as determination of blood alcohol concentration through the drawing of blood from all subjects), unless such a process were conducted as part of a medical services unit, it could be difficult to use this measurement routinely in prevention education.

Criterion five requires that there be adequate means to reduce the problem either through reductions in alcohol exposure or by disconnecting the link between consumption and the undesired consequence. Even if the causal relationship to alcohol can be demonstrated, there must be a potentially effective means to reduce the alcohol contribution.

Problems identified as potential candidates for alcohol prevention trials should meet all five criteria. If, for example, we are uncertain about the causal link between a certain undesired outcome and alcohol, then further basic epidemiological study is needed before the problem can be the target for preventive action. For example, the basic causal involvement of alcohol in crime is unknown, even with evidence that a significant proportion of violent crime victims had been drinking. (See Saltz et al. in this volume). While alcohol prevention is concerned about any problem with potential (but not fully understood) involvement with alcohol, further basic research is necessary before the problem is the target of a community trial.

These criteria emphasize both the problems of measurement in identifying an alcohol problem and the potential for its reduction though purposeful community-level action. Without an adequate standard or measurement of a problem, meaningful scientific evaluation of a program is impossible.

The selection of a social or health problem involving alcohol is also based upon community values, i.e., does the community consider such alcohol-related events or conditions as undesirable or of sufficient concern to mobilize community resources to reduce the problem? Almost all situations or conditions involving alcohol use are incorporated in one way or another into existing community systems. Some may occur so infrequently that they are accepted or tolerated. However, even if the problem occurs infrequently, it may be considered so severe as to be intolerable. For example, alcohol-related birth defects occur quite infrequently (some estimate them to be 1-3 per 1,000 live births [Institute of Medicine, 1989]), but there are many state and community efforts to prevent such birth outcomes via prenatal and community education and health care.

While the actual incidence and prevalence of an alcohol problem are parts of the decision to select targets for prevention, the final decision must reflect community values and norms. This is not to say that community values cannot be shaped by effective education and community mobilization, but education and organizing are effective only if they incorporate the community's existing beliefs and values.

Step 2: Feasibility Assessment

Determining the feasibility of reducing a specific alcohol problem is important and merits more explanation. The potential to reduce a specific alcohol problem involves both scientific and economic considerations.

A prevention trial, to be potentially effective, must be based on sufficient prior research for investigators to know what factors, situations, and inter-actions increase the risk of the problem. We may not know all causal factors, but a determination of risk is necessary to identify those variables that can be changed through purposeful prevention actions to reduce the problem. Our understanding also requires knowledge of variables that influence risk but that are unlikely to be directly changed by a prevention trial. For example, personal disposable income is highly related to alcohol consumption, but is unlikely to be directly manipulated in a prevention trial. On the other hand, alcohol price is related to alcohol consumption and represents a variable that could be manipulated with taxes or retail price regulations.

If we have an adequate means to measure the incidence of a problem, but lack an adequate understanding of the factors associated with the problem to develop effective interventions, then we fail the test of feasibility. For example, since the risk of lung cancer is highly associated with smoking, smoking cessation is a reasonable prevention intervention. In drinking and driving, we know that the number of drivers on the road with elevated blood alcohol levels (BAL) is highly associated with the rate of alcohol-involved crashes. Therefore, efforts to reduce the BAL of drivers passes the test of feasibility. If a prevention effort to reduce a specific alcohol problem fails the test of feasibility, more basic research is needed before this specific alcohol problem should be the target of a prevention trial.

Step 3: Trial Design

Precursors to designing a trial are having a well-defined alcohol problem, having an accurate measurement of current problem levels or prevalence, having assurance that the community believes the alcohol problem requires prevention action, and having sufficient knowledge of risk to develop interventions to pass the feasibility test.

Two major aspects of the trial design phase are intervention design and evaluation design.

Intervention design is based upon existing research concerning risk factors or settings, as well as any previous research (including other evaluated prevention projects) about specific actions or policies. In this phase science meets art in a creative and synergistic manner to produce potentially effective community interventions capable of being evaluated. In general, designing intervention programs requires skills and experiences quite different from the skills and experiences required to do research. For example, professionals who know how to develop training materials and do both targeted and general public training are essential in intervention design.

However, prevention materials and program development must be grounded in existing research and be able to use existing science. This suggests the need for a partnership between basic researchers and program design specialists who can work together productively. For example, scientific knowledge that a specific factor contributes to increased risk of an alcohol problem is not the same as determining the most effective strategy to alter this factor. On the other hand, interesting and stimulating educational materials for community orientation may have no affect on factors that most influence the target alcohol problem.

The most successful prevention strategies to date have employed public policies that affect access to alcohol. The most successful recent example has been raising the minimum purchase age for alcohol (Wagenaar, 1983; Wagenaar and Maybee, 1986; U.S. General Accounting Office, 1987a). Restricted access to alcohol was shown to reduce alcohol-involved traffic crashes for adolescents by between 8 and 20%. The possibility of using the price sensitivity of alcohol to reduce consumers' economic access introduces another system strategy that could reduce alcohol-involved traffic crashes and cirrhosis mortality (Cook and Tauchen, 1982; Coate and Grossman, 1988).

Examples of potential alcohol-problem prevention strategies that could be considered at the local level include:

1. Reducing alcoholic-beverage availability through local zoning of outlets (Wittman, 1986; Wittman and Hilton, 1987).
2. Educating servers of alcohol to institute policies to reduce heavy consumption and reduce blood alcohol levels of patrons (Saltz, 1987, 1989; McKnight, 1987; Russ and Geller, 1987).
3. Changing the form of alcohol availability, such as sale of distilled spirits by the individual drink (Holder and Blose, 1987a; Blose and Holder, 1987a, 1987b), or licensing private individuals to sell wine and/or distilled spirits by the bottle (Wagenaar and Holder, 1991; Holder and Wagenaar, 1990).
4. Increasing retail prices of alcoholic beverages (Cook and Tauchen, 1982; Ornstein and Hanssens, 1983; Levy and Sheflin, 1983; Hoadley, Fuchs, and Holder, 1984; Saffer and Grossman, 1987a).
5. Reducing access of young people to alcohol through increased enforcement of the minimum purchase age (National Highway Traffic Safety Administration, 1982; Wagenaar, 1983, 1986, 1987; U.S. General Accounting Office, 1987a).
6. Educating young people through school-based programs and the general population through the mass media (Moskowitz, 1989; Pentz et al., 1989).
7. Educating drivers about blood alcohol levels and corresponding crash risks (Phelps, 1988; Worden et al., 1989).
8. Establishing curfews to limit hours of alcohol sales to young people (Preusser et al., 1984; Williams, Lund, and Preusser, 1984).
9. Increasing local police enforcement of drinking and driving as a general deterrent (Ross, 1982; Voas and Hause, 1987).
10. Establishing random roadblocks for deterring drinking and driving (Homel, 1988; Voas, 1989).
11. Making loss of license mandatory and increasing punishment for any DUI conviction as a general deterrent (Williams, Lund, and Preusser, 1984; Vingilis et al., 1988).

Evaluation design includes at least four elements, as follows:

1. Outcome Measurement. The problem selection phase described above requires an adequate definition of the alcohol problem. This is not the same as determining the best means to measure the problem over time as a part of evaluation. Here our concern is

with how to undertake a reliable and valid measurement of the
target problem(s). Investigators seek an unbiased assessment of
any changes in the problem.

2. Effectiveness Assessment. Good science requires a determination
of the effect(s) of the prevention intervention; that is, a research
design capable of isolating the effect of the purposeful intervention
on the target. The chapters by Reichardt and Ross in this volume
describe a number of alternative designs to determine effect and
will not be repeated here. However, it is important to underscore
this point: controlled evaluation is an essential component of the
community trial. The research design must be customized to fit
the community situation and interventions planned.

The greatest threat to evaluation is ruling out alternative explanations for any observed changes in the target alcohol problem.
Since community trials are by definition undertaken in the
dynamic ebb and flow of a social, economic, and cultural system,
the challenge to evaluators is how to account for such influences
and effects of other factors while accurately attributing effects to
the intervention itself.

3. Intervening Variable Assessment. While outcome assessment is
concerned with overall program effect or distal outcomes, intervening assessment is concerned with determining the effect of
program activities on short term or intervening factors. For
example, if the final objective is the reduction of alcohol-involved
traffic crashes in a community, then one might be interested in the
distribution of the number of drivers on the road with high blood
alcohol concentrations before, during, and after prevention programs. Since these distributions are known to be related to the
number of actual alcohol-involved crashes (the final outcome
measure), then a determination of any changes in the BAC distribution of drivers gives information about a change in an important
intervening variable. If public norms against drinking and driving
are a part of the causal chain leading to reductions in crashes, then
determining changes in these community values about driving after
or while drinking may be necessary.

4. Process Assessment. Process assessment refers to documenting
the actual level (or dosage) and timing of the intervention. While
specific interventions may be planned, it is essential to understand
how much of the planned intervention was actually implemented
or how the intervention was actually distributed among the target
population, e.g., the number of people or organizations involved.
Documentation assists us in determining the amount of an intervention actually produced in practice so that we can link specific

changes in outcome with levels of actual implementation. Documentation also helps investigators identify problems in design and implementation during and after the prevention trial.

Step 4: Pre-Implementation Research

In the design phase (third phase), investigators may find that adequate research about specific aspects of program activity, measurement, and potential effects is missing. This omission may require small scale research to investigate parts of the design planned. Pre-testing program materials and activities is an example. Others would be pilot testing elements of the trials in small subgroups or in locations other than the target or control communities, or testing outcome measurement through validation using alternative approaches or instruments.

During this phase, experimental or previously untested program elements can be examined and evaluated prior to full scale application. This phase includes activities, sometimes called "formative research," to develop and test new approaches, strategies, and/or materials. An important activity before implementation is estimating potential effectiveness of the planned strategies. This assessment is often accomplished by simple extension of the successes of prior prevention. However, simple extension could be inadequate. For example, the community(ies) involved may have significant differences with the communities used in prior testing, or new trends can occur that will affect outcomes, e.g., changes in economic conditions.

One technology that may help assess long-term effectiveness is computer simulation. Simulation has been used in business, military, and health services planning. It can be used to estimate potential or likely long-term results of specific alcohol problem prevention strategies and interventions. Such estimates, which are only as good as previous research, cannot replace good planning and design. What they can do, however, is complement and assist the introduction of basic research into the planning process. One example of the use of this technology has been described by Holder and Blose (1988). In this prevention planning project, community leaders identified prevention interventions that they preferred to reduce alcohol-involved traffic crashes in San Diego County, California. Each of these interventions was examined through computer simulation, incorporating the best available research and local data. The projections of potential long-term effects of each proposed intervention facilitated the actual discussion and decision making by the community planning group in designing the prevention program.

Step 5: Detailed Project Planning

In the phases prior to this one, investigators develop the overall outline and design of the community trial. Questions of program activity, methods, measurement, and assessment are answered in earlier phases. However, those answers do not constitute the final detailed plan for the community trial.

A detailed project plan is the key to project management and the effective and efficient use of project resources. A timeline for all project activities, specifying the start and duration of each program and evaluation activity, is essential. Since a community prevention trial is a complex mix of program and evaluation activities, personnel, and other resources, a detailed schedule for the life of the project is an essential dimension, not a luxury. Of course, such a plan is expected to be modified and revised amidst the actual dynamics of a community prevention trial.

Step 6: Program Implementation and Evaluation

Three general parts of an actual community trial can be identified as baseline measurement, i.e., pre-implementation, implementation, and post implementation measurement.

Baseline measurement refers to that time when no prevention activities have yet been introduced into the community. This is the time for collecting all baseline measures and determining the level of the target alcohol problems *before* prevention interventions occur.

Implementation is that time after baseline measurement is completed when purposeful prevention activities are undertaken, including any planned community mobilization or organization. During this time in the prevention trial, investigators undertake all planned interventions and alterations of existing natural processes that drive or influence alcohol problems.

If the prevention trial is designed to deliver time-delimited prevention activities, programs, or strategies, the *after implementation* portion of the trial is the period following the end of program activities during which outcome data are collected and program processes documented. If implementations continue through the life of the trial or are designed to be incorporated into existing community structures and processes, there is actually no "after implementation," but the continuous monitoring of process and outcome.

Step 7: Program Effectiveness Assessment and Interpretation

This is the time for documenting overall changes in the levels of target alcohol problems and for conducting analyses to determine whether changes can be appropriately attributed to the prevention interventions. This is also a time for reviewing the program activity documentation and examining the relative contributions of program components. Analysts look at the completeness or actual implementation of each program element; they also assess its contribution to any changes in relevant intervening factors.

In community prevention trial assessment, analysts address not only overall outcomes of the project, i.e., changes in targeted alcohol problems, but also the relative contribution and success of implementation of program elements and the contribution of each to their assigned intervening factors. Therefore, not only should the effect on the target problem be evaluated, but a determination is made of what factors, activities, or processes contributed to the success (or failure) of the trial and how the elements of the prevention intervention(s) worked in practice.

Community prevention trials are specific tests of hypotheses regarding the efficacy of specific interventions to reduce problem levels. They are also valuable sources of information about the elements of success (or failure): what things worked in practice and what did not, and what others can learn from the trial. All of science rests on replication, and regardless of the results of a particular trial, the trial should contribute to the accumulation of scientific knowledge that can be used by other scientists in designing and undertaking future purposeful prevention actions to reduce the level of alcohol problems.

Part VII

Insights, Caveats, and Alternative Research Agendas

To expand the ideas presented in this volume, a select group of experts in prevention and epidemiological research were invited to write brief commentaries on critical issues of interest to them. They offer insights, caveats, and suggestions for basic and applied research that clarify and improve the research agenda for community prevention trials in the alcohol area. They also identify important theoretical, methodological, and pragmatic questions for further discussion.

The first set of four commentaries address issues concerning the intervention process and community participation: the selection of appropriate prevention strategies, outcome variables, and implementation systems. A number of chapters in this volume stimulated these commentaries, particularly the descriptions of previous community-based studies and candidate problems for alcohol research.

The second set of five commentaries focus primarily on methodological issues, particularly on the question of experimental versus quasi-experimental designs. They use as points of departure the chapters by Reichardt, Farquhar and Fortmann, Lasater, Self, and Stout.

PROMOTING COMPREHENSIVE INTERVENTIONS
Lawrence W. Green

Under the conditions of federal funding, health promotion programs that focus on one risk factor such as smoking, alcohol, or illicit drug abuse have the notable advantage of parsimonious and highly-targeted interventions. They concentrate resources where they can, one hopes, have their greatest effect on health outcomes, behavioral change, or risk factors having high priority for federal health policy. They avoid the multiplicity of objectives, the complexity of messages, and the commingling of resources that often confuse the public, if not the investigators seeking to monitor the interventions and to measure their impact.

On the other hand, there are notable advantages of permitting a more comprehensive approach where it is desired by the community, and even encouraging it, although a team of investigators might prefer a more categorical approach.

The most thoroughly documented principle of educational and behavioral change processes in classroom, clinical, and community settings is the effect of engaging learners or target populations actively in the process of assessing their own needs, setting their own priorities, and making a commitment to

Support for preparation of this section was provided by the Henry J. Kaiser Family Foundation. Many of the observations are based on previous work at Johns Hopkins University, and the University of Texas, supported by the National Heart, Lung, and Blood Institute and the National Cancer Institute.

their own goals (Green, 1986). When these conditions precede the development and execution of interventions to facilitate environmental or behavioral change, support for and maintenance of such change tend to be greater.

For community programs this means that the community has to have the opportunity at the outset to identify the priority of alcohol problems relative to its other needs. Seldom will alcohol be the number one problem perceived by the community. Funding agencies interested in reducing alcohol problems must, therefore, face the choice of providing limited funding for a lukewarm alcohol prevention effort or funding a more comprehensive program in which alcohol might be a secondary priority. I believe that experience, if not data, will show that the latter course has been the more prudent. Certainly in school-based programs, teachers will give greater time and effort to a comprehensive prevention program that spans age and grade levels than to sporadic and discontinuous disease-of-the-year projects and curricula.

A second advantage is that programs encompassing a wider range of health problems and issues are likely to gain more sources of support. Comprehensive approaches can be especially helpful when a lead agency that has responsibility for alcohol problems seeks the support of organizations that are more interested in other issues that could be encompassed by a comprehensive agency program. When the organizing strategy for the community is a coalition of organizations, however, comprehensive approaches are less compelling. Coalitions seem to function more efficiently and effectively when they have a single issue around which to rally. Multiple issues clutter the agenda and bring out differences among the collaborating organizations, rather than their commonalty. Coalitions are complicated enough with single issues; adding multiple problems to their agendas can paralyze them.

Various attempts to correlate preventive health practices and risk-taking behaviors have highlighted relationships between smoking, alcohol consumption, and marijuana or other illicit drug use in adolescents and young adults. The consistent correlations and patterned order of uptake among these three behaviors has led to the Gateway concept becoming well established in prevention programs. The Gateway construct that smoking opens the door to alcohol use, which in turn exposes young people to more opportunities and a greater propensity to use illicit drugs, has led to the development of sequential prevention programs in schools and communities. This represents the most common set of targets for comprehensive health education and health promotion programs aimed at substance abuse. Here "comprehensive" may not mean the simultaneous targeting of several risk behaviors in a single program, but rather sequential and coordinated activities across several grade levels or population subgroups stratified by age.

The last justification for comprehensive rather than categorical programs is the idea that a community norm can be established through the cumulative development of a more healthful lifestyle and that new members of the community and new cohorts of young people being socialized will tend to adopt the behaviors modeled by this lifestyle (Becker and Rosenstock, 1989; U.S. Department of Health and Human Services, 1986). The lifestyle notion includes the idea that behavior and conditions of living have an interactive relationship; a family, neighborhood, or community as well as a worksite, institution, or whole society can take on a health-promoting character that involves enduring norms of behavior and environmental conditions conducive to health. This idea is inherent in the World Health Organization's "Healthy Cities" initiative and the Kaiser Family Foundation's community organization approach to health-promotion programming (Green and Kreuter, 1990).

For all their potential advantages, the prospects of demonstrating the effectiveness of comprehensive approaches with the same level of certainty as randomized trials have shown for single interventions will be inherently limited by the nature of comprehensive programs. The very features that make them potentially more effective also tend to conspire against the sanitation of research design.

However messy the data analysis and interpretation might be rendered by quasi-experimental evaluation designs, the end result of comprehensive approaches is likely to be more satisfying to policy makers if not to scientists. In the end, it is a trade-off between rigor and robustness. Cleaner designs and data can be had with more simplistic programs, which lend themselves to greater experimental control, but more robust results with greater policy relevance will be forthcoming from more complex programs, which require more complex designs and analysis.

The first complication of adding dimensions to a program is the problem of sample calculation and statistical power estimation. The minimum sample size required for an evaluation study has to be based on one dependent variable. If the variable of greatest interest to the study's sponsor is one with less variance and greater precision of measurement, then the sample size might be insufficient for other dependent variables of interest.

A second research problem presented by comprehensive programs is the tendency for the various elements to be introduced sequentially, rather than simultaneously. This leads to problems in interpreting intervention effects— e.g., questions about cumulative versus interactive effects. Solutions may be sought through factorial designs, crossover designs, and cross-lagged correlation analysis.

A third set of issues raised by comprehensive programs is quality control in the use of field staff. A single intervention can be highly controlled as to its character and quality of delivery. When the same personnel must deliver multiple interventions, however, their skills may vary across them. This is particularly true where volunteers are used or where indigenous staff, not directly under the control of the researchers, carry out the program and sometimes even the evaluation interviews.

A fourth set of issues, especially in programs for adolescents, relate to informed consent (particularly active parental consent). A program on alcohol-prevention alone might find easy entry and cooperation with schools; but when it adds other elements, such as AIDS education, issues of entry and informed consent can be greatly magnified, with reductions in sample size and biases in study results.

Despite all these potential problems, comprehensive approaches to health education and promotion appear to be worth the bother, both for the program sponsors and for research investigators.

CONFRONTING DRINKING CULTURES
Ernestine Vanderveen

Chapter 6 by Giesbrecht and Pederson describes the implementation of a community based intervention in an imperfect setting. Their honest discussion of the progress and frustrations associated with the effort includes areas and situations that might be approached differently with the benefit of hindsight, the wisdom that comes from experience in real life settings. This is probably best conceptualized as a feasibility study. The people involved will do this again, and they will have benefited a great deal from the field experience gained as they progressed through various phases of the intervention.

Problem perception and problem ownership are concepts that need further discussion. How alcohol problems are perceived and who should be involved in dealing with them are likely to be critical issues in the successful implementation of any community based prevention trial. It is interesting that the community members in Giesbrecht's study viewed excessive alcohol consumption as the problem of only a few people in their community. Yet, the survey indicated that a high proportion of people admitted to heavy drinking; and survey respondents described various complications and consequences of such drinking. However, they did not perceive heavy drinking to be a community problem or even a health problem; it was somebody else's problem.

This situation prompts me to ask several questions: What is a safe level of drinking? How do we operationalize the concept in the context of community norms? If a level of safe drinking could be defined, would it be universally accepted for all drinkers and situations in a given community? Frequently, persons are placed at risk of injury or death directly or indirectly resulting from alcohol used inappropriately relative to the larger drinking context. Individuals who drink while engaged in work or recreational activities where judgment and skills are impaired by alcohol use clearly pose a risk for the safety of others and themselves. The notion of safe drinking levels becomes enormously complicated within the purview of perceived risk. Under some circumstances, no level of alcohol use would be considered safe.

There are undoubtedly numerous reasons why people in a given community may not perceive widespread abusive drinking as a community level problem. Communities that are beset with too many other problems with which they feel powerless to deal may regard alcohol-related health and safety issues as just one more set of problems in a pot of many. Such social ills as crime and unemployment might overshadow or desensitize people to alcohol problems.

Chapter 6 outlines helpful lessons as we ponder and plan clinical trials. There is the matter of a time frame—the long lead time for planning, designing, and implementing an intervention. A crucial factor is the amount of time required for a community to accept new concepts and approaches. An additional consideration is the time needed for the research staff (scientific and administrative) to put all the pieces together for implementing a clinical trial. The creation of a climate for community level intervention cannot be perceived as a short-term or single-shot activity. As is pointed out, over time people can be turned from initial suspicion to more implicit support for alcohol-related interventions.

An important consideration in any intervention is the drinking culture of the community and the norms that comprise that culture. How to avoid adversely tangling with pervasive drinking patterns imbedded in community norms is a critical question that must be addressed during early planning stages of community based interventions. In the study described by Giesbrecht, the staff had an insufficient understanding of what would be involved in dealing with the community's concepts and culture, particularly the drinking culture.

People in the study community perceived prevention as something additional to be done within the treatment milieu. They seemed quite ready to treat a problem that was already there rather than to prevent problems from occurring in the first place. Here we must confront the challenge of translating prevention concepts into meaningful, realistic, and desirable ideas. If we are to be successful in educating decision makers and helping people change attitudes, we probably have to avoid threatening their everyday patterns of social behavior. Yet, those everyday patterns include expressed behaviors of groups and individuals regarding the consumption of alcohol.

The goals of prevention measures need discussion and acceptance by all involved parties before the intervention reaches implementation stage. Questions have been raised about whether it is realistic to encourage everyone to drink less and what that impact would be as opposed to encouraging the higher risk drinkers to reduce their consumption. Perhaps this is not really a dichotomy. On a gross per capita consumption basis, there is already a downward trend nationally. Maybe we could capitalize on this trend and encourage society to continue it—not to abstain, but at least to drink less. If we target total consumption rather than heavy drinkers, will we have a greater impact on the general problem?   This, of course, leaves unanswered another basic question of what should be the key strategy.

To be realistic, very powerful interests are likely to oppose interventions designed to decrease consumption.   Some well planned strategies on how to deal with the beverage industry would seem to be an important consideration in formulating community based intervention plans.   Confrontational approaches are unlikely to produce positive results; and thus, as a very early step, attempts to educate industry leadership maybe useful.

TARGETING CONSUMPTION AS AN ENDPOINT
Thomas C. Harford

Determining the success or failure of an intervention ultimately rests on the quality of the measures used to evaluate the outcome.   The intervention, like the falling tree in the forest, may be soundless if there are no ears to assess its impact.   Equally important, the outcome criteria must represent operationalized objectives that are guided by theory or conceptualizations that command an implicit logic linking antecedents with consequences.

The contextual framework guiding the selection of outcome measures by Saltz and colleagues (Chapter 3) emphasizes the targeted condition as the result of interactions between the environment and the individual.   As a consequence, the search for candidate outcomes focuses on alcohol-related problems rather than individuals at high risk for specific or multiple problems (such as heavy drinkers or alcoholics).   Even assuming a dose-response relationship between alcohol consumption and related problems, a focus on individuals at high risk consumption levels would ignore persons at high-risk for alcohol-related outcomes because of other contributing risk factors (e.g., nutrition, weight, and smoking) as well as persons at risk by virtue of exposure to alcohol.

Following the very thorough review of the current status of the major problem outcomes, however, we are left with only one or two problems in which relationships have been established with alcohol consumption, adequate measurement properties exist, and prevalence rates are of sufficient magnitude for community level interventions.   Alcohol-related highway crashes is judged to be the strongest candidate.   Implicit in the discussion of the validity criteria is the identification of alcohol consumption as a major risk factor for alcohol problems.   This may appear obvious, but many contemporary approaches to prevention confound relationships between alcohol consumption and alcoholism with respect to problem outcomes.

While the authors acknowledge that the measurement of alcohol use in a community represents a crucial mediating variable, its status as a candidate outcome measure is judged as a problem ". . . insofar as its relationship to the sequelae of its consumption has been demonstrated." Except for a few diseases such as, cirrhosis, high blood pressure, and certain cancers, few studies have described the risk of adverse drinking consequences at various levels of intake. In addition, the authors point out that in the literature of drinking and driving, casualties are not solely the province of heavy drinkers and alcoholics. While this may argue against "increased consumption" as a candidate outcome, it is important to recognize that the relationship between alcohol consumption and problems is specified by both the drinking context (e.g., bars) and several individual characteristics (e.g., age, gender, and drinking history).

In my view, the qualifications mentioned by Saltz and colleagues do not seriously impair the candidacy of alcohol consumption level as an important outcome criterion. As the authors note, both aggregate and self-reported alcohol consumption are sensitive to environmental manipulation (e.g., price, availability, legal purchase age); and variables known to specify the nature of the relationship between consumption and problem outcomes can be included in statistical models.

The formidable literature linking tobacco use to disease has implications for alcohol consumption as a possible outcome variable. In this context, it is important to note alcohol's unique contribution to both disease and injury. First, alcohol in excessive doses is poisonous, and even in smaller doses it can have a cumulative effect, contributing to various diseases that may ultimately be fatal. Second, because alcohol can impair perception and judgment, alcohol abuse can cause death and morbidity from a variety of accidents or injuries. From a more general perspective, the literature clearly indicates that increased risks for both illness and injury are associated with increased consumption levels, as reflected in either the incidence of acute intoxication (episodes of heavy consumption) or the level of consumption over a more extended period of time.

For the present, the determination of whether alcohol consumption is an appropriate outcome variable for community intervention studies must be guided by further specification of the conceptual framework for such research.

FOCUSING ON COMMUNITY STRUCTURE AND PROCESS
Marjorie A. Gutman

The essence of the community systems approach to prevention of health problems is the opportunity to intervene at multiple levels of the community and to utilize multiple, presumably interactive and mutually reinforcing, mechanisms for behavior change. One way to understand the community better is to analyze both its *structure* and *process* as a prelude to the design of prevention trials. Community structure is the configuration of components within the system that help define its organic fabric, while the process is the operations by which the components function and interact dynamically over time.

The same criteria distilled from the literature by Holder to define a community can be used to identify and describe its major structural components. These criteria include: geographic coherence, social interaction, fulfillment of necessary functions, and a subjective sense of belonging or identifying with the place and people. An attempt to use these criteria to identify generic components within communities yields multiple units arrayed in four levels of analysis.

The individual is the smallest unit or nucleus in the community system and is the ultimate target of efforts to reduce alcohol problems via community prevention trials. At the next level of analysis, arrayed around the individual, are the multiple small informal groups and larger organizations to which he or she belongs. The next broader level of analysis is the subarea of the community where the individual resides and to which he or she may be strongly attached, such as a neighborhood, housing project, or school catchment area. Within each major subarea are formal organizations and area-wide structures such as health and safety services. The broadest level of analysis is the community in its entirety along with community-wide structures (public and private, formal and informal), including the political, educational, and legal systems, and large "grassroots" organizations.

Structural analysis illustrates that the individual is typically embedded concurrently in groups and organizations at multiple levels, each providing explicit and implicit messages about alcohol use and opportunities and constraints for use. The analysis also raises critical questions for designing community prevention trials to reduce alcohol problems:

1. What are the relevant components in a particular community and what are their characteristics: e.g., consumption levels, outlets, values and norms about alcohol, and socioeconomic status?
2. How homogeneous or heterogeneous are the community components, especially in relation to alcohol use?
3. To what extent are multiple components providing complementary or conflicting messages, regulations, and opportunities pertaining to alcohol use and problems?
4. What are the relevant community-wide structures and their characteristics: e.g., regulations and ideologies about alcohol use?
5. What are the crucial target groups for behavior change in this community?
6. Which individuals and groups are the most powerful or influential for bringing about reductions in alcohol problems?

A central concept used to understand social processes within communities is social norms (Durkheim, 1933; Merton, 1957), generally held standards of behavior against which judgments are made. Group norms can be characterized by the degree of their clarity, consensus about them, adherence, and consensus about relevant sanctions and rewards. In recent years there appear to be clearer, stronger norms about driving under the influence than about other alcohol-related problems, perhaps making this behavior less socially acceptable and, therefore, more amenable to prevention efforts. This raises questions about other alcohol-related impairments, such as family violence, the operation of boats or machinery under the influence, and poor job performance. What norms apply to these impairments, and how amenable are they to prevention efforts?

A paradigm of major small group functions based on the concept of norms applies to component groups and entire communities: forming norms, communicating norms, monitoring behavioral adherence, and imposing sanctions (Secord and Backman, 1964). A crucial task for prevention efforts is to conduct, for each community, a "differential diagnosis" or specially tailored analysis of the relative need to bolster each of these group functions.

Socialization and both formal and informal social control are the major processes used by groups to fulfill their basic normative functions. Socialization is the lifelong process by which individuals learn and internalize norms, values, information, and skills (Clausen et al., 1968; Zigler and Child, 1969). Social control picks up where socialization leaves off, inducing or ensuring compliance with norms (Secord and Backman, 1964). Formal efforts at social control are exercised by formal organizations and bureaucracies, while informal control is exercised by groups such as families and peers.

To attain maximum effectiveness, the design of a prevention trial should consider all of the major functions that communities and component groups could play. Prevention efforts have tended to focus *either* on socialization *or* on one type of social control, but a community-wide trial offers the opportunity to *combine* strong interventions utilizing multiple mechanisms for behavior change. Salient characteristics of the major social processes (see Table 15.1) could help guide the selection of interventions for community trials.

It is, of course, impossible for a community alcohol prevention effort to employ interventions that fully imitate the natural socialization process. However, the more intense the effort, the earlier it is begun, and the more it engages multiple relevant agents, the more likely it is to have a sustained impact. Under some circumstances, prevention socialization may have to reverse previous learning.

Several factors affect the extent to which groups can pressure members to adhere to norms, and how that pressure is applied. These factors include the power structure of groups, their cohesiveness (Festinger et al., 1950), and the degree of alienation experienced by group members (Durkheim, 1951; Merton, 1957).   A community prevention effort will be more successful in reducing alcohol problems if it can identify and mobilize the necessary types of power within target groups.   Change agents should also assess and try to increase the level of group cohesion, or at least recognize that cohesion and alienation can be moderating factors in attempts to enhance conformity to desired norms.

TABLE 15.1
Examples of Characteristics of Community Social Processes

Process	Characteristics

Socialization[1]	▪ begins very early in life
	▪ lifelong duration, but especially during childhood
	▪ high intensity
	▪ major agents
	  - childhood: family, school
	  - adolescence: also peers

Formal Social Control[2]	▪ clear laws, regulations, policies ▪ detection of violations ▪ swift and certain punishment ▪ visibility of entire process ▪ major agents—formal organizations, bureaucracies
Informal Social Control[3]	▪ clear, consistent norms ▪ high degree of consensus ▪ swift, sure sanctions ▪ power—all 6 types (informal, coercive, reward, referent, expert, legitimate) ▪ high group cohesion ▪ low degree of alienation ▪ major agents—informal social groups, such as family, peers

[1]Zigler and Child, 1969.
[2]Moskowitz, 1989.
[3]Secord and Backman, 1964.

In addition, in designing community prevention programs and trials, relationships among the major social processes need to be considered. For example, formal and informal social-control approaches to alcohol problems appear to be interactive (Walsh, 1990; Moskowitz, 1989). Laws and regulations that inhibit alcohol use and abuse may encourage and reinforce social norms in the same direction, probably by making them more explicit and symbolic. Conversely, stronger more widespread social norms against a behavior may provide a better social and political basis for enacting laws and promoting adherence. Moreover, relationships between formal and informal social control may have important sequential properties and "threshold effects" that are still dimly understood (Walsh, 1990). Thus, more stringent laws may be enacted *only after* social norms unfavorable to alcohol abuse have become sufficiently developed. Experience in some states with seatbelt laws, and nationwide with anti-smoking laws and regulations, illustrate this idea.

CLARIFYING CONCEPTS AND TERMINOLOGY
David P. Byar

My background is in cancer research and randomized clinical trials, one of the principal methods used for evaluating treatments for disease. Even though I have worked in the field of clinical trials for some 20 years, but not in the fields of psychology or sociology, I found lots of new terms in the chapter by Reichardt (Chapter 9). For example, he talks about external validity, which is what clinical trialists refer to as generalizability—whether the results can be applied to individuals or groups other than those who were actually studied. As I understand it, internal validity is whether you are getting the right answers and do not have problems with bias, contamination, or compliance to assigned treatments.

Internal and external validity are not necessarily equally important. In the world of randomized clinical trials there is much more interest in first proving that there is some useful effect of a treatment or condition under study; so almost all the concern is for internal validity. Only after such an effect has been demonstrated would one turn attention to the problem of generalizability, which might require a very different study design.

The "nonequivalent group design" is another new term to me. I think it gives itself away by its very name. I have always thought that the purpose of a control group is to be just like the treatment group except for the treatment received. Saying that it is nonequivalent is admitting that there may be serious problems with it. Similarly, the "regression discontinuity design" discussed by Reichardt has serious limitations, making it difficult to imagine a situation where this would be a good choice. First, it requires that very large numbers of units be studied if one is to estimate the regression lines adequately.

Moreover, the interpretation of those regression lines is based on very strong assumptions, and rarely would one be in a position to justify them.

An additional example of terminology new to me is the "interrupted time series." The closest equivalent in assessing medical treatments might be the use of historical patient controls. Unfortunately, subtle biases can arise with this approach; and except in very specialized circumstances, it is inferior to direct randomized comparison between the promising new treatment and the standard one.

Reichardt appears to be somewhat skeptical about using randomized experiments when trying to estimate the effects of community prevention trials. The randomized approach has seldom been used for whole community studies, but there are exceptions such as the Community Intervention Trial for Smoking Cessation (COMMIT) sponsored by the Division of Cancer Prevention and Control at the National Cancer Institute.

I found puzzling Reichardt's conclusion that "all the threats to internal validity of the randomized experiment are also potential threats to the validity of the nonequivalent group design, though in the [latter case] the biases caused by these threats may tend not to be as severe." I would have guessed just the opposite. To be fair, he does mention one important exception that he refers to as the "rival hypothesis of local history," meaning any event that occurs in the control condition but not in the experimental condition or vice versa where the event is not part of the intervention and biases the comparison between the two groups. Perhaps this exception subsumes in one form or another all the usual objections to nonrandomized control groups.

What Reichardt calls "disaggregation" we call "subset analysis;" but we regard it with grave suspicion because of the problem of multiplicity: If you look at enough variables, you are almost sure to find something significant. However, I have spent a lot of time trying to understand the strengths and weaknesses of subset analysis, and I believe that it is a very important activity for explanatory analysis. I, therefore, agree with Reichardt's plea for imagination and creativity in analyzing data.

We make a very useful distinction in medical randomized trials between hypothesis testing and exploratory data analysis. Hypothesis testing refers to looking at the main question a trial was designed to answer. The question has been stated in advance, before the analyst has seen the data, and the probability of a false negative or false positive result has been specified in the trial design. Exploratory data analysis, on the other hand, permits the exercise of creativity. One may ignore the problems of multiple comparisons and selection of subsets of data because the purpose is to generate new hypotheses to be tested in future studies. However, certainty about results derived from exploratory data analysis should not be regarded as being on an equal footing with results of testing the primary hypothesis.

Exploratory data analysis can be very useful in looking for a consistent pattern of meaning in a set of data. It is usually true that if a convincing treatment effect has been demonstrated, there ought to be implications for a lot of other features of the data (like dose-response effects and consistency across subgroups). In simple terms, things should fit together, and if they do not, one ought to start getting rather suspicious of the overall result. Of course, I certainly concur with the need for caveats in exploratory data analysis, saying what the limitations of the analysis are and what uncertainty remains.

Finally, let me turn back to the issue of design options. Although there is doubtless a place for all the designs that Reichardt discusses, I believe that whenever possible one should use randomized experiments for estimating the effects of community prevention trials. Even though randomized trials are difficult to implement, the results of such studies are likely to be more widely believed, and in the long run they may be more cost effective than even a series of studies conducted with weaker designs.

REPLICATING COMMUNITY STUDIES
Laurence S. Freedman

A large part of my work as a statistician has been related to the clinical evaluation of treatments. Two major advances in the last 40 years have been the control of systematic biases in the comparisons of treatments by randomization and the control of random variation by sufficient replication. I would like to emphasize here the concept of replication in the evaluation of community interventions. Much of what we think we know about our world comes from replication. In experimentation with biological systems that we do not fully understand, replication is a fundamental key to predicting the effect of the experiment. In the medical literature a report of the results of treating a series of patients carries much greater weight than a single case report.

Of course, replication in clinical medicine is relatively easy to accomplish when the individual experimental units are people. Replication is more difficult in the evaluation of the components of a community program where the experimental units may be schools or worksites, and even more so in the evaluation of the integrated program itself where the units are whole communities. Nevertheless, in many current studies, a component of a community program is being evaluated among ten or more units with randomization of some units to control. For example, seven such studies of smoking prevention are listed in the National Cancer Institute's directory of prevention trials: four employ schools as the intervention unit, two use school districts, and one uses physicians' offices. In addition there are three such studies of dietary modification (employing churches, physician practices, and worksites) and seven such studies of cancer screening compliance.

Evaluations of the community programs themselves offer a starkly different picture. While most studies have included one or two control communities, these have not usually been selected by randomization. However, there is little point in criticizing this aspect of the designs when the amount of replication is so poor. For example, in community interventions to prevent cardiovascular disease, the numbers of communities included in eight separate projects were two, two, three, three, three, four, five, and six. When there is so little replication, it is nearly impossible to draw reliable *general* conclusions, i.e., conclusions that are likely to hold in communities outside the study.

Sometimes results from these studies are dressed up in a statistical finery that obscures the limitations of the data. For example, data from the Stanford Five City Project (Farquhar et al., 1990) show the decline of smoking in two intervention cities to be greater than in two control cities (Figure 15.1). (Results from the fifth city were not yet available.) There are 16 data points, made up of four time points for each city. The slope and intercept of the regression line is estimated for each city, making eight parameters to be estimated, which leaves eight degrees of freedom for estimating the residual variation. Using this estimate of the residual variation in comparing the average slopes of the intervention cities with the control cities, a significant difference in slopes is found ($P < 0.003$). What does this significant result mean?

First, the validity of the test depends upon the truth of the assumption that in each city there is really a linear decrease in smoking prevalence over time. Although such an assumption is internally unverifiable, it is supported by long-term smoking trends throughout the U.S. over the past 20 years; so we can perhaps let this pass. More importantly, the residual variance as calculated reflects the variation internal to each city (e.g., the sampling variation in the surveys from which the smoking data are derived), *but not the variation between cities*. The test with eight degrees of freedom addresses only the limited question of whether the difference in slopes observed in the Five City Project is real, i.e., is not due to some internal source such as sampling variation in the surveys. However, to make inferences regarding the general effect of the intervention, a more valid approach would be to conduct a t-test, treating the estimated slopes in each city as the raw data. In this study, such a test would have only two degrees of freedom, a number too small for any meaningful analysis.

The aim for all community intervention research must be to find strategies that can be successfully applied over a wide range of communities. This aim itself implies an expansion of the application of community interventions. In any given field the appropriate time for such expansion may not have

FIGURE 15.1

Regression Analysis of Mean Cohort Values for Cities Over Time for Persons Aged 25 Through 74 Years

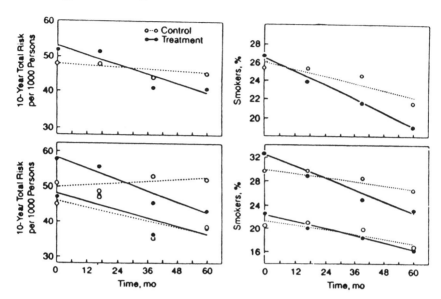

Values for pooled treatment and pooled control cities are shown for 10-year estimated total mortality risk per 1,000 persons (top left, $P < .02$) and for the percentage of smokers (top right, $P < .003$). Mean values for individual cities are also shown (total risk bottom left; percentage of smokers, bottom right).

Source: Farquhar, J. W., Fortmann, S. P., Flora, J. A., Taylor, C. B., Haskell, W. L., Williams, P. T., Maccoby, N., and Wood, P. D. (1990). Effects of Communitywide Education on Cardiovascular Disease Risk Factors: The Stanford Five-City Project. *Journal of the American Medical Association, 264*(3), 359-365. Reprinted with permission.

arrived. For alcohol research, there certainly appears to be a long and uncertain road ahead. In cardiovascular research the time may be much closer. The first stage of expansion, however, should take place under controlled conditions so that a proper evaluation of the chosen strategy can be made. In other words, the first stage of expansion should be in the form of a randomized controlled study involving a dozen or more communities, such as the Community Intervention Trial for Smoking Cessation (COMMIT) (Byar, 1988; Freedman et al., 1990) described earlier. This study was, in fact, deliberately planned as a further step in the broad expansion of community smoking cessation programs.

LEARNING FROM EXPERIENCE
Charles S. Reichardt

Even under the best of circumstances, implementing a field trial for a community intervention program is a difficult undertaking. One way to try to make this task easier is to learn from past experience. The bad news is that we have little experience in conducting field trials of community intervention programs for alcohol abuse prevention. The good news is that we have a relative wealth of experience in conducting field trials of community intervention programs for cardiovascular disease (CVD) and cancer prevention. I wish to comment briefly on the types of methodological questions that alcohol researchers should be asking researchers in these other fields and on the need to report the degree of uncertainty that exists in their studies. Obviously, field trials of community interventions for CVD and cancer prevention should be answering substantive questions, but they also should be teaching us about methodological issues.

In Chapter 5, Lasater describes eight field trials in CVD and cancer prevention. In only one of the eight is the research design a randomized experiment. The other seven studies use nonequivalent group designs. The difference between these two types of design depends on whether or not communities are randomly assigned to treatment and comparison conditions. Because it entails random assignment, the randomized experiment usually is more difficult to implement. But it is not subject to biases due to initial selection differences between the treatment and comparison conditions. In the nonequivalent group design, much attention has been focused on the difficulty of correcting for the biasing effects of initial selection differences (Hausman and Wise, 1985; LaLonde, 1986).

The critical question is whether the advantages of the randomized experiment outweigh its disadvantages in real applications. If the nonequivalent group design provides credible results in field settings, we can avoid the cost and difficulties of randomization. Otherwise we must bite the bullet and stop using the nonequivalent design so extensively. Experience with these two designs in field settings is the only way to answer this central question.

Field trials have well established the importance of process evaluation, documenting the nature of the treatments that are received by both program participants and nonparticipants. From experience we have learned that interventions seldom are implemented as planned (McLaughlin, 1985) and that, even then, they usually change over time. Thus, process evaluation is necessary to help us understand what treatments are actually being received so we can discover what does and does not work. Field trials also are teaching us how to conduct process evaluations, using qualitative as well as quantitative methods (Stake, 1986).

Researchers can assess baseline and outcome measures on the same individuals (a cohort design) or on different individuals (a cross-sectional design). Cohort designs allow a greater number of options for taking account of initial selection differences, but they are susceptible to reactive effects of the baseline measurement. Whether such reactive effects are large or small is an empirical question (Campbell, 1969a); so is the question of what is the best way to adjust for initial selection differences.

Whether we are asking substantive or methodological questions, our answers will be uncertain. Yet, we seldom report our degree of uncertainty as clearly as would be appropriate. For example, estimates of treatment effects in randomized experiments are always subject to uncertainty due to random variability. A confidence interval reveals the degree of uncertainty for a given level of confidence (e.g., 95%). But researchers seldom report confidence intervals. Instead they usually report a point estimate and the results of a statistical significance test.

Consider the difference this can make in interpreting the reported results. A reader might learn, for example, that an alcohol abuse intervention reduced automobile accidents by 20% and that this reduction was significant at the 0.05 level, making it appear as if the 20% reduction were a precise estimate. However, the 95% confidence interval for that reduction in automobile accidents could range from 1% to 39%, more clearly revealing the large degree of uncertainty about the actual size of the effect.

Just as a confidence interval provides a means of representing uncertainty due to random variability, we need to devise ways of representing uncertainty due to other sources (Reichardt and Gollob, 1987). At the very least, we should always provide a narrative description of the uncertainty of our answers. Without such an honest appraisal, we will not be able to provide useful answers to any of the methodological questions raised above. For example, we can not decide whether a nonequivalent group design is as good as a randomized experiment in a given situation without recognizing the degree of uncertainty that accompanies the task of taking account of initial selection differences.

Not to admit the degree of our uncertainty is tantamount to deception. I would argue that in the long run being deceptive is more likely to destroy public confidence in social research and reduce funding than being forthright about the uncertainty of our research. As Artemus Ward put it, "It ain't so much the things we don't know that gets us in trouble. It's the things we know that ain't so."

ANALYZING COMMUNITIES AS COMMUNITIES
Alexander C. Wagenaar

In thinking about intervention trials and their evaluation, the first issue I want to highlight is *change over time*—particularly change over time within communities. We are interested in *community* interventions—changes in the nature and functioning of communities, not changes in selected individuals within the community. The objective of a community intervention (as opposed to interventions in communities) is changing the nature of *community* structures, norms, public policies, and social networks.

Some believe that the community does not exist as a separate entity but is rather inherently an agglomeration of individual people. However, there are many important dimensions to a community that are independent of the individuals within it. A community is much more than the sum of its members. More important than the individuals themselves are:

1. Patterns of interaction between community members
2. Patterns of identification with relevant reference groups
3. The multi-dimensionality of social groups (work, recreation, religious, neighborhood, ethnic, social class)
4. Extant institutional structures
5. The distribution of power throughout the institutional structures and social groups in the community.

Many of the changes in behavior that we hope to effect are very small on the individual level (for example, modest changes in overall alcohol consumption by adults), but, when aggregated over a large population, the benefits in terms of society's burden of morbidity and mortality can be substantial.

Another way to emphasize the importance of communities is to keep units of analysis clear in our minds. The unit of analysis is the *community*, not the individuals within it. This has direct implications for research design, analytic methods, statistical power considerations, and the generalizability of evaluation studies. Research designed solely to assess whether *individuals* change risky behaviors may not optimally inform us of whether the *community* changed as a result of the intervention trial.

Prior to beginning any intervention study, we must have a theory or model about the nature of the outcome variable and its causes and how the intervention is expected to influence the outcome variable. Covariates used in the statistical analyses must be based on such a model. Whether we are from an individual-oriented profession like medicine or a community-oriented profession like public health, whether our disciplinary approach draws from the biological or social sciences, we are all controlling for variance in outcomes due to factors not directly tied to the intervention. The preferred method to control variance is via the research design (e.g., using randomized control groups), but factors not adequately controlled in the design may be controlled statistically in the analysis (e.g., by incorporating covariates into regression or regression-analog models).

The functional form of the expected effects of the intervention over an appropriate time period is very important. We need to think about it at the design stage in terms of our theory. Do we simply expect a sudden, immediate effect that holds constant? Does the magnitude of the effect grow or decay over time; or does it have some more complex shape? If effect patterns are not considered a priori, there is a risk that many alternative models may be tested until one fits well, capitalizing on chance unless the multiple tests are explicitly taken into account when establishing critical p-values. The issue of functional form highlights the importance of monitoring the so-called "dosing schedule" of the intervention and how that schedule relates to our expected effect pattern.

Self mentions that time-series designs require complicated modeling of the baseline event rate. Complex modeling of baseline patterns cannot be avoided if the objective is to identify the causal influence of the intervention. Many less-sophisticated intervention studies have one or only a few baseline observation time-points. As a result, it is difficult to know whether observed post-intervention differences are inconsistent with natural background variation in the outcome measure over time. Such variation may include both systematic patterns and random variation. Naturally occurring "extraneous" events have typically threatened the interpretation of community intervention evaluations. The availability of data over a long baseline period gives us a chance to identify the frequency of such events and the amount of variation in the outcome measure attributable to them.

Time-series research designs do not necessarily require an intervention with a sudden effect that immediately occurs in its entirety. While an abrupt intervention effect maximizes statistical power, there are many other forms of intervention effects that are also best evaluated using time-series models.

TRANSFORMING NOISE INTO SIGNALS
Michael Hennessy

Dr. Stout's chapter (Chapter 8) provides an especially graphic example of the community researcher's inability to emulate the orderly and pristine environment of classical randomized experiments, the theoretical advantages of which are well known and highlighted in the chapter by Howard and Barofsky (Chapter 13).

There are actually two kinds of unplanned events that pose threats to scientific virtue: those orchestrated for good or ill by community members and "random" events that may be confounded with the effects of prevention programs (i.e., the "history" threat to internal validity). As researchers, we tend to emphasize the latter and overlook the former, at least in our research designs. I see little we can do about such rare events except to use comparison communities and long time series of baseline measurements which are both typically recommended as good research practice in this area.

The other sort of unplanned events (the nonrandom ones) are more common because communities are not closed systems, but rather consist of dynamic combinations of different institutions and interest groups. Researchers tend to discuss this problem in terms of the ratio of signal (treatment) to noise (natural variation) and have proposed methods to increase our ability to differentiate between them. These methods include using statistical analyses that have known aggregate rates of error; reducing the variance of one community relative to another (e.g., through pre-randomization matching); amplifying signals relative to noise (e.g., through multiple interventions rather than a single program); or choosing signals that are known to have low noise levels (e.g., particular outcome measures).

All these strategies tend to focus on some aspect of either the noise or the signal to enhance our ability to unambiguously differentiate between the two. Also note that a high proportion of the suggested solutions involve measurement rather than design approaches, in sharp contrast to the prevailing conventional wisdom concerning such research priorities (Light et al., 1990). Thus, the particular challenge for community intervention research is to devise methods for *transforming* the normal background noise of community operation into known, if not manipulable, signals that can be explicitly taken into account.

The very concept of "implementation," "monitoring," or "process" evaluation research would be unnecessary if we believed that the truly important community events were actually random. Although we obviously do not believe this, our current knowledge of how to monitor, classify, and study program implementation and community process more closely approximates folklore than research technology. It is this task of transforming community-level noise into community-level signal—not the fruitless quest for the apparent rigor of the randomized trial in community settings—that is the major methodological issue facing prevention researchers.

Bibliography

Aalen, O. O. (1978). Nonparametric inference for a family of counting processes. *Annals of Statistics, 6*, 701-726.

Aaron, P., & Musto, D. (1981). Temperance and prohibition in America: A historical overview. In M. H. Moore & D. R. Gerstein (Eds.), *Alcohol and public policy: Beyond the shadow of prohibition* (pp. 127-181). Washington, DC: National Academy Press.

ACT UP. (1989, June). *A national AIDS treatment research agenda.* Paper presented at the V International Conference on AIDS, Montreal, Quebec.

Agran, P., & Dunkle, D. (1985). A comparison of reported and unreported noncrash events. *Accident Analysis and Prevention, 17*(1), 7-13.

Aitken, S. S., & Zobeck, T. (1985, Summer). Trends in alcohol-related fatal motor-vehicle accidents for 1983. *Alcohol Health and Research World, 9*(4), 60-62.

Alinsky, S. D. (1946). *Reveille for radicals.* Chicago: University of Chicago Press.

Altman, D., Flora, J. A., Fortmann, S. P., & Farquhar, J. W. (1987, February). The cost-effectiveness of three smoking cessation programs. *The American Journal of Public Health, 77*(2), 162-165.

Altman, D. G., Foster, V., & Rasenick-Douss, L. (1989). Reducing the illegal sale of cigarettes to minors. *Journal of the American Medical Association, 261*, 80-83.

American Medical Association Board of Trustees. (1986). Alcohol advertising, counteradvertising, and depiction in the public media. *Journal of the American Medical Association, 256*, 1485-1488.

Amezcua, C., McAlister, A., Ramirez, A., & Espinoza, R. (1989). Health promotion in a Mexican-American border community: Programma A Su Salud in Eagle Pass, Texas. In N. Bracht (Ed.), *Organizing for community health promotion: A handbook*. Beverly Hills, CA: Sage Publications.

Arensberg, C. M., & Kimball, S. T. (1965). *Culture and community*. New York: Harcourt, Brace, and World, Inc.

Aristizabal, N., Cuello, C., Correa, P., Collazos, T., & Haenszel, W. (1984). The impact of vaginal cytology on cervical risks in Cali, Colombia. *International Journal of Cancer, 34*, 5-9.

Ashley, M. J., & Rankin, J. G. (1988). A public health approach to the prevention of alcohol-related problems. *Annual Review of Public Health, 9*, 233-271.

Atkin, C. K. (1988). Mass communication effects on drinking and driving. *Surgeon General's Workshop on Drunk Driving: Background Papers* (pp. 15-34). Rockville, MD: Office of the Surgeon General.

Babor, T. F., Sanchez-Craig, M., Robertson, I., & Skinner, H. A. (1986). Comments on Griffith Edwards' 'The alcohol dependence syndrome: Concept as a stimulus to enquiry'. *British Journal of Addiction, 81*(2), 185-196.

Bacon, S. (1947). The mobilization of community resources for the attack on alcoholism. *Quarterly Journal of Studies on Alcohol, 8*, 473-497.

Bandura, A. (1977). *Social learning theory*. Englewood Cliffs, NJ: Prentice-Hall.

Bandura, A. (1986). *Social foundations of thought and action: A social cognitive theory*. Englewood Cliffs, NJ: Prentice-Hall.

Barboriak, H., Gruchow, H., & Anderson, A. (1983). Alcohol consumption and the diet-heart controversy. *Alcoholism: Clinical and Experimental Research, 7*(1), 31-34.

Bard, M., & Zacker, J. (1974). Assaultiveness and alcohol use in family disputes. *Criminology, 12*(3), 281-292.

Barnow, B. S., Cain, G. C., & Goldberger, A. S. (1980). Issues in the analysis of selectivity bias. In E. W. Stromsdorfer & G. Farkas (Eds.), *Evaluation studies review annual* (Vol. 5). Newbury Park, CA: Sage Publications.

Beauchamp, D. E. (1980). *Beyond alcoholism: Alcohol and public health policy*. Philadelphia, PA: Temple University Press.

Becker, M. H., & Rosenstock, I. R. (1989). Health promotion, disease prevention, and program retention. In H. E. Freeman & S. Levine (Eds.), *Handbook of medical sociology* (4th ed., pp. 284-305). Englewood Cliffs, NJ: Prentice Hall.

Benfari, R. (1981). The multiple risk factor intervention trial: III. The model for intervention. *Preventive Medicine, 10*, 426-442.

Berk, R. A., Boruch, R. F., Chambers, D. L., Rossi, P. H., & Witte, A. D. (1985, August). Social policy experimentation: A position paper. *Evaluation Review*, *9*(4), 387-429.

Berkowitz, G. S., Kelsey, J. L., LiVolsi, V. A., Holford, T. R., Merino, M. J., Ort, S., O'Connor, T. Z., Goldenberg, I. S., & White, C. (1984). Oral contraceptive use and fibrocystic disease among pre- and post-menopausal women. *American Journal of Epidemiology*, *120*(1), 87-96.

Best, J., Thomson, S., Santi, S., Smith, E., & Brown, K. (1988). Preventing cigarette smoking among school children. *Annual Review of Public Health*, *9*, 161-201.

Blackburn, H., Luepker, R. V., Kline, F. G., Bracht, N., Carlaw, R., Jacobs, D., Mittelmark, M., Stauffer, L., & Taylor, H. L. (1984). The Minnesota Heart Health Program: A research and demonstration project in cardiovascular disease prevention. In J. D. Matarazzo, S. M. Weiss, J. A. Herd, N. E. Miller, & S. M. Weiss (Eds.), *Behavioral health: A handbook of health enhancement and disease prevention* (pp. 1171-1178). New York: John Wiley & Sons.

Blakely, E. J. (Ed.). (1979). *Community development research: Concepts, issues, and strategies*. New York: Human Sciences Press.

Blane, H. T. (1976). Education and the prevention of alcoholism. In B. Kissin & H. Begleiter (Eds.), *The biology of alcoholism* (Vol. IV, pp. 519-578). New York: Plenum Press.

Blane, H. T., & Hewitt, L. (1977). *Mass media, public education and alcohol: A state of the art review*. Prepared for the National Institute on Alcohol Abuse and Alcoholism under Purchase Order NIA-76-12.

Bloom, H. S. (1984, April). Accounting for no-shows in experimental evaluation designs. *Evaluation Review*, *8*(2), 225-246.

Blose, J. O., & Holder, H. D. (1987a). Liquor-by-the-drink and alcohol-related traffic crashes: A natural experiment using time-series analysis. *Journal of Studies on Alcohol*, *48*(1), 52-60.

Blose, J. O., & Holder, H. D. (1987b). Public availability of distilled spirits: Structural and reported consumption changes associated with liquor-by-the-drink. *Journal of Studies on Alcohol*, *48*(4), 371-379.

Blumenthal, M., & Ross, H. L. (1975). Judicial discretion in drinking-driving cases: An empirical study of influences and consequences. In S. Israelstam & S. Lambert (Eds.), *Alcohol, drugs, and traffic safety: Proceedings of the sixth international conference on alcohol, drugs, and traffic safety*. Toronto: Addiction Research Foundation of Ontario.

Botvin, G. (1982). Broadening the focus of smoking prevention strategies. In T. J. Coates, A. R. Peterson, & C. Perry (Eds.), *Promoting adolescent health: A dialog on research and practice* (pp. 137-148). New York: Academic Press.

Box, G. E. P., & Jenkins, G. M. (1970). *Time-series analysis: Forecasting and control.* San Francisco: Holden-Day.

Box, G. E. P., & Tiao, G. C. (1975). Intervention analysis with applications to economic and environmental problems. *Journal of the American Statistical Association, 70,* 70-92.

Bracht, G. H., & Glass, G. V. (1968). The external validity of experiments. *American Educational Research Journal, 5,* 437-474.

Breslow, N. E., & Day, N. E. (1980). *Statistical methods in cancer research: Vol. I. The analysis of case-control studies* (IARC Scientific Publications No. 32). Lyon, France: International Agency for Research on Cancer.

Breslow, N. E., & Day, N. E. (1987). *Statistical methods in cancer research: Vol. II. The design and analysis of cohort studies* (IARC Scientific Publications No. 82). Lyon, France: International Agency for Research on Cancer.

Broders, A. C. (1920). Squamous cell epithelioma of the lip. *Journal of the American Medical Association, 74,* 656-664.

Brownell, K. D., Cohen, R. Y., Stunkard, A. J., Felix, M. R. J., & Cooley, N. B. (1984). Weight loss competitions at the work site: Impact on weight, morale, and cost-effectiveness. *American Journal of Public Health, 74*(11), 1283-1285.

Bruun, K., Edwards, G., Lumio, M., Mäkelä, K., Pan, L., Popham, R. E., Room, R., Schmidt, W., Skog, O.-J., Sulkunen, P., & Österberg, E. (1975). *Alcohol control policies in public health perspective* (Vol. 25). Helsinki: The Finnish Foundation for Alcohol Studies.

Bruvold, W. H., & Rundall, T. G. (1988). A meta-analysis and theoretical review of school based tobacco and alcohol intervention programs. *Psychology and Health, 2,* 53-78.

Bryant, J., & Zillman, D. (Eds.). (1986). *Perspectives on media effects.* Hillsdale, NJ: Lawrence Erlbaum.

Bryk, A. S., & Raudenbush, S. W. (1987). Application of hierarchical linear models to assessing change. *Psychological Bulletin, 101,* 147-158.

Buka, S., & Speare, M. (1990). Rhode Island's community alcohol abuse and injury prevention project. *Evaluating Community Prevention Strategies: Alcohol and Other Drugs* (pp. 15-19). Proceedings of a conference held in San Diego, California, January 11-13, 1990. La Jolla, CA: University of California, San Diego Extension.

Bull, J., & Roberts, B. (1973). Road accident statistics—A comparison of police and hospital information. *Accident Analysis and Prevention, 5,* 45-53.

Byar, D. P. (1988). The design of cancer prevention trials. In H. Scheurlen & R. Kay (Eds.), *Recent results in cancer research: Vol. III. Cancer clinical trials: A critical appraisal* (pp. 34-48). West Germany: Springer-Verlag.

Cahalan, D. (1987). *Understanding America's drinking problem.* San Francisco: Jossey-Bass Publishers.

Cahalan, D., Cisin, I. H., & Crossley, H. M. (1969). *American drinking practices.* New Brunswick, NJ: Rutgers Center of Alcohol Studies.

Cahalan, D., & Room, R. (1974). *Problem drinking among American men.* New Brunswick, NJ: Rutgers Center of Alcohol Studies.

Cain, G. G. (1975). Regression and selection models to improve nonexperimental comparisons. In C. A. Bennett & A. A. Lumsdaine (Eds.), *Evaluation and experiment: Some critical issues in assessing social programs.* New York: Academic Press.

Cairns, F. J., Koelmeyer, T. D., & Smeeton, W. M. I. (1984). Deaths from drowning. *New Zealand Medical Journal, 97,* 65-67.

Cameron, T. (1979, Winter). The impact of drinking-driving countermeasures: A review and evaluation. *Contemporary Drug Problems, 8*(4), 495-565.

Cameron, T. (1982). Drinking and driving among American youth: Beliefs and behaviors. *Drug and Alcohol Dependence, 10,* 1-33.

Campbell, D. T. (1969a). Prospective: Artifact and control. In R. Rosenthal & R. L. Rosnow (Eds.), *Artifact in behavioral research* (pp. 351-382). New York: Academic Press.

Campbell, D. T. (1969b). Reforms as experiments. *American Psychologist, 24,* 409-429.

Campbell, D. T., & Reichardt, C. S. (1991). Problems in assuming the comparability of pre-test and post-test in autoregressive and growth models. In R. E. Snow & D. E. Wiley (Eds.), *Improving inquiry in social science: A volume in honor of Lee J. Cronbach.* Hillsdale, NJ: Lawrence Erlbaum.

Campbell, D. T., & Stanley, J. C. (1966). *Experimental and quasi-experimental designs for research.* Chicago: Rand-McNally.

Carleton, R. A., Lasater, T. M., Assaf, A., Lefebvre, R. C., & McKinlay, S. M. (1987). The Pawtucket Heart Health Program: I. An experiment in population-based disease prevention. *Rhode Island Medical Journal, 70*(12), 533-538.

Casswell, S., & Gilmore, L. (1989, July). An evaluated community action project on alcohol. *Journal of Studies on Alcohol, 50*(4), 339-346.

Casswell, S., Ransom, R., & Gilmore, L. (1990). Evaluation of a mass media campaign for the primary prevention of alcohol-related problems. *Health Promotion International, 5*(1), 9-17.

Center for Science in the Public Interest. (1990). *State alcohol taxes: Case studies of the impact of higher excise taxes in 14 states and the District of Columbia: Raising revenues and reducing alcohol-related problems.* Washington, DC: Author.

Cherpitel, C. J. S. (1988, November). Alcohol consumption and casualties: A comparison of two emergency room populations. *British Journal of Addiction, 83*(11), 1299-1307.

Clarke, E. A., & Anderson, T. W. (1979). Does screening by "pap" smear help prevent cervical cancer? A case-control study. *Lancet, ii*, 1-4.

Clausen, J. A., Brim, O. G., Jr., Inkeles, A., Lippitt, R., Maccoby, E. E., & Smith, M. B. (1968). *Socialization and society.* Boston: Little, Brown and Company.

Coate, D., & Grossman, M. (1988). Effects of alcoholic beverage prices and legal drinking ages on youth alcohol use. *Journal of Law and Economics, 31*, 145-171.

Colditz, G., Branch, L., Lipnick, R., Willett, W., Rosner, B., Posner, B., & Hennekens, C. (1985). Moderate alcohol and decreased cardiovascular mortality in an elderly cohort. *American Heart Journal, 109*(4), 886-889.

Collette, H. J. A., Day, N. E., Rombach, J. J., & deWaard, F. (1984). Evaluation of screening for breast cancer in a non-randomized study (The DOM Project) by means of a case-control study. *Lancet, i*, 1224-1226.

Colon, I., & Cutter, H. (1983). The relationship of beer consumption and state alcohol and motor vehicle policies to fatal accidents. *Journal of Safety Research, 14*, 83-89.

Combs-Orme, T., Taylor, J. R., Scott, E. B., & Holmes, S. J. (1983, November). Violent deaths among alcoholics. *Journal of Studies on Alcohol, 44*(6), 938-949.

Cook, P. J. (1981). The effect of liquor taxes on drinking, cirrhosis, and auto accidents. In M. H. Moore & D. R. Gerstein (Eds.), *Alcohol and public policy: Beyond the shadow of prohibition* (pp. 255-285). Washington, DC: National Academy Press.

Cook, P. J. (1987). The impact of distilled-spirits taxes on consumption, auto fatalities, and cirrhosis mortality. In H. D. Holder (Ed.), *Control issues in alcohol abuse prevention: Strategies for states and communities* (pp. 159-167). Greenwich, CT: JAI Press Inc.

Cook, P. J., & Tauchen, G. (1982). The effect of liquor taxes on heavy drinking. *Bell Journal of Economics, 13*(4), 379-390.

Cook, T. D. (1985). Postpositivist critical multiplism. In R. L. Shotland & M. M. Mark (Eds.), *Social science and social policy* (pp. 21-62). Newbury Park, CA: Sage Publications.

Cook, T. D., & Campbell, D. T. (1979). *Quasi-experimentation: Design and analysis issues for field settings.* Boston: Houghton Mifflin Company.

Cordelia, A. (1985, March). Alcohol and property crime: Exploring the causal nexus. *Journal of Studies on Alcohol, 46*(2), 161-171.

Cordray, D. S. (1986). Quasi-experimental analysis: A mixture of methods and judgment. In W. M. K. Trochim (Ed.), *Advances in quasi-experimental design and analysis* (New Direction for Program Evaluation, No. 31, pp. 9-27). San Francisco: Jossey-Bass.

Council on Scientific Affairs. (1983). Automobile related injuries. *Journal of the American Medical Association, 249*(23), 3216-3222.

Cox, D. R. (1957). The use of a concomitant variable in selecting an experimental design. *Biometrika, 44*, 150-158.

Cox, D. R. (1975). Partial likelihood. *Biometrika, 62*, 269-276.

Criqui, M. (1990). The reduction of coronary heart disease with light to moderate alcohol consumption: Effect or artifact? *British Journal of Addiction, 85*(7), 854-857.

Criteria for approval of new drugs for advanced metastatic breast cancer: Few hard answers, but there are endpoints other than survival. (1989, September). *The Clinical Cancer Letter, 12*, 1-3.

Cronbach, L. J. (1982). *Designing evaluations of educational and social programs.* San Francisco: Jossey-Bass.

Cronbach, L. J., & Snow, R. E. (1981). *Aptitudes and instructional methods* (2nd ed.). New York: Irvington.

Crow, K. E., & Greenway, R. M. (1989). The metabolic effects of alcohol on the liver. In K. E. Crow & R. D. Batt (Eds.), *Human metabolism of alcohol* (Vol. III, pp. 3-18). Boca Raton, FL: CRC Press.

Dahl, R. A. (1961). *Who governs? Democracy and power in an American city.* New Haven, CT: Yale University Press.

de Lint, J., & Schmidt, W. (1968, December). The distribution of alcohol consumption in Ontario. *Quarterly Journal of Studies on Alcohol, 29*(4), 968-973.

Del Priore, L. (1987). Geomapping tools for market analysis. *Marketing/Communications, 12*, 91-94.

Department of Health and Human Services, Public Health Service. (1990, May 21). Expanded availability of investigational new drugs through a parallel track mechanism for people with AIDS and HIV-related disease. *Federal Register* (pp. 20856-20860). Washington, DC: U.S. Government Printing Office.

Department of Transportation. (1989). *Alcohol involvement in fatal traffic crashes 1987* (Department of Transportation Document HS-807-401). Washington, DC: National Technical Information Service.

DeVita, Moertel engage in debate over release of Levamisole results. (1990, February 16). *The Cancer Letter, 16,* 5-8.

Dielman, T. E. (1989). *Pooled cross-sectional and time series data analysis.* New York: Marcel Dekker.

Domhoff, G. W. (1978). *Who really rules? New Haven and community power reexamined.* New Brunswick, NJ: Transaction Books.

Domhoff, G. W. (1980). *Power structure research.* Beverly Hills: Sage Publications.

Domhoff, G. W. (1983). *Who rules America now? A view for the '80s.* New York: Simon & Schuster, Inc.

Durkheim, E. (1933). *The division of labor in society.* New York: Macmillan.

Durkheim, E. (1951). *Suicide* (J. Spaulding and G. Simpson, Trans.). Glencoe, IL: The Free Press.

Durkheim, E. (1964). *The division of labor in society* (George Simpson, Trans.). New York: The Free Press.

Dyer, A. R., Stamler, J., Oglesby, P., Lepper, M., Shekelle, R. B., McKean, H., & Garside, D. (1980). Alcohol consumption and 17 year mortality in the Chicago Western Electric Company study. *Preventive Medicine, 9,* 78-90.

Ebeling, K., & Nischan, P. (1987). Screening for lung cancer—results from a case-control study. *International Journal of Cancer, 40,* 141-144.

Edwards, G. (1986, April). The alcohol dependence syndrome: A concept as stimulus to enquiry. *British Journal of Addiction, 81*(2), 171-183.

Egger, G., Fitzgerald, W., Frape, G., Monaem, A., Rubinstein, P., Tyler, C., & McKay, B. (1983). Results of a large scale media antismoking campaign: North Coast "Quit for Life" programme. *British Medical Journal, 286,* 1125-1128.

Elliot, D. (1987). Self-reported driving while under the influence of alcohol/ drugs and the risk of alcohol/drug-related accidents. *Alcohol, Drugs, and Driving, 3*(3-4), 31-43.

Evans, L. (1987). Young drivers involvement in severe car crashes. *Alcohol, Drugs, and Driving, 3*(3-4), 63-78.

Farquhar, J. W. (1978). The community based model of lifestyle intervention trials. *American Journal of Epidemiology, 108,* 103-111.

Farquhar, J. W., Flora, J. A., Good, L., & Fortmann, S. P. (1985, March 13). *Integrated comprehensive health promotion programs.* Monograph prepared for the Kaiser Family Foundation.

Farquhar, J. W., Fortmann, S. P., Flora, J. A., & Maccoby, N. (1991). Methods of communication to influence behavior. In W. Holland, R. Detels, & G. Knox (Eds.), *Oxford textbook of public health* (Vol. 2, 1991). New York: Oxford University Press.

Farquhar, J. W., Fortmann, S. P., Flora, J. A., Taylor, C. B., Haskell, W. L., Williams, P. T., Maccoby, N., & Wood, P. D. (1990). Effects of community-wide education on cardiovascular disease risk factors: The Stanford Five-City Project. *Journal of the American Medical Association, 264*(3), 359-365.

Farquhar, J. W., Fortmann, S. P., Maccoby, N., Haskell, W. L., Williams, P. T., Flora, J. A., Taylor, C. B., Brown, B. W., Jr., Solomon, D. S., & Hulley, S. B. (1985). The Stanford Five-City Project: Design and methods. *American Journal of Epidemiology, 122*(2), 323-334.

Farquhar, J. W., Maccoby, N., & Solomon, D. (1984). Community applications of behavioral medicine. In W. D. Gentry (Ed.), *Handbook of behavioral medicine* (pp. 437-478). New York: Guilford Press.

Farquhar, J. W., Maccoby, N., Wood, P. D., Alexander, J. K., Breitrose, H., Brown, B. W., Haskell, W. L., McAlister, A. L., Meyer, A. J., Nash, J. D., & Stern, M. P. (1977). Community education for cardiovascular health. *Lancet, i,* 1192-1195.

Farris, R., Malone, T. B., & Kirkpatrick, M. (1977, September). *A comparison of alcohol involvement in exposed and injured drivers* (Final Report #DOT HS 802-555). Washington, DC: National Highway Traffic Safety Administration.

Feinstein, A. R. (1973). Clinical biostatistics: XX. The epidemiologic trohoc, the ablative risk ratio, and 'retrospective' research. *Clinical Pharmacological Therapy, 14,* 291-307.

Feinstein, A. R. (1985). Experimental requirements and scientific principles in case-control studies. *Journal of Chronic Diseases, 38*(2), 127-133.

Feinstein, A. R., & Horwitz, R. I. (1978). A critique of the statistical evidence associating estrogens with endometrial cancer. *Cancer Research, 38,* 4001-4005.

Feldman, J. G., Carter, A. C., Nicastri, A. D., & Hosat, S. T. (1981). Breast self-examination, relationship to stage of breast cancer at diagnosis. *Cancer, 47*(11), 2740-2745.

Feldt, L. S. (1958). A comparison of the precision of three experimental designs employing a concomitant variable. *Psychometrika, 23,* 335-353.

Felix, M. R. J., Stunkard, A. J., Cohen, R. Y., & Cooley, N. B. (1985). Health promotion at the worksite. 1. A process for establishing programs. *Preventive Medicine, 14*(1), 99-108.

Fell, J. (1983a, November). *Alcohol involvement in U.S. traffic accidents: Where it is changing* (#DOT HS 806-733). Washington, DC: National Highway Traffic Safety Administration, National Center for Statistics and Analysis.

Fell, J. (1983b). Tracking the alcohol involvement problem in U.S. highway crashes. *27th Annual Proceedings, American Association for Automotive Medicine* (pp. 23-42).

Fell, J., & Nash, C. (1989). The nature of the alcohol problem in U.S. fatal crashes. *Health Education Quarterly, 16*(3), 335-343.

Ferrence, R., Truscott, S., & Whitehead, P. (1986). Drinking and the prevention of coronary heart disease: Findings, issues, and public health policy. *Journal of Studies on Alcohol, 47*(5), 394-408.

Festinger, L., Schachter, S., & Back, K. (1950). *Social pressures in informal groups: Study of human factors in housing.* New York: Harper and Row.

Fetterman, D. M. (1982). Ibsen's baths: Reactivity and insensitivity. *Educational Evaluation and Policy Analysis, 4,* 261- 279.

Fillmore, K. M. (1987, January). Prevalence, incidence and chronicity of drinking patterns and problems among men as a function of age: A longitudinal and cohort analysis. *British Journal of Addiction, 82*(1), 77-83.

Fingarette, H. (1988). *Heavy drinking: The myth of alcoholism as a disease.* Berkeley, CA: University of California Press.

Finney, J. W., & Moos, R. H. (1986, March). Matching patients with treatments: Conceptual and methodological issues. *Journal of Studies on Alcohol, 47*(2), 122-134.

Flay, B. R. (1985). What we know about the social influences approach to smoking prevention: Review and recommendations. *Prevention research: Deterring drug abuse among children and adolescents* (Research 63 Monograph Series, USDHHS Pub. No. (ADM) 85-1334). Washington, DC: National Institute on Drug Abuse.

Flay, B. R. (1986, September). Efficacy and effectiveness trials (and other phases of research) in the development of health promotion programs. *Preventive Medicine, 15*(5), 451-474.

Flay, B. R. (1987). Mass media and smoking cessation: A critical review. *The American Journal of Public Health, 77*(2), 153-160.

Foster, R. S., Lang, S. P., Costanza, M. C., Worden, J. K., Haines, C. R., & Yates, J. W. (1978). Breast self-examination practices and breast cancer stage. *New England Journal of Medicine, 229,* 265-270.

Fraser, G., Anderson, J., Goldberg, R., Jacobs, D., & Blackburn, H. (1983). The effect of alcohol on serum high density lipoprotein: A controlled experiment. *Atherosclerosis, 46*(3), 275-286.

Freedman, L. S., Green, S. B., & Byar, D. P. (1990). Assessing the gain in efficiency due to matching in a community intervention study. *Statistics in Medicine, 9*(8), 943-952.

Freilich, M. (1963). Toward an operational definition of community. *Rural Sociology, 28,* 117-127.

Freimuth, V., Hammond, S., & Stein, J. (1988). Health advertising: Prevention for profit. *American Journal of Public Health, 78*(5), 557-561.

Friedman, L. M., Furberg, C. D., & DeMets, D. L. (1981). *Fundamentals of clinical trials*. Boston, MA: John Wright, PSG, Inc.

Fuller, R. K., Lee, K. K., & Gordis, E. (1988, April). Validity of self-report in alcoholism research: Results of a Veterans Administration cooperative study. *Alcoholism: Clinical and Experimental Research*, *12*(2), 201-205.

Gallagher, J. E. (with reporting by McDonald, J. F., & Winbush, D.) (1990, March 5). Under fire from all sides: Cigarette makers are assailed for targeting the young. *Time*, page 41.

Gardner, R. (1984). Can geodemographics simplify media planning? *Marketing and Media Decisions*, *19*, 66-68 and 79-82.

GCP Study Group. (1988). The German cardiovascular prevention study (GCP): Design and methods. *European Heart Journal*, *9*, 1058-1066.

Gerbner, G., Gross, L., Morgan, M., & Signorielli, N. (1982). Charting the mainstream: Television's contributions to political orientations. *Journal of Communication*, *32*, 100-127.

Gerbner, G., Gross, L., Morgan, M., & Signorielli, N. (1984). Political correlates of television viewing. *Public Opinion Quarterly*, *48*, 283-300.

Giesbrecht, N. (1987, October 18-22). *Alcohol-related problems, community agenda and prevention initiatives*. Paper presented at the 115th Annual Meeting of the American Public Health Association, New Orleans, LA.

Giesbrecht, N., & Douglas, R. R. (1990). The demonstration project and comprehensive community programming: Dilemmas in preventing alcohol-related problems. *Contemporary Drug Problems*, *17*(3), 421-459.

Giesbrecht, N., Holder, H. D., & Wood, L. (1990). Longitudinal analysis of the impact of a prevention project on local alcohol sales. (unpublished manuscript)

Giesbrecht, N., & Pranovi, P. (1986). Prevention agenda in the context of drinking cultures. In N. Giesbrecht & A. E. Cox (Eds.), *Prevention: Alcohol and the environment* (pp. 43-57). Toronto, Ontario: Addiction Research Foundation.

Giesbrecht, N., Pranovi, P., & Wood, L. (1990). Impediments to changing local drinking practices: Lessons from a prevention project. In N. Giesbrecht, P. Conley, R. W. Denniston, L. Gliksman, H. Holder, A. Pederson, R. Room, & M. Shain (Eds.), *Research, action, and the community: Experiences in the prevention of alcohol and other drug problems* (OSAP Prevention Monograph No. 4, pp. 161-182). Rockville, MD: Office for Substance Abuse Prevention.

Glanz, K., & Mullis, R. M. (1988). Environmental interventions to promote healthy eating: A review of models, programs, and evidence. *Health Education Quarterly*, *15*, 395-415.

Glaser, F. B., Mendelson, J., Mäkelä, K., Room, R., Uchtenhagen, A., Moser, J., Heitman, L., & Charles-Nicholas, A. (1987, October). The future of the word 'alcoholism'. *British Journal of Addiction, 82*(10), 1061-1071.

Glass, G. V. (1988). Quasi-experiments: The case of interrupted time series. In R. M. Jaeger (Ed.), *Complementary methods for research in education* (pp. 445-464). Washington, DC: American Educational Research Association.

Glass, G. V., Willson, V. L., & Gottman, J. M. (1975). *Design and analysis of time-series experiments*. Boulder, CO: Colorado Associated University Press.

Gleiberman, L., & Harburg, E. (1986). Alcohol usage and blood pressure: A review. *Human Biology, 58*(1), 1-31.

Goldberger, A. S. (1972). *Selection bias in evaluating treatment effects: Some formal illustrations* (Discussion Paper 123-72). Madison, WI: University of Wisconsin, Institute for Research on Poverty.

Goodstadt, M. S. (1989). Drug education: The prevention issues. *The Journal of Drug Education, 19*(3), 197-208.

Goplen, A. (1982, June). Alcohol and cardiovascular disease. *The Globe,* pp. 10-12.

Gove, W. R., Hughes, M., & Geerken, M. (1985). Are uniform crime reports a valid indicator of the index crimes? An affirmative answer with minor qualifications. *Criminology, 23*(3), 451-501.

Grant, B., Noble, J., & Malin, H. (1986). Decline in liver cirrhosis mortality and components of change: United States, 1973-1983. *Alcohol Health and Research World, 10*(3), 66-69.

Green, L. W. (1986). The theory of participation: A qualitative analysis of its expression in national and international health policies. In W. Ward (Ed.), *Advances in health education and promotion,* 1(Part A), pp. 211-236.

Green, L. W., & Kreuter, M. W. (1990). Health promotion as a public health strategy for the 1990s. *Annual Review of Public Health, 11,* 319-334.

Green, L. W., & McAlister, A. L. (1984). Macro-intervention to support health behavior: Some theoretical perspectives and practical reflections. *Health Education Quarterly, 11*(3), 322-339.

Greenberg, S. W. (1981). Alcohol and crime: A methodological critique of the literature. In J. J. Collins Jr. (Ed.), *Drinking and crime: Perspectives on the relationships between alcohol consumption and criminal behavior* (pp. 70-109). New York: The Guilford Press.

Greenwald, P., & Caban, C. (1986). A strategy for cancer prevention and control research. *Bulletin of The World Health Organization, 64,* 73-78.

Greenwald, P., & Cullen, J. W. (1985). The new emphasis in cancer control. *Journal of the National Cancer Institute, 74*(3), 543-551.

Greenwald, P., Cullen, J. W., & McKenna, J. W. (1987). Cancer prevention and control: From research through applications. *Journal of the National Cancer Institute, 79*(2), 389-400.

Greenwald, P., Nasca, P. C., Lawrence, C. E., Horton, J., McGarrah, R. P., Gabrile, T., & Carlton, K. (1978). Estimated effect of breast self-examination and routine physical examinations on breast cancer mortality. *New England Journal of Medicine, 299*, 271-273.

Grosser, C. F. (1973). *New directions in community organization: From enabling to advocacy.* New York: Praeger Publishers.

Grossman, M. (1988). *Health economics of prevention of alcohol-related problems.* Paper presented at the workshop on Health Economics of Prevention and Treatment of Alcohol-Related Problems, Washington, DC: National Insititute on Alcohol Abuse and Alcoholism.

Grossman, M., Coate, D., & Arluck, G. M. (1987). Price sensitivity of alcoholic beverages in the U.S.: Youth alcohol consumption. In H. Holder (Ed.), *Control issues in alcohol abuse prevention: Strategies for states and communities* (pp. 169-198). Greenwich, CT: JAI Press.

Grube, J. W., & Morgan, M. (1986). *Smoking, drinking and other drug use among Dublin post-primary school pupils* (Paper #132). Dublin: The Economic and Social Research Institute.

Gruchow, H., Hoffman, R., Anderson, A., & Barboriak, J. (1982). Effects of drinking patterns on the relationship between alcohol and coronary occlusion. *Atherosclerosis, 43*, 393-404.

Gruenewald, P. J. (1989, June 12). *A choice model of alcohol consumption.* Paper presented at the annual meeting of the Research Society on Alcoholism, Beaver Creek, CO.

Gruenewald, P. J. (1990). *Baseline data for California tax initiative* (NIAAA Grant 3 RO1 AA08395-02S1A2). Berkeley, CA: Pacific Institute for Research and Evaluation.

Gruenewald, P. J., Stewart, K., & Klitzner, M. (1990, January). Alcohol use and the appearance of alcohol problems among first offender drunk drivers. *British Journal of Addiction, 85*(1), 107-117.

Guralnik, D. B. (Ed.) (1982). *Webster's new world dictionary of the American language.* New York: Warner Books.

Gusfield, J. R. (1975). Categories of ownership and responsibility in social issues: Alcohol abuse and automobile use. *Journal of Drug Issues, 5*, 285-303.

Gutzwiller, F., Nater, B., & Martin, J. (1985, July). Community-based primary prevention of cardiovascular disease in Switzerland: Methods and results of the national research program (NRP 1A). *Preventive Medicine, 14*(4), 482-491.

Haberman, P. W., & Baden, M. M. (1978). *Alcohol, other drugs and violent death*. New York: Oxford University Press, Inc.

Hansen, W. B., Johnson, C. A., Flay, B. R., Graham, J. W., & Sobel, J. (1988). Affective and social influences approaches to the prevention of multiple substance abuse among seventh grade students: Results from Project SMART. *Preventive Medicine, 17*, 135-154.

Hasin, D., Grant, B., & Harford, T. (1990). Male and female differences in liver cirrhosis mortality in the United States, 1961-1985. *Journal of Studies on Alcohol, 51*(2), 123-129.

Hausman, J. A., & Wise, D. A. (Eds.) (1985). *Social experimentation*. Chicago: University of Chicago Press.

Heckman, J. J., & Robb, R. (1985). Alternative methods for evaluating the impact of interventions. In J. J. Heckman & B. Singer (Eds.), *Longitudinal analysis of labor market data* (pp. 156-245). New York: Cambridge University Press.

Heeren, T., Smith, R., Morelock, S., & Hingson, R. (1985). Surrogate measures of alcohol involvement in fatal crashes: Are conventional indicators adequate? *Journal of Safety Research, 16*, 127-134.

Hillery, G. A., Jr. (1955). Definitions of community: Areas of agreement. *Rural Sociology, 20*, 111-123.

Hillery, G. A., Jr. (1963). Villages, cities, and total institutions. *American Sociological Review, 28*, 779-791.

Hillery, G. A., Jr. (1972). Selected issues in community theory. *Rural Sociology, 37*, 534-552.

Hillery, G. A., Jr. (1982). *A research odyssey: Developing and testing a community theory*. New Brunswick: Transaction Books.

Hilton, M. E. (1989, May). What I would most like to know: How many alcoholics are there in the United States? *British Journal of Addiction, 84*(5), 459-460.

Hingson, R., Heeren, T., Mangione, T., Morelock, S., & Mucatel, M. (1982). Teenage driving after using marijuana or drinking and traffic accident involvement. *Journal of Safety Research, 13*, 33-37.

Hingson, R., & Howland, J. (1987). Alcohol as a risk factor for injury or death resulting from accidental falls: A review of the literature. *Journal of Studies on Alcohol, 48*(3), 212-219.

Hingson, R., & Howland, J. (1990). Use of laws to deter drinking and driving. *Alcohol and Health Research World, 14*(1), 36-43.

Hingson, R., Howland, J., Morelock, S., & Heeren, T. (1988). Legal interventions to reduce drunken driving and related fatalities among youthful drivers. *Accident Analysis and Prevention, 4*(2), 87-98.

Hoadley, J. F., Fuchs, B. C., & Holder, H. D. (1984). The effect of alcohol beverage restrictions on consumption: A 25-year longitudinal analysis. *American Journal of Drug and Alcohol Abuse, 10*, 375-401.

Hochheimer, J. L. (1981). Reducing alcohol abuse: A critical review of educational strategies. In M. H. Moore & D. R. Gerstein (Eds.), *Alcohol and public policy: Beyond the shadow of prohibition* (pp. 286-335). Washington, DC: National Academy Press.

Holden, C. (1988). NCI may evaluate "alternative therapy". *Science, 241*, 1285-1286.

Holder, H. D. (Ed.). (1987). *Control issues in alcohol abuse prevention: Strategies for states and communities.* Greenwich, CT: JAI Press, Inc.

Holder, H. D., & Blose, J. O. (1983). Prevention of alcohol-related traffic problems: Computer simulation of alternative strategies. *Journal of Safety Research, 14*(3), 115-129.

Holder, H. D., & Blose, J. O. (1985). Impact of changes in distilled spirits availability on alcohol distribution. *Alcohol, 2*(3), 541-544.

Holder, H. D., & Blose, J. O. (1987a, June). Impact of changes in distilled spirits availability on apparent consumption: A time series analysis of liquor-by-the-drink. *British Journal of Addiction, 82*(6), 623-631.

Holder, H. D., & Blose, J. O. (1987b). Reduction of community alcohol problems: Computer simulation experiments in three counties. *Journal of Studies on Alcohol, 48*(2), 124-135.

Holder, H. D., & Blose, J. O. (1988). Community planning and the prevention of alcohol involved traffic problems: An application of computer simulation technology. *Evaluation and Program Planning, 11*(3), 267-277.

Holder, H. D., & Giesbrecht, N. (1990). Perspectives on the community in action research. In N. Giesbrecht, P. Conley, R. W. Denniston, L. Gliksman, H. Holder, A. Pederson, R. Room, & M. Shain (Eds.), *Research, action, and the community: Experiences in the prevention of alcohol and other drug problems* (OSAP Prevention Monograph No. 4, pp. 27-40). Rockville, MD: Office for Substance Abuse Prevention.

Holder, H. D., & Wagenaar, A. C. (1990, December). Effects of the elimination of a state monopoly on distilled spirits' retail sales: A time-series analysis of Iowa. *British Journal of Addiction, 85*(12), 1615-1625.

Holder, H. D., & Wallack, L. M. (1986). Contemporary perspectives for preventing alcohol problems: An empirically-derived model. *Journal of Public Health Policy, 7*(3), 324-339.

Homel, R. (1988). *Policing and punishing the drinking driver: A study of general and specific deterence.* New York: Springer-Verlag.

Honkanen, R., Ertama, L., Kuosmanen, P., Linnoila, M., Alha, A., & Visuri, T. (1983). The role of alcohol in accidental falls. *Journal of Studies on Alcohol, 44*(2), 231-245.

Howard, J. (1984). *Breast self examination: Issues for research: Proceedings of the working group meeting to explore issues in breast self examination* (Bethesda, MD, April 19-20, 1982). Bethesda, MD: National Cancer Institute, Division of Cancer Prevention and Control, Health Promotion Sciences Branch.

Howard, J., Ganikos, M. L., & Taylor, J. A. (1990). Alcohol prevention research: Confronting the challenge. In R. R. Watson (Ed.), *Drug and alcohol abuse prevention* (pp. 1-18). Clifton, NJ: Humana Press.

Howard, J., Whittemore, A. S., Hoover, J. J., Panos, M., & Aspirin Myocardial Infarction Study Research Group (1982). How blind was the patient blind in AMIS? *Clinical Pharmacology and Therapeutics, 32,* 543-553.

Howland, J., & Hingson, R. (1987, Sept-Oct). Alcohol as a risk factor for injuries or death due to fires or burns: Review of the literature. *Public Health Reports, 102*(5), 475-483.

Howland, J., & Hingson, R. (1988). Alcohol as a risk factor for drownings: A review of the literature (1950-1985). *Accident Analysis and Prevention, 20*(1), 19-25.

Huguley, C. M., & Brown, R. L. (1981). The value of breast self-examination. *Cancer, 47*(5), 989-995.

Hume, D., & Fitzgerald, E. (1985). Chemical tests for intoxication: What do the numbers really mean? *Analytical Chemistry, 57*(8), 876A-886A.

Hunter, F. (1952). *Community power structure: A study of decision makers.* Chapel Hill: University of North Carolina Press.

Hunter, F. (1980). *Community power succession: Atlanta's policy-makers revisited.* Chapel Hill: University of North Carolina Press.

Hyman, H., & Sheatsley, P. (1947). Some reasons why information campaigns fail. *Public Opinion Quarterly, 11,* 412-423.

Institute of Medicine, Division of Mental Health and Behavioral Medicine. (1989). *Prevention and treatment of alcohol problems: Research opportunities.* Washington, DC: National Academy Press.

Jellinek, E. M. (1959, June). Estimating the prevalence of alcoholism: Modified values in the Jellinek formula and an alternative approach. *Quarterly Journal of Studies in Alcohol, 20*(2), 261-269.

Jones, A. (1982). How breathing techniques can influence the results of breath-alcohol analysis. *Medicine, Science, and the Law, 22*(4), 275-280.

Joreskog, K. G., & Sorbom, D. (1988). *LISREL 7: A guide to the program and applications.* Chicago: SPSS, Inc.

Judd, C. M., & Kenny, D. A. (1981). *Estimating the effects of social interventions.* New York: Cambridge University Press.

Kalbfleisch, J. D., & Prentice, R. L. (1980). *The statistical analysis of failure time data.* New York: John Wiley.

Karpf, R., & Williams, A. (1983). Teenage drivers and motor vehicle deaths. *Accident Analysis and Prevention*, *15*(1), 55-63.

Kaufman, D., Rosenberg, L., Helmrich, S., & Shapiro, S. (1985). Alcoholic beverages and myiocardial infarction in young men. *American Journal of Epidemiology*, *121*(4), 548-554.

Kendell, R. E. (1987). Drinking sensibly (The first Benno Pollak Lecture). *British Journal of Addiction*, *82*(12), 1279-1288.

Keys, A. (1980). *Seven countries: A multivariate analysis of death and coronary heart disease*. Cambridge, MA: Harvard University Press.

Killen, J. D. (1985). Prevention of adolescent tobacco smoking: The social pressure resistance training approach. *Journal of Child Psychology and Psychiatry*, *26*, 7-15.

Killen, J. D., Telch, M. J., Robinson, T. N., Maccoby, N., Taylor, C. B., & Farquhar, J. W. (1988). Cardiovascular disease risk reduction for tenth graders: A multiple factor school-based approach, *Journal of the American Medical Association*, *260*, 1728-1733.

Kinal, D. (1984, September 14). Dip into several segmentation schemes to paint accurate picture of marketplace. *Marketing News*, p. 32.

Kinder, B. N. (1975). Attitudes toward alcohol and drug abuse. II. Experimental data, mass media research, and methodological considerations. *International Journal of the Addictions*, *10*, 1035-1054.

King, A. C., Flora, J. A., Fortmann, S. P., & Taylor, C. B. (1987). Smokers' challenge: Immediate and long-term findings of a community smoking cessation contest. *American Journal of Public Health*, *77*(10), 1340-1341.

Klein, T. (1986). *A method for estimating posterior BAC distributions for persons involved in fatal traffic accidents* (DOT HS-807-094). Washington, DC: National Highway Traffic Administration.

Knupfer, G. (1966). Some methodological problems in the epidemiology of alcoholic beverage usage: Definition of amount of intake. *American Journal of Public Health*, *56*, 237-242.

Knupfer, G. (1987, June). New directions for survey research in the study of alcoholic beverage consumption. *British Journal of Addiction*, *82*(6), 583-585.

Kornitzer, M., & Rose, G. (1985, May). WHO European collaborative trial of multifactorial prevention of coronary heart disease. *Preventive Medicine*, *14*(3), 272-278.

Kotler, P., & Zaltman, G. (1971). Social marketing: An approach to planned social change. *Journal of Marketing*, *35*, 3-12.

Kraemer, H. C., & Thiemann, S. (1987). *How many subjects? Statistical power analysis in research*. Newbury Park, CA: Sage Publications.

Kramer, R. M., & Specht, H. (Eds.) (1983). *Readings in community organization practice* (3rd ed.). Englewood Cliffs, NJ: Prentice-Hall, Inc.

Kreitman, N. (1986, June). Alcohol consumption and the prevention paradox. *British Journal of Addiction, 81*(3), 353-363.

Kuusi, P. (1957). *Alcohol sales experiment in rural Finland*. Helsinki: The Finnish Foundation for Alcohol Studies.

La Vecchia, C., Franceschi, S., DeCarli, A., Fasoli, M., Gentile, A., & Tognoni, G. (1984). 'Pap' smear and the risk of cervical neoplasia: Quantitative estimates from a case-control study. *Lancet, ii*, 779-782.

LaLonde, R. J. (1986). Evaluating the econometric evaluations of training programs with experimental data. *American Economic Review, 76*, 604-620.

Lang, A. R., Goeckner, D. J., Adesso, V. J., & Marlatt, G. A. (1975). Effects of alcohol on aggression in male social drinkers. *Journal of Abnormal Psychology, 84*(5), 508-518.

Lasater, T., Abrams, D., Artz, L., Beaudin, P., Cabrera, L., Elder, J., Ferreira, A., Knisley, P., Peterson, G., Rodrigues, A., Rosenberg, P., Snow, R., & Carleton, R. (1984). Lay volunteer delivery of a community-based cardiovascular risk factor change program: The Pawtucket experiment. In J. D. Matarazzo, S. M. Weiss, J. A. Herd, N. E. Miller, & S. M. Weiss (Eds.), *Behavioral health: A handbook of health enhancement and disease prevention* (pp. 1166-1170). New York: John Wiley & Sons.

Last, J. M. (Ed.) (1983). *A dictionary of epidemiology*. New York: Oxford University Press.

Lauffer, A. (1981). The practice of social planning. In N. Gilbert & H. Specht (Eds.), *Handbook of the social services* (pp. 583-597). Englewood Cliffs, NJ: Prentice-Hall.

Ledermann, S. (1956). *Alcool, alcoolisme, alcoolisation* [Alcohol, alcoholism, alcoholization] (Vol. 1). Paris, France: Presses Universitaires de France.

Ledermann, S. (1964). *Alcool, alcoolisme, alcoolisation* [Alcohol, alcoholism, alcoholization] (Vol. 2). Mortalité, morbidité, accidents du travail. (Institut National d'Études Démographiques, Travaux et Documents, Cahier n 41). Paris, France: Presses Universitaires de France.

Lefebvre, R. C., & Flora, J. A. (1988). Social marketing and public health intervention. *Health Education Quarterly, 15*(3), 299-315.

Lelbach, W. K. (1974). Organic pathology related to volume and pattern of alcohol use. In R. J. Gibbins, Y. Israel, H. Kalant, R. E. Popham, W. Schmidt, & R. G. Smart (Eds.), *Research advances in alcohol and drug problems* (Vol. 1, pp. 93-198). New York: John Wiley and Sons.

Lenke, L. (1975). *Valdbrott och alkohol: En studie i misshandelsbrottslighetens utveckling* [Violent crime and alcohol: A study of the developments in assaultive crime]. Stockholm: University of Stockholm, Department of Criminology.

Lesser, J., & Hughes, M. (1986). The generalizability of psychographic market segments across geographic locations. *Journal of Marketing, 50,* 18-27.

Levy, D., & Sheflin, N. (1983, November). New evidence on controlling alcohol use through price. *Journal of Studies on Alcohol, 44*(6), 929-937.

Levy, D., & Sheflin, N. (1985). The demand for alcoholic beverages: An aggregate time-series analysis. *Journal of Public Policy and Marketing, 4,* 47-54.

Levy, P., Voas, R., Johnson, P., & Klein, T. (1978). An evaluation of the Department of Transportation's alcohol safety action projects. *Journal of Safety Research, 10*(4), 162-176.

Liang, K.-Y., & Zeger, S. L. (1986). Longitudinal data analysis using generalized linear models. *Biometrika, 73,* 13-22.

Light, R., Singer, J., & Willett, J. (1990). *By design: Planning research in higher education.* Cambridge, MA: Harvard University Press.

Linet, M. S., & Brookmeyer, R. (1987). Use of cancer controls in case-control cancer studies. *American Journal of Epidemiology, 125*(1), 1-11.

Lipsey, M. W. (1990). *Design sensitivity: Statistical power for experimental research.* Newbury Park, CA: Sage Publications, Inc.

Lipsey, M. W., Cordray, D. S., & Berger, D. E. (1981, June). Evaluation of a juvenile diversion program: Using multiple lines of evidence. *Evaluation Review, 5*(3), 283-306.

Livingston, I. (1985). Alcohol consumption and hypertension: A review with suggested implications. *Journal of the National Medical Association, 72*(2), 129-135.

Lord, F. M. (1967). A paradox in the interpretation of group comparisons. *Psychological Bulletin, 68,* 304-305.

Lowenfels, A., & Zevola, S. (1989). Alcohol and breast cancer: An overview. *Alcoholism: Clinical and Experimental Research, 13*(1), 109-111.

Lubin, J. H. (1986). Extension of analytic methods for nested and population-based incident case-control studies. *Journal of Chronic Diseases, 39*(5), 379-388.

Lubin, J. H., & Hartge, P. (1984). Excluding controls: Misapplications in case-control studies. *American Journal of Epidemiology, 120*(5), 791-793.

Luepker, R. V., Johnson, C. A., Murray, D. M., & Pechacek, T. F. (1983). Prevention of cigarette smoking: Three year follow-up of an education program for youth. *Journal of Behavioral Medicine, 6*, 53-62.

Maas, M., & Harris, S. (1984). Police recording of road accident in-patients. *Accident Analysis and Prevention, 16*(3), 167-184.

MacAndrew, C., & Edgerton, R. B. (1969). *Drunken comportment: A social explanation.* Chicago: Aldine Publishing Company.

Maccoby, N., Farquhar, J. W., Wood, P. D., & Alexander, J. (1977). Reducing the risk of cardiovascular disease: Effects of a community-based campaign on knowledge and behavior. *Journal of Community Health, 3*, 100-114.

Macgregor, J. E., Moss, S. M., Parkin, D. M., & Day, N. E. (1985). A case-control study of cervical cancer screening in Northeast Scotland. *British Medical Journal, 290*, 1543-1546.

Mäkelä, K. (1978). Level of consumption and social consequences of drinking. In Y. Israel, et al. (Eds.) *Research advances in alcohol and drug problems* (Vol. 4, pp. 303-348). New York: Plenum Press.

Mäkelä, K. (1980, Winter). Differential effects of restricting the supply of alcohol: Studies of a strike in Finnish liquor stores. *Journal of Drug Issues, 10*(1), 131-144.

Mäkelä, K., & Room, R. (1985). *Alcohol policy and the rights of the drunkard.* Paper presented at the 30th International Institute on the Prevention and Treatment of Alcoholism, Athens, Greece, May 27 - June 2, 1984.

Mäkelä, K., Room, R., Single, E., Sulkunen, P., Walsh, B., Bunce, R., Cahannes, M., Cameron, T., Giesbrecht, N., de Lint, J., Mäkinen, H., Morgan, P., Mosher, J., Moskalewicz, J., Müller, R., Österberg, E., Wald, I., & Walsh, D. (1981). *Alcohol, society and the state, Volume 1: A comparative study of alcohol control.* Toronto: Addiction Research Foundation.

Malin, H., Coakley, J., Kaelber, C., Munch, N., & Holland, W. (1982). An epidemiologic perspective on alcohol use and abuse in the United States. In National Institute on Alcohol Abuse and Alcoholism, *Alcohol consumption and related problems* (Alcohol and Health Monograph No. 1, DHHS Pub. No. ADM 82-1190, pp. 99-153). Washington, DC: Superintendent of Documents, U.S. Government Printing Office.

Maloy, B. F. (1984). Viewpoint of the United States Brewers Association, Inc. In H. D. Holder & J. B. Hallan (Eds.), *Control issues in alcohol abuse prevention: Local, state and national designs for the '80s* (pp. 191-194). Chapel Hill, NC: The Human Ecology Institute.

Mann, R., & Anglin, L. (1988). The relationship between alcohol-related traffic fatalities and per capita consumption of alcohol, Ontario, 1957-1983. *Accident Analysis and Prevention, 20*(6), 441-446.

Manning, W. G., Keeler, E. B., Newhouse, J. P., Sloss, E. M., & Wasserman, J. (1989). The taxes of sin: Do smokers and drinkers pay their way? *Journal of the American Medical Association, 261,* 1604-1609.

Mark, M. M. (1990). From program theory to *tests* of program theory. In L. Bickman (Ed.) *Advances in program theory* (New Directions in Program Evaluation, No. 47) (pp. 37-51). San Francisco: Jossey-Bass.

Marlatt, G. A. (1982). Relapse prevention: A self-control program for the treatment of addictive behaviors. In R. B. Stuart (Ed.), *Adherence, compliance and generalization in behavioral medicine* (pp. 329-378). New York: Brunner/Mazel Inc.

Marmot, M. (1984). Alcohol and coronary heart disease. *International Journal of Epidemiology, 113*(2), 160-167.

Mason, A., & McBay, A. (1984). Ethanol, marijuana, and other drug use in 600 drivers killed in single-vehicle crashes in North Carolina, 1978-1981. *Journal of Forensic Sciences, 29*(4), 987-1026.

Massachusetts Medical Society. (1990). Alcohol-related mortality and years of potential life lost 1987—United States, 1990. *Morbidity and Mortality Weekly Report, 39*(11), 174-178.

Mausner, J. S., & Kramer, S. (1985). *Epidemiology: An introductory text* (pp. 10-12). Philadelphia: W. B. Saunders.

Maxwell, B., & Jacobson, M. (1989). *Marketing disease to Hispanics: The selling of alcohol, tobacco and junk foods.* Washington, DC: Center for Science in the Public Interest.

Mayhew, D., Donelson, A., Beirness, D., & Simpson, H. (1986). Youth, alcohol and relative risk of crash involvement. *Accident Analysis and Prevention, 18*(4), 273-287.

McAlister, A. L., & Green, L. W. (1985). Health promotion. In R. Michels (Ed.), *Psychiatry* (Vol. 2., pp. 1-7). New York: Basic Books.

McAlister, A. L., Perry, C., & Maccoby, N. (1979). Adolescent smoking: Onset and prevention. *Pediatrics, 63,* 650-658.

McAlister, A., Ramirez, A., Amezcua, C., Pulley, L., Stern, M., & Mercado, S. (1992). Smoking cessation in Texas-Mexico border communities: A quasi-experimental panel study. *American Journal of Health Promotion, 6*(4), 274-279.

McCarty, D., & Argeriou, M. (1988, January). Rearrest following residential treatment for repeat offender drunken drivers. *Journal of Studies on Alcohol, 49*(1), 1-6.

McCarty, D., Poore, M., Mills, K. C., & Morrison, S. (1983). Direct-mail techniques and the prevention of alcohol-related problems among college students. *Journal of Studies on Alcohol, 44*(1), 162-170.

McCleary, R., & Hay, R. A. (1980). *Applied time series analysis.* Newbury Park, CA: Sage Publications, Inc.

McCord, W., & McCord, J. (1962). A longitudinal study of the personality of alcoholics. In D. J. Pittman & C. R. Synder (Eds.), *Society, culture, and drinking patterns*. New York: John Wiley & Sons.

McCullagh, P. (1983). Quasi-likelihood functions. *Annals of Statistics, 11*, 59-67.

McGavran, E. G. (1963). Facing reality in public health. *Key Issues in the Prevention of Alcoholism* (pp. 55-61). Proceedings of the Northeast States Conference on Key Isues in the Prevention of Alcoholism held in Pittsburgh, PA, October 22-24, 1962. Sponsored by the Pennsylvania Department of Health, Harrisburg, PA.

McGraw, S. A., McKinlay, S. M., McClements, L., Lasater, T. M., Assaf, A., & Carleton, R. A. (1989). Methods in program evaluation: The process evaluation system of the Pawtucket Heart Health Program. *Evaluation Review, 3*(5), 459-483.

McKeown-Eyssen, G. E., & Thomas, D. C. (1985). Sample size determination in case-control studies: The influence of the distribution of exposure. *Journal of Chronic Diseases, 38*(7), 559-568.

McKinlay, S. M., Carleton, R. A., McKenney, J. L., & Assaf, A. R. (1989). A new approach to surveillance for acute myocardial infarction: Reproducibility and cost efficiency. *International Journal of Epidemiology, 18*(1), 67-75.

McKnight, A. J. (1987). *Development and field test of a responsible alcohol service program. Volume I: Research findings* (Report No. DOT HA 807 221). Washington, DC: U.S. Department of Transportation, National Highway Traffic Safety Administration.

McKnight, A. J. (1991). Factors influencing the effectiveness of server-intervention education. *Journal of Studies on Alcohol, 52*(5), 389-397.

McLaughlin, J. K., Blot, W. J., Mehl, E. S., & Mandel, J. S. (1985). Problems in the use of dead controls in case-control studies: I—General results. *American Journal of Epidemiology, 121*(1), 131-139.

McLaughlin, M. W. (1985). Implementation realities and evaluation design. In R. L. Shotland & M. M. Mark (Eds.), *Social science and social policy* (pp. 96-120). Newbury Park, CA: Sage Publications.

Meinert, C. L. (1986). *Clinical trials: Design, conduct and analysis*. New York: Oxford Press.

Mendelson, J. (1987, October). Problem thinking. *British Journal of Addiction, 82*(10), 1062-1063.

Merton, R. K. (1957). *Social theory and social structure*. Glencoe, IL: The Free Press.

Meyer, A. J., & Henderson, J. B. (1974). Multiple risk factor reduction in the prevention of cardiovascular disease. *Preventive Medicine, 3*, 225-236.

Michaelson, G. (1988). Niche marketing in the trenches. *Marketing/ Communications*, *13*, 19-24.

Midanik, E. (1982). Validity of self-reported alcohol consumption and alcohol problems. *British Journal of Addiction*, *77*, 357-382.

Mierley, M. C., & Baker, S. P. (1983). Fatal house fires in an urban population. *Journal of the American Medical Association*, *249*, 1466-1468.

Mills, C. W. (1956). *The power elite*. New York: Oxford University Press.

Mills, K. C., & McCarty, D. (1983, Winter). A data based alcohol abuse prevention program in a university setting. *Journal of Alcohol and Drug Education*, *28*(2), 15-27.

Moertel, C. G., Fleming, T. R., Rubin, J., Kvols, L. K., Sarna, G., Koch, R., Currie, V. E., Young, C. W., Jones, S. E., & Davignon, J. P. (1982). A clinical trial of Amygdalin (Laetrile) in the treatment of human cancer. *New England Journal of Medicine*, *306*, 201-206.

Mogford, M. (1983). *An analysis of boating fatalities in Ontario, 1980-1983*. Ontario: Ministry of Natural Resources.

Mohr, L. B. (1988). *Impact analysis for program evaluation*. Chicago: Dorsey.

Moore, M. H., & Gerstein, D. R. (Eds.). (1981). *Alcohol and public policy: Beyond the shadow of prohibition*. Washington, DC: National Academy Press.

Moore, R., & Pearson, T. (1986). Moderate alcohol consumption and coronary artery disease. *Medicine*, *65*(4), 242-267.

Morgan, P. A. (1988, Summer). Power, politics and public health: The political power of the alcohol beverage industry. *Journal of Public Health Policy*, *9*(2), 177-197.

Mosher, J. F., & Colman, V. (1989). *Alcohol beverage control in a public health perspective: A handbook for action*. San Rafael, CA: Marin Institute for the Prevention of Alcohol and Other Drug Problems.

Mosher, J. F., & Jernigan, D. H. (1989). New directions in alcohol policy. *Annual Review of Public Health*, *10*, 245-279.

Moskowitz, J. M. (1989). The primary prevention of alcohol problems: A critical review of the research literature. *Journal of Studies on Alcohol*, *50*(1), 54-88.

Moskowitz, J. M., & Jones, R. (1988). Alcohol and drug problems in the schools: Results of a national survey of school administrators. *Journal of Studies on Alcohol*, *49*(4), 299-305.

Mullis, R. M., Hunt, M. K., Foster, M., Hachfeld, L., Lansing, D., Synder, T., & Pirie, P. (1987). The shop smart for your health grocery program. *Journal of Nutrition Education*, *19*, 225-228.

Mullis, R. M., & Pirie, P. (1988). Lean meats make the grade: A collaborative nutrition education program. *Journal of the American Dietary Association, 88,* 191.

Myers, C. A., Hovell, M. F., Elder, J. P., & Hall, J. A. (1991). Paradoxical effects of blood alcohol concentration charts. *Preventive Medicine, 20*(3), 431-435.

National Cancer Institute. (1986). *Technical report: Cancer awareness survey, Wave II.* Bethesda, MD: Office of Cancer Communications.

National Heart, Lung, and Blood Institute. (1984). [Community Cardiovascular Surveillance Pilot Study Data.] Unpublished data.

National Heart, Lung, and Blood Institute. (1987). *Guidelines for demonstration and education research grants.* Washington, DC: U.S. Government Printing Office.

National Highway Traffic Safety Administration. (1982). *Evaluation of minimum drinking age laws using the national electronic injury surveillance system.* Washington, DC: Author.

National Institute on Alcohol Abuse and Alcoholism & Office for Substance Abuse Prevention. (1990). *Community-based research on the prevention of alcohol-related problems* (RFA-AA-91-01). Rockville, MD: Alcohol, Drug Abuse, and Mental Health Administration.

National Transportation Safety Board. (1985). *Recreational boating safety and alcohol* (NTSB /55-83/02). Washington, DC: Author.

Nelson, J. P. (1988). *Effects of regulation on alcoholic beverage consumption: Regression diagnostics and influential data.* University Park, PA: Pennsylvania State University, Department of Economics.

Neuman, W. (1982). Television and American culture: The mass medium and the pluralist audience. *Public Opinion Quarterly, 46,* 471-487.

Noordzij, P. (1983). Measuring the extent of the drinking and driving problem. *Accident Analysis and Prevention, 15*(6), 407-414.

Nörstrom, T. (1987, June). The abolition of the Swedish alcohol rationing system: Effects on consumption distribution and cirrhosis mortality. *British Journal of Addiction, 82*(6), 633-641.

Office of Substance Abuse Prevention. (1984). *Evaluation of the OSAP demonstration grant program: Current status and planned activities.* Unpublished manuscript.

Office on Smoking and Health. (1989). *Reducing the health consequences of smoking: 25 years of progress: A report of the Surgeon General, 1989* (DHHS Publication No. (CDC) 89-8411). Rockville, MD: Centers for Disease Control.

Olsen, G., Mandel, J., Gibson, R., Wattenberg, L., & Schuman, L. (1989). A case-control study of pancreatic cancer and cigarettes, alcohol, coffee, and diet. *American Journal of Public Health, 79*(8), 1016-1019.

Olsen, M., Canan, P., & Hennessy, M. (1985). A value based community assessment process. *Sociological Methods and Research*, *13*(3), 325-361.

Olson, M. (1965). *The logic of collective action*. Cambridge, MA: Harvard University Press.

O'Malley, P. M., & Wagenaar, A. C. (1991, September). Effects of minimum drinking age laws on alcohol use, related behaviors, and traffic crash involvement among American youth: 1976-1987. *Journal of Studies on Alcohol*, *52*(5), 478-491.

O'Neill, B., Williams, A., & Dubowski, K. (1983). Variability in blood alcohol concentrations: Implications for estimating individual results. *Journal of Studies on Alcohol*, *44*(2), 222-230.

Ornstein, S. K., & Hanssens, D. M. (1983). *Alcohol control laws and the consumption of distilled spirits and beer*. Working paper, Research Program in Competition and Business Policy, Graduate School of Management, University of California at Los Angeles.

Osborn, R. (1987). Micro marketing into the niches: The eye of the stranger. *Marketing/Communications*, *12*, 57-72.

Oshima, A., Hirata, N., Ubukata, T., Umeda, K., & Fujimoto, I. (1986). Evaluation of a mass screening program for stomach cancer with a case-control study design. *International Journal of Cancer*, *38*, 829-833.

Paddock, R. C. (1989, November 10). Stiff "nickel-a-drink" tax on alcohol proposed by coalition. *Los Angeles Times*, p. A3.

Palca, J. (1989). AIDS drug trials enter new age. *Science*, *246*, 19-21.

Parker, D. A., & Harman, M. S. (1978, March). The distribution of consumption model of prevention of alcohol problems: A critical assessment. *Journal of Studies on Alcohol*, *39*(3), 377-399.

Pechacek, T. F. (1987). A randomized community trial for smoking cessation. In M. Aoki, S. Hisamichi, & S. Tominaga (Eds.), *Proceedings of the Sixth World Conference on Smoking and Health*. Tokyo, Japan: Elsevier Science Publishing Company.

Pederson, A., Roxburgh, S., & Wood, L. (1990). Conducting community action research. In N. Giesbrecht, P. Conley, R. W. Denniston, L. Gliksman, H. Holder, A. Pederson, R. Room, & M. Shain (Eds.), *Research, action, and the community: Experiences in the prevention of alcohol and other drug problems* (OSAP Prevention Monograph No. 4, pp. 265-285). Rockville, MD: Office for Substance Abuse Prevention.

Peele, S. (1989). *Diseasing of America: Addiction treatment out of control*. Lexington, MA: Lexington Books.

Pelz, D., & Schuman, S. (1971). Are young drivers really more dangerous after controlling for exposure and experience? *Journal of Safety Research*, *3*(2), 68-79.

Pentz, M. A., Cormack, C., Flay, B., Hansen, W. B., & Johnson, C. A. (1986). Balancing program and research integrity in community drug abuse prevention: Project STAR Approach. *Journal of School Health*, *56*, 389-393.

Pentz, M. A., Dwyer, J. H., MacKinnon, D. P., Flay, B. R., Hansen, W. B., Wang, E. Y. I., & Johnson, C. A. (1989). A multicommunity trial for primary prevention of adolescent drug abuse: Effects on drug use prevalence. *Journal of the American Medical Association*, *261*(22), 3259-3266.

Pernanen, K. (1976). Alcohol and crimes of violence. In B. Kissin & H. Begleiter (Eds.), *The biology of alcoholism: Volume 4. Social aspects of alcoholism* (pp. 351-444). New York: Plenum Press.

Pernanen, K. (1981). Theoretical aspects of the relationship between alcohol use and crime. In J. J. Collins, Jr. (Ed.), *Drinking and crime: Perspectives on the relationships between alcohol consumption and criminal behavior* (pp. 1-69). New York: The Guilford Press.

Peterson, P. L., & McKirnan, D. J. (1989, June). *Gay identity, alcohol use, and AIDS risk behavior*. Paper presented at the V International Conference on AIDS, Montreal, Quebec.

Petersson, B., Trell, E., Krentz, P., & Hook, B. (1984). Major determinants of premature mortality in middle-aged urban males. *American Journal of Epidemiology*, *120*(2), 265-272.

Phelps, C. (1988). Alcohol taxes and highway safety. In J. Graham (Ed.), *Preventing automobile injury: New findings from evaluation research* (pp. 197-219). Dover, MA: Auburn House Publishing Company.

Pleuckhahn, V. D. (1982, May). Alcohol consumption and death by drowning in adults. *Journal of Studies on Alcohol*, *43*(5), 445-452.

Poikolainen, K. (1983). Inebriation and mortality. *International Journal of Epidemiology*, *12*(2), 151-155.

Polsby, N. W. (1963). *Community power and political theory*. New Haven, CT: Yale University Press.

Polsby, N. W. (1980). *Community power and political theory: A further look at problems of evidence and inference* (2nd ed.). New Haven, CT: Yale University Press.

Popham, R., Schmidt, W., & Israelstam, S. (1984). Heavy alcohol consumption and physical health problems. *Recent Advances in Alcohol and Drug Problems Number 8*. New York: Plenum Press.

Poplin, D. E. (1979). *Communities: A survey of theories and methods of research*. New York: MacMillan Publishing Company, Inc.

Prentice, R. L., Yoshimoto, Y., & Mason, M. W. (1988). Relationship of cigarette smoking and radiation exposures to cancer mortality in Hiroshima and Nagasaki. *Journal of the National Cancer Institute*, *70*, 611-622.

Press, E., Walker, J., & Crawford, I. (1968). An interstate drowning study. *American Journal of Public Health, 58*, 2275-2289.

Preusser, D. F., Williams, A. R., Zador, P. L., & Blomberg, R. D. (1984). The effect of curfew laws on motor vehicle crashes. *Law and Policy, 6*(1), 115-128.

Public Health Service. (1983). Blood alcohol concentration among young drivers—United States, 1982. *Morbidity and Mortality Weekly Report, 32*(25), 646-648.

Public Health Service. (1985). Alcohol related premature mortality—United States, 1980. *Morbidity and Mortality Weekly Report, 34*(32), 493-495.

Puska, P., Nissinen, A., Tuomilehto, J., Salonen, J. T., Koskela, K., McAlister, A., Kottke, T. E., Maccoby, N., & Farquhar, J. W. (1985). The community-based strategy to prevent coronary heart disease: Conclusions from the ten years of the North Karelia Project. *Annual Review of Public Health, 6*, 147-93.

Puska, P., Tuomilehto, J., Salonen, J., Nissinen, A., Virtamo, J., Börkqvist, S., Koskela, K., Neittaanmaki, L., Takalo, T., Kottke, T. E., Maki, J., Sipila, P., & Varvickko, P. (1981). *The North Karelia Project: Evaluation of a comprehensive community programme for control of cardiovascular diseases from 1972-1977 in North Karelia, Finland.* World Health Organization Regional Office for Europe, Copenhagen: Public Health in Europe, WHO/EURO Monograph Series.

Putnam, S. (1990). Planning, development and process issues in the Rhode Island alcohol-related inquiry prevention project. In N. Giesbrecht, P. Conley, R. W. Denniston, L. Gliksman, H. Holder, A. Pederson, R. Room, & M. Shain (Eds.), *Research, action, and the community: Experiences in the prevention of alcohol and other drug problems* (OSAP Prevention Monograph No. 4, pp. 183-195). Rockville, MD: U.S. Department of Health and Human Services, Office of Substance Abuse Prevention.

Ramirez, A. G., & McAlister, A. L. (1988). Mass media campaign—A Su Salud. *Preventive Medicine, 17*, 608-621.

Rankin, J. G., & Ashley, M. J. (1986). Alcohol-related health problems and their prevention. In J. M. Last (Ed.), *Maxcy-Rosenau, public health and preventive medicine* (pp. 1039-1073). Norwalk, CT: Appleton-Century-Crofts.

Rapp, S., & Collins, T. (1987). Conversing with prime prospects. *Marketing/Communications, 12*, 74-80.

Ravenholt, R. (1984). Addiction mortality in the United States, 1980: Tobacco, alcohol, and other substances. *Population and Development Review, 10*(4), 697-724.

Redfield, R. (1955). *The little community: Viewpoints for the study of a human whole.* Uppsala and Stockholm: Almqvist and Wiksells Boktryckeri AB.

Reichardt, C. S. (1979). The statistical analysis of data from nonequivalent group designs. In T. D. Cook & D. T. Campbell (Eds.), *Quasi-experimentation: Design and analysis issues for field settings* (pp. 147-205). Chicago: Rand McNally.

Reichardt, C. S., & Gollob, H. F. (1987). Taking uncertainty into account when estimating effects. In M. M. Mark & R. L. Shotland (Eds.), *Multiple methods for program evaluation* (New Directions for Program Evaluation, No. 35, pp. 7-22). San Francisco: Jossey-Bass.

Reichardt, C. S., & Gollob, H. F. (1989, February). Ruling out threats to validity. *Evaluation Review, 13*(1), 3-17.

Reinarman, C. (1988). The social construction of an alcohol problem. *Theory and Society, 17,* 91-120.

Report on Burton's IAT due in June; NCI could be more open, OTA says. (1990, February 9). *The Cancer Letter, 16,* 5-6.

Rhode Island Department of Health. (1989a). *Final report of the Rhode Island community alcohol abuse and injury prevention project, Volume I: Description and process evaluation.* Providence, RI: Rhode Island Department of Health.

Rhode Island Department of Health. (1989b). *Final report of the Rhode Island community alcohol abuse and injury prevention project, Volume II: Statistical outcome evaluation.* Providence, RI: Rhode Island Department of Health.

Rice, B. (1984). The role of state alcoholic beverage control in alcohol abuse prevention. In H. D. Holder & J. B. Hallen (Eds.), *Control issues in alcohol abuse prevention: Local, state, and national designs for the '80s.* Proceedings of a conference held in Charleston, SC on September 27-29, 1981. Columbia, SC: South Carolina Commission on Alcohol and Drug Abuse.

Riche, M. F. (1989). Psychographics for the 1990s. *American Demographics, 11,* 18-23.

Rindskopf, D. (1986). New developments in selection modeling for quasi-experimentation. In W. M. K. Trochim (Ed.), *Advances in quasi-experimental design and analysis* (New Directions for Program Evaluation, No. 31, pp. 79-89). San Francisco: Jossey-Bass.

Ritson, E. G. (1985). *Community response to alcohol-related problems: Review of an international study* (Public Health Papers No. 81). Geneva, Switzerland: World Health Organization.

Robertson, L. (1980). Crash involvement of teenaged drivers when driver education is eliminated from high school. *American Journal of Public Health, 70*(6), 599-603.

Robertson, L., Rich, R., & Ross, H. L. (1973). Jail sentences for driving while intoxicated in Chicago: A judicial policy that failed. *Law and Society Review, 8*, 55-67.

Roizen, J. (1982). Estimating alcohol involvement in serious events. In National Institute on Alcohol Abuse and Alcoholism, *Alcohol consumption and related problems* (Alcohol and Health Monograph No. 1, DDHS Pub. No. ADM 82-1190). Washington, DC: U.S. Government Printing Office.

Roizen, J., & Schneberk, D. (1977). Alcohol and crime. In M. Aarens, T. Cameron, J. Roizen, R. Roizen, R. Room, D. Schnerberk, & D. Wingard (Eds.), *Alcohol, casualties and crime* (pp. 289-465). Berkeley, CA: Social Research Group.

Room, R. (1977). Measurement and distribution of drinking patterns and problems in general populations. In G. Edwards, M. M. Gross, M. Keller, J. Moser, & R. Room (Eds.), *Alcohol-related disabilities* (pp. 61-87). Geneva, Switzerland: World Health Organization.

Room, R. (1980a, Spring). Concepts and strategies in the prevention of alcohol-related problems. *Contemporary Drug Problems, 9*(1), 9-47.

Room, R. (1980b). Treatment-seeking populations and larger realities. In G. Edwards & M. Grant (Eds.), *Alcoholism treatment in transition* (pp. 205-224). London: Croom Helm.

Room, R. (1983). Alcohol and crime: Behavioral aspects. In S. H. Kadish (Ed.), *Encyclopedia of crime and justice* (Vol. 1). New York: Free Press.

Room, R. (1984). Alcohol control and public health. *Annual Review of Public Health, 5*, 293-317.

Room, R. (1989). Developments in evaluating programs to prevent alcohol problems. In R. Ray & R. W. Pickens (Eds.), *Proceedings of the Indo-U.S. Symposium on Alcohol and Drug Abuse* (NIMHANS Publication No. 20, pp. 275-283). Bangalore, India: National Institute of Mental Health and Neuro Sciences.

Room, R. (1990). Community action and alcohol problems: The demonstration project as an unstable mixture. In N. Giesbrecht, P. Conley, R. W. Denniston, L. Gliksman, H. Holder, A. Pederson, R. Room, & M. Shain (Eds.), *Research, action, and the community: Experiences in the prevention of alcohol and other drug problems* (OSAP Prevention Monograph No. 4, pp. 1-25). Rockville, MD: Office for Substance Abuse Prevention.

Room, R., & Collins, G. (Eds.). (1983). *Alcohol and disinhibition: Nature and meaning of the link* (Research Monograph No. 12). (Proceedings of a conference, February 11-13, 1981, Berkeley/Oakland, CA.) Rockville, MD: National Institute on Alcohol Abuse and Alcoholism.

Rootman, I., & Moser, J. (1985). *Community response to alcohol-related problems: A World Health Organization project monograph* (DHHS Publication No. (ADM) 85-1371). Washington, DC: U.S. Government Printing Office.

Rose, G. (1981, June 6). Strategy of prevention: Lessons from cardiovascular disease. *British Medical Journal, 282,* 1847-1851.

Rose, G. (1985). Sick individuals and sick populations. *International Journal of Epidemiology, 14,* 32-38.

Ross, H. L. (1973). Law, science and accidents: The British Road Safety Act of 1967. *Journal of Legal Studies, 2,* 1-78.

Ross, H. L. (1976). The neutralization of severe penalties: Some traffic law studies. *Law and Society Review, 10,* 403-413.

Ross, H. L. (1977). Deterrence regained: The Cheshire constabulary's 'breathalyser blitz'. *Journal of Legal Studies, 6,* 241-249.

Ross, H. L. (1982). *Deterring the drinking driver: Legal policy and social control.* Lexington, MA: D.C. Heath and Company.

Ross, H. L. (1990). Drinking and driving: Beyond the criminal approach. *Alcohol Health and Research World, 14*(1), 58-62.

Ross, H. L., Campbell, D. T., & Glass, G. V. (1970). Determining the social effects of a legal reform. In S. S. Nagel (Ed.), *Law and social change* (pp. 15-32). Newbury Park, CA: Sage Publications.

Ross, H. L., Howard, J. M., Ganikos, M. L., & Taylor, E. D. (1991). Drunk driving among American Blacks and Hispanics. *Accident Analysis and Prevention, 23*(1), 1-11.

Ross, H. L., & McCleary, R. (1983, December). Methods for studying the impact of drunk-driving laws. *Accident Analysis and Prevention, 15*(6), 415-428.

Ross, H. L., McCleary, R., & Epperlein, T. (1981). Deterrence of drinking and driving in France: An evaluation of the law of July 12, 1978. *Law and Society Review, 16,* 345-374.

Ross, H. L., McCleary, R., & LaFree, G. (1990). Can mandatory jail laws deter drunk driving? The Arizona case. *Journal of Criminal Law and Criminology, 81,* 156-170.

Ross, H. L., & Voas, R. (1989). *The new Philadelphia story: The effects of severe punishment for drunk driving.* Washington, DC: AAA Foundation for Traffic Safety.

Rossouw, J. E., Jooste, P. L., Kotze, J. P., & Jordaan, P. C. J. (1981). The control of hypertension in two communities: An interim evaluation. *South African Medical Journal, 60,* 208-212.

Rothman, K. J. (1986). *Modern epidemiology* (pp. 51-76). Boston, MA: Little, Brown and Company.

Rothman, J., & Tropman, J. E. (1987). Models of community organization and macro practice perspectives: Their mixing and phasing. In Fred M. Cox, et al. (Eds.), *Strategies of community organization*. Itasca, IL: F. E. Peacock Publishers, Inc.

Rubin, D. B. (1977). Assignment to treatment group on the basis of a covariate. *Journal of Educational Statistics, 2,* 1-26.

Rubin, I. (1983). Function and structure of community: Conceptual and theoretical analyses. In R. Warren & L. Lyon (Eds.), *New perspectives on the American community*. Homewood, IL: The Dorsey Press.

Rush, B. R., Gliksman, L., & Brook, R. (1986). Alcohol availability, alcohol consumption, and alcohol-related damage. I. The distribution of consumption model. *Journal of Studies on Alcohol, 47*(1), 1-10.

Russ, N. W., & Geller, E. S. (1987, August). Training bar personnel to prevent drunk driving: A field evaluation. *American Journal of Public Health, 77*(8), 952-954.

Sackett, D. L. (1979). Bias in analytic research. *Journal of Chronic Diseases, 32,* 51-63.

Saffer, H., & Grossman, M. (1987a, June). Beer taxes, the legal drinking age, and youth motor vehicle fatalities. *Journal of Legal Studies, 16,* 351-374.

Saffer, H., & Grossman, M. (1987b). Drinking age laws and highway mortality rates: Cause and effect. *Economic Inquiry, 25*(3), 403-417.

Sallis, J. F., Hill, R. D., Fortmann, S. P., & Flora, J. A. (1986). Health behavior change at the worksite: Cardiovascular risk reduction. *Progress in Behavior Modification, 20,* 161-197.

Saltz, R. F. (1987). The roles of bars and restaurants in preventing alcohol-impaired driving: An evaluation of server intervention. *Evaluation and Health Professions, 10,* 5-27.

Saltz, R. F. (1989a). Research needs and opportunities in server intervention programs. *Health Education Quarterly, 16*(3), 429-438.

Saltz, R. F. (1989b). Server intervention and responsible beverage service programs. *Surgeon General's workshop on drunk driving: Background papers* (pp. 169-179). Rockville, MD: U.S. Department of Health and Human Services, Public Health Service, Office of the Surgeon General.

Sanchez-Craig, M. (1984). *A therapist's manual for secondary prevention of alcohol problems: Procedures for teaching moderate drinking and abstinence*. Toronto: Addiction Research Foundation.

SAS Institute, Inc. (1984). *SAS/ETS users guide* (Version 5 ed.). Cary, NC: Author.

Sasco, A. J., Day, N. E., & Walter, S. D. (1986). Case-control studies for the evaluation of screening. *Journal of Chronic Diseases, 39*(5), 399-405.

Saunders, J., Walters, J., Davies, P., & Paton, A. (1981). A 20-year prospective study of cirrhosis. *British Medical Journal, 282*, 263-266.

Schaps, E., DiBartolo, R., Moskowitz, J., Palley, C. S., & Churgin, S. (1981, Winter). A review of 127 drug abuse prevention program evaluations. *Journal of Drug Issues, 11*(1), 17-43.

Schenker, S. (1984). Alcoholic liver disease: Evaluation of natural history and prognostic factors. *Hepatology, 4*(1), 365-435.

Schlesselman, J. J. (1982). Basic concepts in the assessment of risk. In J. J. Schlesselman & P. D. Stoley (Eds.), *Case-control studies design conduct analysis* (pp. 27-68). New York: Oxford University Press.

Schmidt, W. (1980). Effects of alcohol consumption on health. *Journal of Public Health Policy, 1*(1), 25-40.

Schmidt, W., & Popham, R. E. (1978, March). The single distribution theory of alcohol consumption: A rejoinder to the critique of Parker and Harman. *Journal of Studies on Alcohol, 39*(3), 400-419.

Schmidt, W., & Popham, R. E. (1981). Alcohol consumption and ischemic heart disease: Some evidence from population studies. *British Journal of Addiction, 76*, 407-417.

Secord, P. F., & Backman, C. W. (1964). *Social psychology.* New York: McGraw Hill.

Secretary of Health and Human Services. (1987). *Sixth special report to the U.S. Congress on alcohol and health* (DHHS Publication No. (ADM) 87-1519). Rockville, MD: U.S. Department of Health and Human Services, National Institute on Alcohol Abuse and Alcoholism.

Secretary of Health and Human Services. (1990). *Seventh special report to the U.S. Congress on alcohol and health* (DHHS Publication No. (ADM) 90-1656). Rockville, MD: U.S. Department of Health and Human Services, National Institute on Alcohol Abuse and Alcoholism.

Seeley, J. R. (1960). Death by liver cirrhosis and the price of beverage alcohol. *Canadian Medical Association Journal, 83*, 1361-1366.

Selvanathan, A. E. (1988). Alcohol consumption in the UK, 1955-85: A system-wide analysis. *Applied Economics, 20*, 1071-1086.

Senie, R. T., Rosen, R. P., Lesser, M. L., & Kinne, D. W. (1981). Breast self-examination and medical examination related to breast cancer stage. *American Journal of Public Health, 71*(6), 583-590.

Settle, R., & Alreck, P. (1987). Knowing the consumer inside and out. *Marketing/Communications, 12*, 49-56.

Shaper, A. G. (1990). Alcohol and mortality: A review of prospective studies. *British Journal of Addiction, 85*(7), 837-847.

Shea, S. (1992, July). *New York State Healthy Heart Program: An interim report.* New York: State Department of Health.

Shilts, R. (1987). *And the band played on: Politics, people, and the AIDS epidemic.* New York: St. Martin's Press.

Shore, E. R., Gregory, T., & Tatlock, L. (1991). College students' reactions to a designated driver program: An exploratory study. *Journal of Alcohol and Drug Education, 37*(1), 1-6.

Signorielli, N. (1986, Summer). Selective television viewing: A limited possibility. *Journal of Communication, 36*(3), 64-76.

Simonton, D. K. (1977). Cross-sectional time-series experiments: Some suggested statistical analyses. *Psychological Bulletin, 84,* 489-502.

Siscovick, D., Weiss, N., & Fox, N. (1986). Moderate alcohol consumption and primary cardiac arrest. *American Journal of Epidemiology, 123*(3), 499-503.

Skinner, H. A. (1981). Primary syndromes of alcohol abuse: Their measurement and correlates. *British Journal of Addiction, 76,* 63-76.

Skinner, H. A., & Allen, B. A. (1982). Alcohol dependence syndrome: Measurement and validation. *Journal of Abnormal Psychology, 91,* 199-207.

Skinner, H. A., & Horn, J. L. (1984). *Alcohol dependence scale user's guide.* Toronto: Addiction Research Foundation.

Skog, O.-J. (1980, Winter). Social interaction and the distribution of alcohol consumption. *Journal of Drug Issues, 10*(1), 71-92.

Skog, O.-J. (1983). *The collectivity of drinking cultures: A theory of the distribution of alcohol consumption* (SIFA, Mimeograph No. 69). Oslo: National Institute for Alcohol Research.

Skog, O.-J. (1985, March). The collectivity of drinking cultures: A theory of the distribution of alcohol consumption. *British Journal of Addiction, 80*(1), 83-99.

Skog, O.-J. (1989, February 8). *Epidemiology of alcohol use, alcoholism, and their implications.* Paper presented at the Addiction Research Foundation, 40th Anniversary Scientific Lecture Series, Toronto, Ontario, Canada.

Smith, A. H., Pearce, N. E., & Callas, P. W. (1988). Cancer case-control studies with other cancers as controls. *International Journal of Epidemiology, 17*(2), 298-306.

Smith, E. M., & Burns, T. L. (1985). The effects of breast self-examination in a population-based cancer registry: A report of differences in extent of disease. *Cancer, 55*(2), 432-437.

Smith, E. M., Francis, A. M., & Polissar, L. (1980). The effect of breast self-exam practices and physical examination on extent of disease at diagnosis. *Preventive Medicine, 9,* 409-417.

Smith, M. L., Gabriel, R., Schoot, J., & Padia, W. L. (1976). Evaluation of the effects of outward bound. In G. V. Glass (Ed.), *Evaluation studies review annual* (Vol. 1, pp. 400-421). Newbury Park, CA: Sage Publications.

Smith, R. T. (1976). The legal and illegal markets for taxed goods: Pure theory and an application to state government taxation of distilled spirits. *Journal of Law and Economics, 19,* 393-429.

Specter, M. (1989, July 9). Remarkable summit on AIDS research. *The Washington Post,* p. A10.

Specter, M. (1990, March 9). AIDS group will resume Compound Q study. *Washington Post,* p. A3.

Spitzer, W. D. (1985). Ideas and words: Two dimensions for debates on case-controlling [Editorial]. *Journal of Chronic Diseases, 38*(7), 541-542.

Stake, R. E. (1986). *Quieting reform: Social science and social action in an urban youth program.* Urbana, IL: University of Illinois Press.

Stall, R., McKusick, L., Wiley, J., Coates, T. J., & Ostrow, D. G. (1986). Alcohol and drug use during sexual activity and compliance with safe sex guidelines for AIDS: The AIDS behavioral research project. *Health Education Quarterly, 13,* 359-371.

Stampfer, M., Colditz, G., Willett, W., Speizer, F., & Hennekens, C. (1985). A prospective study of moderate alcohol consumption and the risk of coronary disease and stroke in women. *New England Journal of Medicine, 319*(5), 267-273.

Stephens, C. J. (1985). *A study of alcohol use and injuries among emergency room patients.* Prepared by Alcohol Research Group, Medical Research Institute of San Francisco for the Symposium: Statistics on Alcohol-Related Casualties, Toronto, Canada, August 12-16, 1985.

Stephens, C. J. (1987). Alcohol consumption and casualties: Drinking in the event. *Drug and Alcohol Dependence, 20,* 115-127.

Stewart, K., Epstein, L. G., Gruenewald, P., Laurence, S., & Roth, T. (1987). *The California first DUI offender evaluation project final report.* Prepared for the California Office of Traffic Safety. Bethesda, MD: Pacific Institute for Research and Evaluation.

Stoneall, L. (1983). *Country life, city life: Five theories of community.* New York: Praeger Scientific.

Stoto, M. A. (1988). Dealing with uncertainty: Statistics for an aging population. *American Statistician, 42,* 103-110.

Stromsdorfer, E. W., & Farkas, G. (1980). *Evaluation studies review annual* (Vol. 5). Newbury Park, CA: Sage Publications.

Surgeon General's Workshop on Drunk Driving: Background Papers. (1989). Rockville, MD: U.S. Department of Health and Human Services, Public Health Service, Office of the Surgeon General (Washington, DC, December 14-16, 1988).

Surgeon General's Workshop on Drunk Driving: Proceedings. (1989). Rockville, MD: U.S. Department of Health and Human Services, Public Health Service, Office of the Surgeon General (Washington, DC, December 14-16, 1988).

Swaminathan, H., & Algina, J. (1977). Analysis of quasi-experimental time-series designs. *Journal of Multivariate Behavioral Research, 12,* 111-131.

Takala, H. (1973). Alkoholstrejkens inverkan pa uppdagad brottslighet [The effect of the alcohol strike on reported crime]. *Alkoholpolitik, 36,* 14-16.

Telch, M. J., Killen, J. D., McAlister, A. L., Perry, C. L., & Maccoby, N. (1982). Long-term follow-up of a pilot project on smoking prevention with adolescents. *Journal of Behavioral Medicine, 5*(1), 1-8.

Telch, M. J., Miller, L. M., Killen, J. D., Cooke, S., & Maccoby, N. (1990). Social influences approach to smoking prevention: The effects of videotape delivery with and without same-age peer leader participation. *Addictive Behaviors, 15*(1), 21-28.

Terris, M. (1967). The epidemiology of cirrhosis of the liver: National mortality data. *American Journal of Public Health, 57,* 2076-2088.

Thistlethwaite, D. L., & Campbell, D. T. (1960). Regression-discontinuity analysis: An alternative to the ex-post-facto experiment. *Journal of Educational Psychology, 51,* 309-317.

Thorarisson, A. A. (1979, July). Mortality among men alcoholics in Iceland, 1951-74. *Journal of Studies on Alcohol, 40*(7), 704-718.

Thornton, J., Symes, C., & Heaton, K. (1983). Moderate alcohol intake reduces bile cholesterol saturation and raises hdl cholesterol. *Lancet, ii,* 819-822.

Tobler, N. (1986). Meta-analysis of 143 adolescent drug prevention programs: Quantitative outcome results of program participants compared to a control or comparison group. *Journal of Drug Issues, 16,* 537-567.

Tonnies, F. (1957). *Community and society* [Gemeinschaft und Gesellschaft] (C. P. Loomis, Ed. and Trans.). East Lansing, MI: Michigan State University Press.

Townsend, B. (1985). Psychographic glitter and gold. *American Demographics, 7,* 22-29.

Trier, H. (1983). Fire fatalities and deaths from burns in Denmark. *Medical Science and Law, 23,* 116-120.

Trochim, W. M. K. (1984). *Research designs for program evaluation: The regression-discontinuity approach.* Newbury Park, CA: Sage Publications, Inc.

Truett, J., Cornfield, J., & Kannel, W. A. (1967). Multivariate analysis of the risk of coronary heart disease in Framingham. *Journal of Chronic Diseases, 20,* 511.

Tuomilehto, J., Geboers, J., Salonen, J. K., Nissinen, A., Kuulasmaa, K., & Puska, P. (1986). Decline in cardiovascular mortality in North Karelia and other parts of Finland. *British Medical Journal, 293*, 1068-1071.

U.S. Department of Health and Human Services. (1986). *Integration of risk factor interventions*. Washington, DC: Office of Disease Prevention and Health Promotion, Public Health Service.

U.S. Department of Health and Human Services. (1989). *Reducing the health consequences of smoking: 25 years of progress: A report of the Surgeon General* (DHHS Publication No. (CDC) 89-8411, p. 502). Rockville, MD: Office on Smoking and Health.

U.S. Department of Health and Human Services/NCEP. (1988). *Current status of blood cholesterol measurement in clinical laboratories in the United States: A report from the laboratory standardization panel of the national cholesterol education program* (NIH Publication No. 88-2928). Bethesda, MD: National Cholesterol Education Program.

U.S. General Accounting Office. (1987a). *Drinking-age laws: An evaluation synthesis of their impact on highway safety*. Report to the Chairman, Subcommittee on Investigations and Oversight, Committee on Public Works and Transportation, House of Representatives. Washington, DC: U.S. Superintendent of Documents.

U.S. General Accounting Office. (1987b). *Drug abuse prevention: Further efforts needed to identify programs that work* (GAO/HRD-88-26). Washington, DC: U.S. Government Printing Office.

U.S. General Accounting Office. (1989). *Alcohol warning labels: Current rules may allow health warnings to go unnoticed* (GAO/HRD-89-118). Washington, DC: Author.

U.S. Preventive Services Task Force (Report of). (1989). *Guide to clinical preventive services* (Prepublication copy, pp. 182-189).

University of California, San Diego Extension. (1990). *Evaluating community prevention strategies: Alcohol and other drugs*. Proceedings of a conference held in San Diego, California, January 11-13, 1990. La Jolla, CA: University of California, San Diego Extension.

Valdiserri, R. O., Lyter, D., Leviton, L. C., Callahan, C. M., Kingsley, L. A., & Rinaldo, C. R. (1988, July). Variables influencing condom use in a cohort of gay and bisexual men. *American Journal of Public Health, 78*(7), 801-805.

Verbeek, A. L. M., Hendriks, J. H., Holland, R., Mravunac, M., Sturmans, F., & Day, N. E. (1984). Reduction of breast cancer mortality through mass screening with modern mammography: First results of the Nijmegen Project 1975-1981. *Lancet, i*, 1222-1224.

Vingilis, E., Blefgen, H., Lei, H., Sykora, K., & Mann, R. (1988). An evaluation of the deterrent impact on Ontario's 12-hour license suspension law. *Accident Analysis and Prevention, 20*(1), 9-17.

Voas, R.B. (1989). *Sobriety check points, an evaluation*. Paper presented at the 11th Triannual Meeting of the International Committee on Alcohol, Drugs, and Traffic Safety, Chicago, IL.

Voas, R. B., & Hause, J. M. (1987). Deterring the drinking driver: The Stockton experience. *Accident Analysis & Prevention, 19*(2), 81-90.

Wagenaar, A. (1983). *Alcohol, young drivers, and traffic accidents: Effects of minimum-age laws*. Lexington, MA: Lexington Books.

Wagenaar, A. C. (1986). Preventing highway crashes by raising the legal minimum age for drinking: The Michigan experience six years later. *Journal of Safety Research, 17*(3), 101-109.

Wagenaar, A. C. (1987). Effects of minimum drinking age on alcohol-related traffic crashes: The Michigan experience five years later. In H. D. Holder (Ed.), *Control Issues in Alcohol Abuse Prevention: Strategies for States and Communities* (pp. 119-131). Greenwich, CT: JAI Press.

Wagenaar, A. (1990). Valuative criteria to guide prevention planners. *Evaluating Community Prevention Strategies: Alcohol and Other Drugs* (pp. 39-42). Proceedings of a conference held in San Diego, California, January 11-13, 1990. La Jolla, CA: University of California, San Diego Extension.

Wagenaar, A. C., & Holder, H. D. (1991). A change from public to private sale of wine: Results from natural experiments in Iowa and West Virginia. *Journal of Studies on Alcohol, 52*(2), 162-173.

Wagenaar, A., & Maybee, R. (1986). The legal minimum drinking age in Texas: Effects of an increase from 18 to 19. *Journal of Safety Research, 17*(4), 165-176.

Wallack, L. M. (1983). Mass media campaigns in a hostile environment: Advertising as anti-health education. *Journal of Alcohol and Drug Education, 28*(2), 51-63.

Wallack, L. M. (1984a). Drinking and driving: Toward a broader understanding of the role of mass media. *Journal of Public Health Policy, 5*(4), 471-496.

Wallack, L. M. (1984b). Practical issues, ethical concerns, and future directions in the prevention of alcohol-related problems. *Journal of Primary Prevention, 4*(4), 199-224.

Wallack, L. M. (1984-1985). A community approach to the prevention of alcohol-related problems: The San Francisco experience. *International Quarterly of Community Health Education, 5*(2), 85-102.

Wallack, L. M., & Barrows, D. C. (1981). *Preventing alcohol problems in California: Evaluation of the three year "Winners" Program*. Berkeley, CA: Social Research Group, School of Public Health, University of California.

Wallack, L., & Barrows, D. C. (1982-1983). Evaluating primary prevention: The California "Winners" Alcohol Program. *International Quarterly of Community Health Education, 3*(4), 307-336.

Wallack, L., Breed, W., & Cruz, J. (1987). Alcohol on prime-time television. *Journal of Studies on Alcohol, 48*(1), 33-38.

Wallack, L., & Wallerstein, N. (1987). Health education and prevention: Designing community initiatives. *International Quarterly of Community Health Education, 7*(4), 319-342.

Waller, J. A. (1972). Nonhighway injury fatalities—I. The role of alcohol and problem drinking, drugs, and medical impairment. *Journal of Chronic Diseases, 25*, 33-45.

Walsh, D. C. (1990). The shifting boundaries of alcohol policy. *Health Affairs, 9*(2), 48-62.

Warren, R. L. (1983). A community model. In R. M. Kramer & H. Specht (Eds.), *Readings in community organization practice* (3rd ed.). Engelwood Cliffs, NJ: Prentice-Hall, Inc.

Warren, R. L., & Lyon, L. (Eds.). (1983). *New perspectives on the American community.* Homewood, IL: The Dorsey Press.

Watts, R. K., & Rabow, J. (1983). Alcohol availability and alcohol-related problems in 213 California cities. *Alcoholism: Clinical and Experimental Research, 7*(1), 47-58.

Weber, M. (1964). *The city* (Don Martindale and Gertrude Neuwirth, Ed. and Trans.) New York: Collier Books.

Webster, J. G. (1986, Summer). Audience behavior in the new media environment. *Journal of Communication, 36*(3), 77-91.

Wedderburn, R. W. M. (1974). Quasi-likelihood functions, generalized linear models, and the Gauss-Newton method. *Biometrika, 61*, 439-447.

Weil, A. (1988). *Health and healing: Understanding conventional and alternative medicine.* Boston, MA: Houghton Mifflin Company.

Weiss, N. S. (1983). Control definition in case-control studies of the efficacy of screening and diagnostic testing. *American Journal of Epidemiology, 118*(4), 457-460.

Welte, J. W., & Abel, E. L. (1989). Homicide: Drinking by the victim. *Journal of Studies on Alcohol, 50*(3), 197-201.

Wheeler, F. C., Lackland, D. P., Mace, M. L., Reddick, A., Hogelin, G., & Remington, P. L. (1991). Evaluating South Carolina's community cardiovascular disease prevention project. *Public Health Reports, 105*(5), 536-542.

Whitehead, J. T., & Lab, S. P. (1989). A meta-analysis of juvenile correctional treatment. *Journal of Research in Crime and Delinquency, 26*, 276-295.

Williams, A. (1985). Nighttime driving and fatal crash involvement of teenagers. *Accident Analysis and Prevention, 17*(1), 1-5.

Williams, A., & Karpf, R. (1984). Teenage drivers and fatal crash responsibility. *Law and Policy*, *6*(1), 156-169.

Williams, A., Lund, A., & Preusser, D. (1984). *Night driving curfews in New York and Louisiana*. Washington, DC: Insurance Institute for Highway Safety.

Williams, A., Lund, A., & Preusser, D. (1986). Drinking and driving among high school students. *International Journal of the Addictions*, *21*(6), 643-655.

Williams, G., Grant, B., Stinson, F., Zobeck, T., Aitken, S., & Noble, J. (1988). Trends in alcohol related morbidity and mortality. *Public Health Reports*, *103*(6), 592-597.

Williams, G. D., Stinson, F. S., Parker, D. A., Harford, T. C., & Noble, J. (1987, Spring). Demographic trends, alcohol abuse and alcoholism 1985-1995. *Alcohol Health and Research World*, *11*(3), 80-83.

Wittman, F. (1982). Current status of research demonstration programs in the primary prevention of alcohol problems. *Prevention, intervention and treatment: Concerns and models* (Alcohol and Health Monograph No. 3, DHHS Publication (ADM) 82-1192, pp. 3-57). Washington, DC: U.S. Government Printing Office.

Wittman, F. (1983). *Local regulation of alcohol availability in selected California communities: Introduction and summary of findings*. Berkeley, CA: Prevention Research Group, Institute of Epidemiology and Behavioral Medicine, Medical Research Institute of San Francisco.

Wittman, F. (1985). Community perspectives on the prevention of alcohol problems. *Framework for Community Initiatives: Preventing Alcohol-Related Problems in California* (pp. 77-94). Sacramento, CA: Department of Alcohol and Drug Problems, State of California Health and Welfare Agency.

Wittman, F. (1986). Regulation of availability as a focus for community-level prevention planning. In A. Cox and N. Giesbrecht (Eds.) *Prevention, alcohol and the environment—Issues, constituencies, and strategies*. Toronto, Canada: The Addiction Research Foundation.

Wittman, F., & Hilton, M. (1987). Uses of planning and zoning ordinances to regulate alcohol outlets in California cities. In H. Holder (Ed.), *Control issues in alcohol abuse prevention: Strategies for states and communities* (pp. 337-366). Greenwich, CT: JAI Press.

Wolfinger, R. E. (1974). *The politics of progress*. Englewood Cliffs, NJ: Prentice-Hall, Inc.

Worden, J. K., Flynn, B. S., Merrill, D. G., Waller, J. A., & Haugh, L. D. (1989). Preventing alcohol-impaired driving through community self-regulation. *American Journal of Public Health*, *79*(3), 287-291.

Wortman, P. M., Reichardt, C. S., & St. Pierre, R. G. (1978, May). The first year of the Educational Voucher Demonstration: A secondary analysis of student achievement test scores. *Evaluation Quarterly*, *2*(2), 193-214.

Wyllie, A., Casswell, S., & Stewart, J. (1989, June). The response of New Zealand boys to corporate and sponsorship alcohol advertising on television. *British Journal of Addiction*, *84*(6), 639-646.

Yeaton, W. H., Wortman, P. M., & Langberg, N. (1983). Differential attrition: Estimating the effect of crossovers on the evaluation of a medical technology. *Evaluation Review*, *7*, 831-840.

Young, T. K., & Hershfield, E. S. (1986). A case-control study to evaluate the effectiveness of mass neonatal BCG vaccination among Canadian Indians. *American Journal of Public Health*, *76*(7), 783-786.

Zeger, S. L. (1988). A regression model for time series of counts. *Biometrika*, *75*, 621-629.

Zigler, E., & Child, I. L. (1969). Socialization. In G. Lindzey & E. Aronson (Eds.), *The handbook of social psychology* (Vol. I). Reading, MA: Addison-Wesley Publishing Company.

Zobeck, T. (1986, July). Trends in alcohol-related fatal traffic accidents, United States: 1977-1984. *Surveillance Report #1. Alcohol Epidemiologic Data System.* Rockville, MD: National Institute on Alcohol Abuse and Alcoholism.

Zucker, R. (1968, December). Sex-role identity patterns and drinking behavior of adolescents. *Quarterly Journal of Studies on Alcohol*, *29*(4A), 868-884.

Zylman, R. (1974). A critical evaluation of the literature on alcohol involvement in highway deaths. *Accident Analysis and Prevention*, *6*, 163-204.

Contributors

Cornelia J. Baines, M.D.
University of Toronto
Toronto, Ontario
Canada

Ivan Barofsky, Ph.D.
Francis Scott Key Medical Center
Baltimore, MD

David P. Byar, Ph.D.
National Cancer Institute
Bethesda, MD

Elizabeth Edmundson, Ph.D.
University of Texas Health Science
  Center
Houston, TX

John W. Farquhar, M.D.
Stanford University School of
  Medicine
Palo Alto, CA

Stephen P. Fortmann, M.D.
Stanford University School of
  Medicine
Palo Alto, CA

Laurence S. Freedman, M.A.
National Institutes of Health
Bethesda, MD

Norman Giesbrecht, Ph.D.
Addiction Research Foundation
Toronto, Ontario
Canada

Lawrence W. Green, Dr.P.H.	University of British Columbia Vancouver, British Columbia Canada
Paul J. Gruenewald, Ph.D.	Prevention Research Center Berkeley, CA
Marjorie A. Gutman, Ph.D.	The Robert Wood Johnson Foundation Princeton, NJ
Thomas C. Harford, Ph.D.	National Institute on Alcohol Abuse and Alcoholism Rockville, MD
Michael Hennessy, Ph.D.	Prevention Research Center Berkeley, CA
Harold D. Holder, Ph.D.	Prevention Research Center Berkeley, CA
Jan M. Howard, Ph.D.	National Institute on Alcohol Abuse and Alcoholism Rockville, MD
Thomas M. Lasater, Ph.D.	Memorial Hospital of Rhode Island Pawtucket, RI
Alfred McAlister, Ph.D.	University of Texas Health Science Center Houston, TX
Ann Pederson, M.A.	University of Toronto Toronto, Ontario Canada
Charles S. Reichardt, Ph.D.	University of Denver Denver, CO
H. Laurence Ross	University of New Mexico Albuquerque, NM
Robert F. Saltz, Ph.D.	Prevention Research Center Berkeley, CA
Steven G. Self, Ph.D.	Fred Hutchinson Cancer Research Center Seattle, WA

Robert L. Stout, Ph.D.	Butler Hospital Providence, RI
Ernestine Vanderveen, Ph.D.	National Institute on Alcohol Abuse and Alcoholism Rockville, MD
Alexander C. Wagenaar, Ph.D.	University of Minnesota Minneapolis, MN

Index

About the Editors

HAROLD D. HOLDER is Director of the Prevention Research Center, one of 14 national alcohol research centers and the only one specializing in prevention. He is the editor of *Control Issues in Alcohol Abuse Prevention: Strategies for States and Communities* (1987).

JAN M. HOWARD is Chief, Prevention Research Branch, Division of Clinical and Prevention Research, National Institute on Alcohol Abuse and Alcoholism. She is the co-editor of *Humanizing Health Care* (1975).